Rifaximin: A Poorly Absorbed Antibiotic

Rifaximin: A Poorly Absorbed Antibiotic

Pharmacology and Clinical Use

Editor

C. Scarpignato *Parma, Italy*

28 figures, 5 in color, and 43 tables, 2005

KARGER

Basel · Freiburg · Paris · London · New York · Bangalore · Bangkok · Singapore · Tokyo · Sydney

Carmelo Scarpignato, MD, DSc (Hons), PharmD (h.c.), FCP, FACG
Laboratory of Clinical Pharmacology
School of Medicine and Dentistry
University of Parma
Via Volturno, 39
43100 Parma (Italy)

Reprint of 'Chemotherapy' (ISSN 0009-3157)
Vol. 51 Suppl. 1, 2005

Library of Congress Cataloging-in-Publication Data

Rifaximin, a poorly absorbed antibiotic : pharmacology and clinical use / editor, C. Scarpignato.
p. ; cm.
Reprint of Chemotherapy ; v. 51, suppl. 1.
Includes bibliographical references and index.
ISBN 3-8055-7917-9 (hard cover : alk. paper)
1. Rifamycins.
[DNLM: 1. Gastrointestinal Diseases–drug therapy. 2. Anti-Infective Agents–therapeutic use. 3. Gastrointestinal Agents–therapeutic use. 4. Gastrointestinal Tract–microbiology. 5. Gastrointestinal Tract–physiopathology. 6. Rifamycins–therapeutic use.] I. Scarpignato, C. II. Chemotherapy.
RM666.R57R525 2005
616.3′3061–dc22
2005001673

Bibliographic Indices. This publication is listed in bibliographic services, including Current Contents® and Index Medicus.

Drug Dosage. The authors and the publisher have exerted every effort to ensure that drug selection and dosage set forth in this text are in accord with current recommendations and practice at the time of publication. However, in view of ongoing research, changes in government regulations, and the constant flow of information relating to drug therapy and drug reactions, the reader is urged to check the package insert for each drug for any change in indications and dosage and for added warnings and precautions. This is particularly important when the recommended agent is a new and/or infrequently employed drug.

www.karger.com
Printed in Switzerland on acid-free paper by Reinhardt Druck, Basel
ISBN 3–8055–7917–9

Contents

Foreword

In this era of antibiotic famine – only five new antibiotics in the industry pipeline – it is refreshing to read about new clinical applications for an old drug. Rifaximin is a semisynthetic rifamycin which is nonabsorbable from the gastrointestinal tract. It has been available in Europe and other countries for several years, and has recently been approved for treatment of traveler's diarrhea in the USA. This supplement brings together all of the available microbiology, pharmacology and clinical aspects of this drug in a series of well-referenced and scholarly articles, ably edited by Professor C. Scarpignato.

Given its broad spectrum of antimicrobial activity, rifaximin has been used with success in the treatment of infectious diarrhea, hepatic encephalopathy, small intestinal bacterial overgrowth, inflammatory bowel disease, and colonic diverticular disease. All of these conditions, with the exception of infectious diarrhea, involve native components of the intestinal microflora. Several other conditions are under study including *Clostridium difficile* antibiotic-associated diarrhea and *Helicobacter pylori* infection.

The intestinal microflora has gained prominence in recent years as the source of beneficial as well as nefarious activities. On the positive side, the flora is responsible for establishing immunity at the intestinal wall level, and through the gastrointestinal-associated lymphoid tissue this immune function is disseminated throughout other mucosal surfaces as well. Yet, a super-'hygienic' individual who has a limited intestinal flora in infancy may be subject to food allergy and atopic diseases such as asthma in childhood and later life. The microflora assists in digesting foodstuffs and supports good nutrition in the individual. On the other hand, for animals and humans consuming a minimal diet, the flora may inhibit absorption; suppression of the microflora by antibiotics in this setting can improve absorption and increase growth. This observation has been used, and abused, widely in animal husbandry in some countries where poorly absorbed antibiotics have been added to animal feed in order to increase weight and add muscle.

Suppression of the microflora with antibiotics has been used to benefit the host in several conditions which are prime opportunities for rifaximin's activity. During the course of elective colorectal surgery, inadvertent spillage of intestinal contents can lead to wound infection, peritonitis and intra-abdominal abscess. Such complications are seen in approximately 40% of patients undergoing colon resection without antibiotic protection. By suppressing the microflora before surgery with nonabsorbable antibiotics, the postoperative wound infection rate can be reduced to 5–10%. Clearly, this presents a target of opportunity for rifaximin, and some studies have already shown benefit in this setting.

One of the most vexing clinical problems facing many hospitals in this era is antibiotic-associated diarrhea caused by a constituent of the microflora, *C. difficile*. In North America, hospital-wide epidemics are raging in many hospitals, including highly lethal outbreaks in Canada, which have raised intense public awareness. The current treatments with vancomycin and metronidazole are clearly wanting, not only for reduced efficacy as seen in the recent outbreaks with attributable mortalities of 15–20%, but also for the high relapse rate, averaging 20%. Rifaximin shows early promise as a substitute therapy, and we await more clinical trials to establish definitive efficacy.

Other clinical conditions in which suppression of the microflora would exert benefits to the host include inflammatory bowel disease, hepatic encephalopathy, prevention of spontaneous bacterial peritonitis in cirrhosis, and treatment of a most unwelcome member of the gastric microflora, *H. pylori*.

Despite the impressive body of work chronicled in this publication, some questions remain about rifaximin's role in our therapeutic arsenal. Most importantly, we need large and carefully controlled clinical trials in many of the promising areas discussed in this issue. These research clinical trials must pass muster by the licensing authorities of the European Union and North America, since these agencies often set the standards for the rest of world to follow. Because rifaximin is related to rifamycin, a compound which has been associated in the past with antimicrobial resistance, high vigilance must be exerted to watch for such trends. The reports of infrequent resistance to rifaximin in clinical trials have been reassuring, but we must assume a posture of watchful waiting in this area. Regarding treatment of infectious diarrhea, some failures in invasive diarrheas caused by *Campylobacter* have been noted in early trials. This concern must be settled by more studies with a broad array of diarrheal pathogens including the invasive strains.

In spite of some reservations, the overall message about rifaximin is very positive. It is a remarkably active antimicrobial agent which has the highly desirable property of little or no absorption from the gastrointestinal tract. Potential uses that capitalize on these attributes have been recorded in this exciting collection of articles. We look forward with great anticipation to more clinical trials to establish definitive efficacy in several promising areas.

Sherwood L. Gorbach, MD
Professor of Medicine and Public Health
Tufts University School of Medicine
Editor, *Clinical Infectious Diseases*

Preface

The flora of the gastrointestinal (GI) tract is complex and should be considered as a functionally active organ, the full potential of which remains to be elucidated. Each individual has about 10^{12} viable bacteria per gram of large bowel content, which is equivalent to more bacteria in one person's gut than there have ever been humans on the planet. This ecosystem is vast, both quantitatively and in terms of diversity, with the presence of at least 400–500 different species. Taking into account that a single organism displays a huge metabolic capability, the metabolic activity of the entire GI flora is immense. The magnitude of this 'organ' is even more evident if one considers that the total number of genes contained in the microflora is about 50–100 times that in the human genome.

A relationship between the normal flora and the host immune system exists with a mutual dependency between the two. A successful coexistence with a complex microflora presents a particular challenge to the immune system of the host. On the one hand, the host needs to avoid an overly aggressive response to this microbial population that would lead to the elimination of beneficial organisms and would almost certainly result in inflammation and extensive tissue damage. On the other hand, the capability to limit the spread of bacteria from the lumen into underlying tissues and to mount an effective response to intestinal pathogens needs to be maintained. A weakness of the intestinal 'mucosal barrier' would leave the host highly vulnerable to a wide range of intestinal pathogens. This kind of relationship between the GI flora and gut function (and dysfunction) has only recently become to be appreciated. The re-emergence of interest in the pathogenic role of gut bacteria in GI diseases has been fuelled in part by the recognition of the potential value of antibiotics and probiotics as therapeutic modalities.

The proliferation of antibacterial agents has made the choice of antibiotics increasingly complex. General considerations in selecting an antibiotic therapy include (1) the identity and susceptibility pattern of the infecting organisms, (2) the anatomic localization of the infection, (3) the antimicrobial spectrum of the drug, and (4) its pharmacokinetic properties. Other important considerations include the possible selection of resistant organisms, interactions with other drugs, toxicity and cost. The anatomic location of the GI infection influences the selection of the antimicrobial agent and the route of administration. For instance, oral administration of poorly absorbable agents is a suitable approach when enteric bacteria represent the therapeutic target. Nonabsorbed oral antibiotic therapy, unlike systemically available antibiotics, allows localized enteric targeting of pathogens and is associated with a minimal risk of systemic toxicity or side effects. Provided that nonabsorbed antibiotics are as effective as systemically absorbed drugs for the target illness, their safety and tolerability profiles may render them more appropriate for certain patient groups, such as young children, pregnant or lactating women, and the elderly, among whom side effects are a particular concern.

Rifaximin is a poorly absorbed antibiotic, which was first described in 1982 and introduced into the Italian market 5 years later. Taking into account its excellent activity against a broad range of enteropathogens, the first 'logical' indication for this GI-targeted antibiotic was the treatment of infectious diarrhea in both adults and children. However, the appreciation of the pathogenic role of gut bacteria in several organic and functional GI diseases has increasingly broadened its clinical use, which is now extended to hepatic encephalopathy, small intestine bacterial overgrowth, inflammatory bowel disease and colonic diverticular disease. Potential indications include the irritable bowel syndrome and chronic constipation, *Clostridium difficile* infection and bowel preparation before colorectal surgery.

After almost 20 years of extensive clinical use, new exciting developments have been made and novel therapeutic applications are being explored. It is therefore a timely moment to review both the present and future clinical use of rifaximin and the pharmacology behind it. Unlike some other publications in the field, this issue is not the result of any national or international symposium. It represents the collection of 12 commissioned monographic reviews, generously offered by 30 internationally renowned scientists, all of whom have significantly contributed to this new knowledge, in order to provide a glimpse of what may lie ahead. I am indebted to all of them for having accepted to share their knowledge with us and for having provided me with excellent manuscripts despite their many daily commitments.

I would like to thank Mr. Peter Roth and Ms. Nadine Schwald of S. Karger AG for their excellent cooperation during the publication of this supplement. I would also like to acknowledge the help of Dr. Antonella Ferrieri in collecting the manuscripts for this issue, nagging authors to submit their papers and interacting with the editor. Moreover I am grateful to Alfa Wassermann (Bologna, Italy) for backing the publication costs. Last but not least, my sincere gratitude goes to Dr. Giuseppe D'Ambrosio at the Alfa Wassermann, International Division (Milan, Italy), who rendered this publication possible. He did show a never failing enthusiasm from the very beginning and did make huge efforts to render this volume available to the medical community.

Carmelo Scarpignato, MD, DSc (Hons), PharmD (h.c.), FCP, FACG
Professor of Pharmacology & Therapeutics
Associate Professor of Gastroenterology
School of Medicine & Dentistry
University of Parma, Italy

Scarpignato C (ed): Rifaximin: A Poorly Absorbed Antibiotic.
Pharmacology and Clinical Use.

The Pathogenesis of Gastrointestinal Bacterial Overgrowth

Einar Husebye

Clinic of Medicine, Hospital of Buskerud HF, Drammen, and Division of Medicine, Ullevaal University Hospital of Oslo, Oslo, Norway

Abstract

The normal indigenous intestinal microflora consists of about 10^{15} bacteria that under physiological conditions reside mainly in the lower gastrointestinal tract. Bacterial overgrowth implies abnormal bacterial colonization of the upper gut, resulting from failure of specific defense mechanisms restricting colonization under physiological conditions. At present two types of bacterial overgrowth with defined pathogenesis can be distinguished: (1) gastric overgrowth with upper respiratory tract microflora resulting from selective failure of the gastric acid barrier, and (2) gastrointestinal overgrowth with Gram-negative bacilli (enteric bacteria) resulting from failure of intestinal clearance. *Helicobacter pylori*-induced gastritis of the oxyntic mucosa is the main cause of acquired failure of the gastric acid barrier, which is common among the healthy elderly. Intestinal clearance may fail as the result of impaired intestinal peristalsis or anatomical abnormalities that alter luminal flow. Impaired peristalsis is associated with conditions interfering with intestinal neuromuscular function including myopathic, neuropathic, autoimmune, infectious, inflammatory, metabolic, endocrine, and neoplastic diseases. Anatomical abnormalities are mainly the result of gastrointestinal surgery, intestinal diverticula or fistula. Combined failure of intestinal clearance and the gastric acid barrier results in more severe colonization with Gram-negative bacilli. Gram-negative bacilli are uncommon in the upper gut of otherwise healthy individuals with gastric hypochlorhydria, being acquired (*H. pylori*) or drug-induced. Significant bacterial overgrowth with Gram-negative bacilli is a rational in the search for an explanation to optimize clinical management. The clinical significance of colonization with upper respiratory tract microflora remains unclear. Translocation of live bacteria, their metabolic products, or antigens from a small bowel colonized by Gram-negative bacilli play a role in the pathogenesis of spontaneous bacterial peritonitis in hepatic disease and in certain types of sepsis, indicating that further studies can point to new patient populations with potential benefit from medical treatment.

Introduction

The oral cavity and the lower gastrointestinal tract are densely colonized by bacteria with counts exceeding 10^9 colony-forming units (CFU)/ml, whereas the density in the stomach and proximal small bowel is normally below 10^5 CFU/ml (fig. 1). Bacterial density increases through the ileum to approximately 2 log below cecal counts in the distal ileum. Bacterial overgrowth implies abnormal bacterial colonization of the upper gut.

There is also a segmental distribution of the types of bacteria. Strict anaerobic species are normally confined to the oral cavity and the colon, habitats they densely colonize and predominate [1–5] (fig. 1). Bacteria indigenous to the upper respiratory tract (URT flora) and anaerobic bacteria of oral origin are swallowed with saliva and recovered from the upper gut at densities below 10^5 CFU/ml. Under physiological conditions, they are considered transitory rather than indigenous to the upper gut. Facultative anaerobic bacteria are usually confined to the distal small bowel and colon, but transient species entering the gut with nutrients are occasionally recovered from the healthy upper gut at low counts.

When the mechanisms restricting bacterial colonization in the upper gut fail, due to disease or dysfunction, bacterial overgrowth develops. The segmental distribution may be gastric, intestinal or both depending on the type of failure. The consequences for the host vary from none to life-threatening complications, caused by severe water and electrolyte deficiencies and septic manifestations.

Definition of Bacterial Overgrowth

The predominant quotation in the literature is purely quantitative with 10^5 CFU/ml of small intestinal aspirate as a limit [2, 6–8]. In symptomatic bacterial overgrowth, Gram-negative bacilli are present in the small intestine, making the flora 'colonic-like' [2, 7]. The term 'bacterial overgrowth syndrome' has been used to define bacterial overgrowth leading to clinical symptoms [7], without reference to the pathogenesis of the disorder.

In the present review, an increase in bacterial density above 10^5 CFU/ml of small intestinal aspirate is considered the general definition of bacterial overgrowth, in accordance with the current standard [2, 6–8]. Based on this definition, recent data make it possible to distinguish between two types of bacterial overgrowth with distinct pathogenesis, microflora and clinical presentation: bacterial overgrowth with URT flora and with Gram-negative bacilli, respectively (table 1). With cultures from both the stomach and small intestine, the segmental distribution can also be defined. Unless the segment is specified, bacterial overgrowth is synonymous with small intestinal bacterial overgrowth.

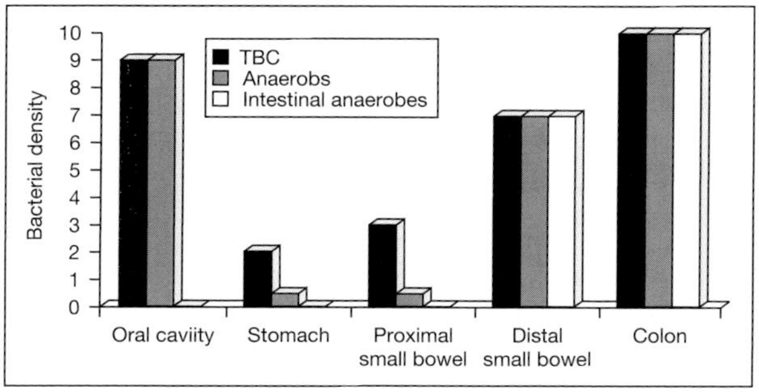

Fig. 1. The density of bacteria along the gastrointestinal tract of man is shown schematically based on data from references 1–5 in the text. Density is given by $\log_{10}$CFU/ml of luminal contents in the fasting state. TBC = Total bacterial count.

Table 1. Developing the concept of bacterial overgrowth[a]

Type	URT flora	GNB
Pathogenesis	Failure of the gastric acid barrier	Failure of intestinal clearance
Etiology	*H. pylori*-induced atrophy of gastric mucosa, drug-induced etc.	Failure of small bowel motility or intestinal anatomical abnormality
Bacteria	Mainly Gram-positive bacteria	Enterobacteriacea In severe forms strict anaerobic species of colonic type
Tracer species	α-hemolytic streptococci	*E. coli* ± *Bacteroides fragilis* group
Location and extent	Gastric stomach Similar flora present in duodenum and proximal jejunum	Small intestine, segmental or global Backwards colonization of the stomach in severe forms

Features of the two main types of bacterial overgrowth, defined by the underlying pathogenesis. See text for details of the failure required to alter the microflora of the upper gut, and the diseases and clinical conditions that can lead to failure of the gastric acid barrier and intestinal clearance, respectively.

GNB = Gram-negative bacilli.

[a]$>10^5$ CFU/ml of fasting luminal contents.

Testing for Bacterial Overgrowth

Culture of intestinal contents is the gold standard for detecting bacterial overgrowth [2, 7, 9]. This technique allows both segmental localization and the identification required to distinguish between URT and Gram-negative bacilli, respectively. The labor intensity and cost, however, make its clinical use difficult.

Of the indirect tests the ^{13}C or ^{14}C-*d*-xylose or lactulose breath test and the glucose, lactose or lactulose hydrogen breath tests are available alternatives. These tests are in general developed to recognize Gram-negative bacilli rather than URT overgrowth. There are, however, pitfalls involved.

Rapid intestinal transit may result in a false-positive breath test, in particular when hyperosmolar nonabsorbable substrates are used. A false-negative outcome in patients with culture-proven Gram-negative bacilli in the upper gut further query the sensitivity and usefulness of breath tests for clinical practice [10–13]. Positive microbial culture from small intestine is thus advantageous when major alterations of clinical management are considered.

The Main Defense Mechanisms

The pathogenesis of bacterial overgrowth is reviewed by considering separately the consequences of failure of the two main defense mechanisms in the upper gut responsible for the two types of bacterial overgrowth (table 1): the gastric acid barrier and intestinal clearance. The significance of oral bacterial carriage, degree of illness, malnutrition and immunological disorders will also be addressed.

The Gastric Acid Barrier

Defining the Gastric Acid Barrier

Gastric acid can be quantified by the capacity of secretion (peak or maximal acid output) or by the concentration of H_3O^+ ions generating the acidity of gastric juice (pH). It is the acidity that regulates microbial growth [1, 14–16], which is further emphasized by the observation that bacterial counts in the stomach correlate with basal but not with peak acid output [17]. Failure of the basal acid secretion that determines fasting gastric pH is therefore of particular importance. Accordingly, patients with a preserved ability to secrete acid in response to maximal stimulation may still have fasting hypochlorhydria [18].

At pH 4 most bacteria are killed within 30 min, and at physiological luminal pH, 99% of bacteria are killed within 5 min [14]. Certain bacteria, like lactobacilli, are more acid-resistant, and some microbes survive the hostile gastric environment by colonizing luminal niches at the mucosal surface, protected by gastric bicarbonate secretion. This is the case for *Helicobacter pylori*, related spiral-shaped bacteria, and particular fungi [5]. Although the gastric acid barrier is acidic enough to kill all bacteria ingested, dynamic changes of gastric pH and emptying related to the intake of nutrients explain survival through the gastrointestinal tract. Passage of live bacteria is physiological, and a prerequisite for maintaining a normal indigenous gut microflora [19].

Reduced gastric acidity with pH 3–5 during and just after meal intake [1] and the rapid initial phase of gastric emptying [20] both contribute to the gastric passage of live bacteria. The meal-induced increase of bacteria in the stomach and upper small bowel disappears about 1 h after meal intake, when gastric emptying is slower and gastric pH has returned towards fasting levels [1]. This occurs hours before the recurrence of the migrating motor complex in the upper gut [21], a motility pattern associated with luminal clearance of the small bowel [12, 22, 23] (see below).

The short-lasting temporal variations in gastric pH in concert with the migrating motor complex during fasting [24] are less likely to result in significant changes in gastric microflora, although the secretory component [24, 25] of the migrating motor complex contributes to intestinal clearance.

There are also segmental variations of intragastric acidity. Because the antrum is usually empty in the fasting state, local pH is substantially influenced by duodenogastric reflux and also by other factors [26] making this location less suitable for reliable measurements of the gastric acid barrier. The fundic reservoir, however, is capable of acidifying considerable amounts of refluxate. If, for example, 10 ml of duodenal chyme at pH 7 refluxes into a fundic reservoir of 50 ml gastric juice at pH 2.00, the increase to pH 2.08 is negligible in terms of microbial growth. The pH of fundic aspirate is thus a robust indicator of fasting gastric acidity with respect to the control of luminal microbial growth.

There is also a gradient from the low luminal pH through the mucus layer, under which gastric bicarbonate secretion maintains neutral conditions. Mechanically, this is explained by the acid secretion occurring like small finger-like ejections penetrating the thick gel-like mucus layer into the gastric lumen [27].

Bacterial colonization of the mucosal surface by, for example, *H. pylori*, other spiral-formed bacteria, and fungi reflect the microbial ability to pass the mucus layer and to adhere, rather than a failure of host defense. Accordingly, in developing countries with poor hygienic conditions, the great majority of people are colonized by *H. pylori* from early childhood [28, 29], whereas the prevalence in industrial countries is steadily falling with improved standards of living [29]. This type of colonization thus differs from bacterial overgrowth of the lumen that reflects microbial adaptation to the failure of host defense.

In the present review the gastric lumen is confined to the habitat above the mucus layer, for which the pH of fasting gastric juice is the major defense mechanism against bacterial colonization. This defense mechanism is henceforth denoted the gastric acid barrier.

Testing the Gastric Acid Barrier

The gastric acid barrier is tested by measuring the acidity of gastric aspirate or by an intragastric pH probe [30]. Serial aspirations during fasting over 24 h [31] gave results comparable to those obtained by intragastric pH probes during 24 h with four meals [30]. The average 24-hour pH is thus mainly determined by the fasting pH, confirming the importance of basal acid secretion in this regard. The ease and superior data acquisition when using an intragastric pH probe connected to a portable data logger make this test attractive [30], but it is expensive, time-consuming, uncomfortable for the patient, and requires expertise.

Measurement of pH in gastric juice aspired during endoscopy can be used as a rough albeit robust indicator of the gastric acid barrier. In 29 consecutive outpatients undergoing routine endoscopy, aspirates were collected from the fundic reservoir by entry of the stomach and again before withdrawal of the endoscope [32]. The increase from the first to the second aspiration was only 0.22 pH units (range −0.99 to 1.39). For the 24 patients with fasting gastric pH < 4, the mean was pH 1.87, which fits in well with the average intragastric pH 1.98 observed during 24-hour recordings in healthy individuals eating four meals [33]. The mean + 2 SD was pH 2.95 [32], corresponding to the recommended upper limit of pH 3 for normal pH of fasting gastric aspirates [1, 14, 34, 35].

A single aspirate from the fundus during fasting is also a valid indicator. Fasting gastric aspirates were obtained from 51 patients participating in an acid secretion study (unpubl. data kindly provided by L. Blomquist at the Karolinska Hospital, Stockholm, Sweden). In 26 of 51 patients pH > 3 was found in the first aspirate after intubation. The average of the four succeeding basal aspirates taken at 15 min intervals showed 100% agreement: the same 26 patients had at least one of four succeeding samples with elevated pH, using pH 3 as a cutoff. The clinical relevance of this limit is confirmed by the correlation between bacterial counts and time of pH > 3 from 24-hour pH recordings [36].

Measuring pH in fundic juice aspired when entering the stomach during endoscopy is thus a simple, robust, and valid means of testing the gastric acid barrier, and pH > 3 indicates failure.

Failure of the Gastric Acid Barrier

Causes of Failure of the Gastric Acid Barrier

Drug-Induced Inhibition of Acid Secretion

H2-Receptor Blockers

Although H_2-receptor blockade markedly inhibits maximal acid output, the reduction of gastric acidity is modest because basal output remains and tolerance develops during chronic use [37]. With a standard dosage of cimetidine of 800 mg [38] or nizatidine of 300 mg [36] gastric pH will increase modestly to about pH 2 in gastric aspirate [36, 38], which is too acidic to allow for clinically significant bacterial colonization of the stomach. Increased bacterial density in gastric juice has been reported during H_2-receptor blockade in some studies [17, 35, 39, 40], although others have found no significant change [34, 36]. The limited effect of H_2-receptor blockers that explains this discrepancy was clearly shown in a recent comparison with proton pump inhibitors [38].

Proton Pump Inhibitors

Proton pump inhibitors are potent inhibitors of gastric acid secretion, resulting in an increase of gastric pH that interferes significantly with the gastric acid barrier. It is now well established that *H. pylori* is of major importance for the magnitude of this response, an effect that relates to the extension of the gastritis into the gastric corpus [41]. In *H. pylori*-negative individuals, 20 mg of omeprazole daily increases gastric pH about 2 pH units to pH 3–4 [42] (fig. 2). This results in a 50–100-fold increase of bacterial density in the stomach [43]. In *H. pylori*-positive individuals, however, the same dose will raise gastric pH by about 4 pH units to pH 5–6, which will almost completely abolish the gastric acid barrier. Accordingly, the bacterial density increases more than 1,000-fold [42, 43]. Comparable results were obtained by Sharma et al. [44] when 30 mg of omeprazole was given to healthy volunteers without knowing their *Helicobacter* status. Based on the available literature, figure 3 shows how the density of bacteria in the stomach increases with gastric pH, to reach a plateau of about 10^8 CFU/ml beyond pH 6.

H. pylori *Colonization*

When the gastritis induced by *H. pylori* is confined to the antrum, the increase of gastrin and the reduction of somatostatin released by the G and D cells in the antrum, respectively, will increase the drive for acid secretion from the preserved oxyntic mucosa [45]. This increased acid secretion contributes to the development of duodenal ulcer and maintains the gastric acid barrier.

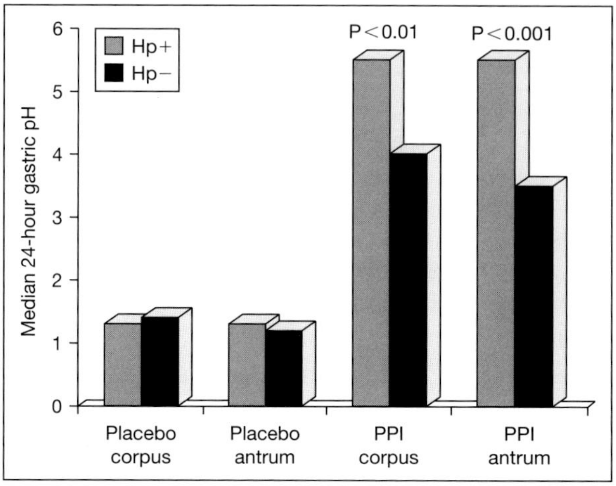

Fig. 2. Median gastric pH is elevated about 2 log by 20 mg of omeprazole in *H.* pylori-negative healthy subjects, and by 4 log in *H. pylori*-positive ones [based on data from 42]. Hp = *H. pylori*; PPI = proton pump inhibitor.

In another subpopulation, the *Helicobacter* gastritis extends into the corpus resulting in atrophy of the oxyntic mucosa and reduced acid secretion. It is not yet clear to which extent these manifestations reflect different stages or different courses of *Helicobacter*-induced gastritis [41, 45]. *H. pylori* thus emerges as the main cause of acquired gastric hypochlorhydria [46–48].

The Role of Aging

Achlorhydria, implying reduced peak acid output, was found in only 17.5% of 348 patients above 70 years of age [49]. Evidence for elevated gastric pH, however, was found in 82% of 657 patients above 65 years using the azuresin test: achlorhydria in 68% and hypochlorhydria in 14% [50]. Differences in techniques and definitions explain this divergence. Elevated fasting gastric pH is thus prevalent in the elderly. Accordingly, in healthy old people >75 years of age, 80% had hypochlorhydria defined as fasting gastric pH > 3 with average gastric pH of 6.6 (Husebye et al. in fig. 3) [32].

The observation that gastric acid secretion declines with age [49, 50] is biased because of the influence of *H. pylori*. Accordingly, the reduction of acid secretion in the elderly is a cohort effect caused by *H. pylori*-associated atrophic gastritis of the oxyntic mucosa [46–48]. In *H. pylori*-negative individuals, gastric acid secretion persists during aging [46, 48, 51, 52] in the absence of autonomic diseases and other conditions interfering with acid secretion [53].

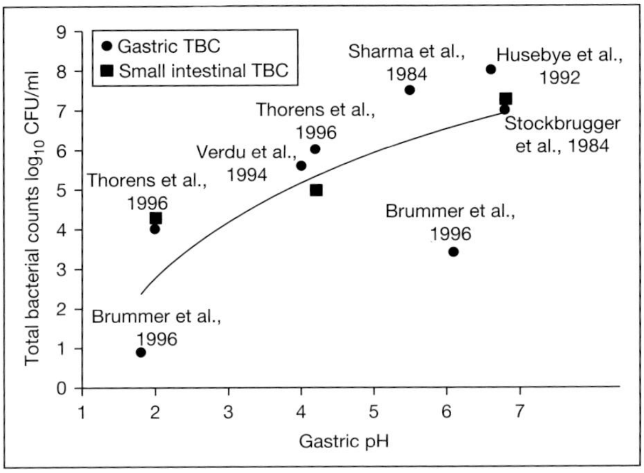

Fig. 3. The relationship between gastric pH and total bacterial counts in the stomach is shown by studies of patient populations and healthy volunteers with different gastric pH levels. Verdu et al. [43], 1994: *H. pylori*-negative healthy subjects on omeprazole 20 mg. Sharma et al. [44], 1984: Healthy individuals on omeprazole 30 mg. Thorens et al. [38], 1996: Patients on omeprazole 20 mg or cimetidine 800 mg (lower pH). Brummer et al. [36], 1996: Patients on omeprazole 20 mg or nizatidine 300 mg (lower pH). Stockbrugger et al. [17], 1984: Patients with pernicious anemia. Husebye et al. [32], 1992: Healthy old individuals with hypochlorhydria related to gastritis. Thorens et al. and Stockbrugger et al. also give data for duodenal cultures; corresponding values are found at the same pH as for gastric TBC. Logarithmic trend line for gastric bacterial counts is given.

Autoimmune Disease

Pernicious anemia is the classical autoimmune disease associated with immunologically mediated injury of the oxyntic mucosa resulting in achlorhydria [52]. Parietal cell antibodies are also present in other autoimmune diseases [52, 53] and immunopathies [54] that can be associated with hypo- or achlorhydria.

Malnutrition and Degree of Illness

Malnutrition per se is associated with both gastric hypochlorhydria and bacterial overgrowth with both URT flora and Gram-negative bacilli [55]. The degree of illness, which determines oral colonization with Gram-negative bacilli [56], contributes to this change of microflora in severe malnutrition. Accordingly, when severely malnourished children were nourished, the gastric Gram-negative colonization disappeared after initial treatment, before gastric acidity was restored [55]. Malnutrition, therefore, induces Gram-negative colonization of the upper gut through mechanisms other than the failure of the gastric acid barrier. This observation concurs with other studies showing that gastric hypochlorhydria per se does not lead to Gram-negative colonization of the stomach [32, 34, 40, 44].

Surgery

Gastric surgery reducing acid secretion is associated with gastric bacterial overgrowth with URT flora corresponding to the degree of pH elevation, and in a proportion of patients also Gram-negative bacilli, depending on the type of surgery [16, 57, 58]. Greenlee et al. [59] carefully examined the influence of different types of gastric acid-reducing surgery on the microflora of the upper gut in dogs. Gastrectomy and truncal vagotomy resulted in 100–1,000 times higher concentrations of bacteria in the upper jejunum. After proximal gastric vagotomy, however, resulting in a similar elevation of gastric pH, no change of jejunal microflora was found [59]. The same pattern is seen in clinical studies [16, 58, 60]. Changes of the anatomy and the parasympathetic innervation of the antroduodenal region after surgery may interfere with motility and clearance, and thus predispose to colonization with Gram-negative bacilli in the small bowel.

Consequences for the Gastric Microflora

Gastric Acidity and the Density of the Gastric Microflora

There is a close correlation between gastric acidity and the density of bacteria in the stomach. At fasting gastric pH < 3, gastric aspirate will be sterile or contain less than 10^3–10^4 CFU/ml [1, 14, 61–63]. With an elevation of gastric pH, bacterial counts increase to a plateau of about 10^6–10^8 CFU/ml at pH 6–7.5 [1, 62–64] (see fig. 3). This was recently reviewed in further detail by Yeomans et al. [65].

Gastric Acidity and the Composition of the Gastric Microflora

In healthy individuals URT flora multiplies in gastric aspirate during treatment with antisecretory compounds and in particular proton pump inhibitors [34, 40, 44]. This concerns viridans streptococci, coagulase-negative staphylococci, *Haemophilus* sp., diphtheroids, *Moraxella* sp., lactobacilli, and other streptococci, most of which are Gram-positive bacteria. With dedicated measures anaerobic species of oral origin are also recovered [66].

Gram-negative bacilli are in general not recovered or only occasionally and at low counts in studies of healthy individuals on acid inhibitors [34, 40, 43, 44] (table 2). This pattern has also been shown in healthy old people with hypochlorhydria secondary to chronic gastritis, of whom the great majority only harbored URT flora despite gastric pH > 6 [32].

In patient populations with gastric hypochlorhydria, as discussed above, Gram-negative bacilli are recovered in a minor proportion. This concerns

Table 2. Degree and cause of failure of the gastric acid barrier and gastric microflora in density and composition

Gastric pH	Cause	Gastric bacterial density	Gastric microflora
2–3(4)	H_2 blockers	No or mild increase $<10^{3-5}$ CFU/ml	Sterile or URT (5–10% GNB in patients)
3–4	PPI in Hp− healthy subjects	Moderate increase 10^{4-6} CFU/ml	URT
	PPI in Hp− patients[a]		URT (10–25% GNB)
4–6	Moderate Hp gastritis[b]	Marked increase 10^{5-7} CFU/ml	URT
	Incomplete proximal vagotomy		URT (10% GNB)
	PPI in Hp+ healthy subjects		URT
	PPI in Hp+ patients		URT (10–30% GNB)
	Peptic ulcer surgery		URT (10–50% GNB)[c]
6–7.5	Advanced Hp gastritis[d]	Maximum increase 10^{8-9} CFU/ml	URT
	Peptic ulcer surgery		URT (10–50% GNB)
	Autoimmune atrophic gastritis		URT (20–30% GNB)

GNB = Gram-negative bacilli; PPI = proton pump inhibitor; Hp = *H. pylori.*
[a]Patients with peptic ulcer disease and reflux esophagitis.
[b]Early stage of atrophic corpus gastritis of limited extension (less common).
[c]The prevalence of Gram-negative bacilli colonization depends on the type of surgery (see text).
[d]Atrophic corpus gastritis (prevalent in the elderly due to the high prevalence and duration of *H. pylori* colonization in this age cohort).

10–30% of patients on acid inhibitors, in particular proton pump inhibitors [36, 39, 67], 10–50% after gastric ulcer surgery depending on the type of surgery [16, 57, 58], and about 30% of patients with pernicious anemia (table 2). The Gram-negative bacilli most frequently reported are *Escherichia coli, Klebsiella* sp., and *Proteus* sp., belonging to the Enterobacteriacea. This type of colonization is hard to explain only with increased gastric pH.

Patients with peptic ulcer disease have mucosal injury and may develop fibrosis in the antroduodenal region and changes in mucosal defense and motility [68] that may contribute to a shift from URT flora to Gram-negative bacilli when on proton pump inhibitors. Moreover, 41% of patients with reflux disease have delayed gastric emptying [69], a delay that is considerable in some patients, suggesting an underlying motility disorder [70].

To predict the type of gastric microflora in patients with elevated gastric pH, the presence of local structural and functional changes that may result from diseases requiring acid inhibition [36, 39, 67], nutritional status [55], degree of illness [56], and concurrent diseases or drugs that may interfere with gastrointestinal motility [71] must be considered. It should be recalled that when such factors are present, acid inhibition may promote colonization with Gram-negative bacilli in the upper gut. In a detailed prospective study of patients with late radiation enteropathy, concurrent failure of the gastric acid barrier was found to aggravate significantly the bacterial overgrowth with Gram-negative bacilli resulting from failure of intestinal peristalsis [12]. Accordingly, jejunal bacterial overgrowth was promoted by concurrent hypochlorhydria in patients with progressive systemic sclerosis [72].

Summary of Failure of the Gastric Acid Barrier: Gastric Bacterial Overgrowth

Selective failure of the gastric acid barrier, as seen in otherwise healthy individuals on proton pump inhibitors or with *H. pylori*-induced corpus gastritis, results in gastric colonization of swallowed oropharyngeal bacteria. In otherwise healthy subjects this will be mainly Gram-positive bacteria belonging to the URT flora and strict anaerobic bacteria of oral origin.

Gastric acid is the main defense mechanism against gastric bacterial overgrowth, and the density of bacteria correlates to intragastric acidity, as shown in figure 3 and table 2, depending mainly on basal acid output. A significant increase in bacterial density is seen when fasting gastric acidity exceeds pH 3, the upper normal limit for pH in fasting gastric juice aspired during endoscopy. Bacterial density peaks at 10^8–10^9 CFU/ml of gastric juice at pH 6–7.5.

H. pylori is now recognized as the main cause of selective gastric hypochlorhydria, which today is highly prevalent (more than 50%) in the normal elderly population of western countries and predominant in developing countries with prevalence often exceeding 90%. The influence of proton pump inhibitors on gastric pH and microflora is enhanced in the presence of *H. pylori* (fig. 2). H_2-receptor blockers have less effect on gastric acidity, remaining below pH 3, and thus on gastric microflora.

Concurrent colonization by Gram-negative bacilli occurs in some patients with failure of the gastric acid barrier, suggesting additional deficiencies of host defense: abnormal oral flora, malnutrition, general illness, or diseases or medication interfering with intestinal peristalsis and clearance. This type of microflora is also seen in 10–30% of patients on acid inhibitors, for which mucosal injury and functional changes related to peptic ulcer and reflux disease may be responsible.

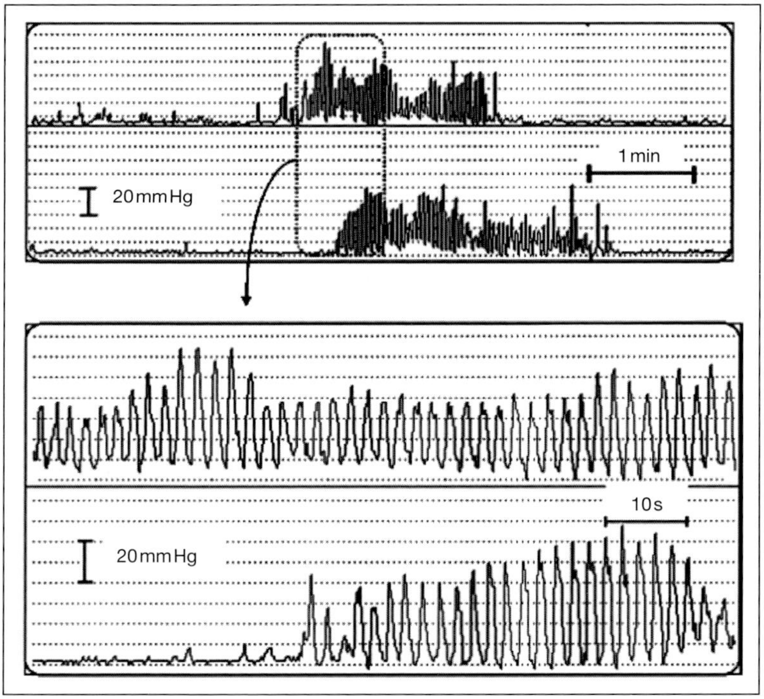

Fig. 4. The normal nocturnal migrating motor complex (MMC) recorded in the duodenum (upper tracing) and proximal jejunum (lower tracing) of a 91-year-old healthy woman. A short period is shown in high resolution in the lower panel. Phase III is preceded by phase II with some contractile activity, usually limited during sleep, and succeeded by contractile quiescence, phase I. The sequence of phase III-I-II-III constitutes one MMC cycle, and recurs during fasting (modified with permission from Husebye and Engedal [79]).

Consequences for the Intestinal Microflora

The consequences of a failure of the gastric acid barrier for the intestinal microflora emerge from studies of healthy individuals and patient populations with other important defense mechanisms against bacterial colonization intact.

Intestinal Microflora in Healthy Individuals with Gastric Hypochlorhydria

Drug-Induced Inhibition of Acid Secretion

Shindo et al. [66] treated 19 healthy volunteers with omeprazole 20 mg, cultured gastric and jejunal aspirate, and determined gastric pH and bile acid metabolism. Although motility studies were not performed, it can be assumed that intestinal migrating motor complexes were normal [21] (fig. 4). Bacterial colonization was defined by species density exceeding 10^5 CFU/0.5 ml, and only reported for those exceeding this limit.

Omeprazole resulted in an increase in URT flora, without a significant shift towards Gram-negative bacilli colonization. Two subjects had *E. coli* colonization in jejunal aspirates before treatment. Eleven showed colonization during treatment, all by a single species: *Bacteroides vulgatus* (n = 4) and *Bacteroides uniformis* (n = 1), *Eubacterium parvum* (n = 2) and *Eubacterium lentum* (n = 1), *Lactobacillus bifidus* (n = 2), and *Corynebacterium granulosum* (n = 1). These are anaerobic and aerobic bacteria that may colonize the oropharyngeal habitat. The *Bacteroides* spp. are, however, of the intestinal type, although they are not obligatorily intestinal as is *Bacteroides fragilis* [73]. It is notable that Shindo et al. [74] also reported significant jejunal colonization by intestinal types of anaerobes in healthy individuals during cimetidine treatment, which they explained by a shift to neutral pH in gastric juice [74]. Significant jejunal colonization by *E. coli* was found in 7 of 53 individuals before and in 4 individuals only during treatment with H_2 blocker. The same species as reported during omeprazole treatment [66] were recovered [74], mostly bacteria of oropharyngeal origin.

Significant colonization by *E. coli* in 13% [74] and 21% [66] of the healthy subjects prior to treatment may suggest oral carriage for reasons unrelated to gastrointestinal structure and function. H_2-receptor blockers elevate gastric pH only modestly, regardless of *H. pylori*, and fasting gastric pH < 3 should be expected [36, 38], which does not lead to major changes of gastric or duodenal microflora in healthy individuals [34, 36, 38–40]. Moreover, colonization by strict anaerobic bacteria of intestinal type in the proximal small bowel has thus far been associated with stasis of the small bowel [12, 75] and co-colonization by coliforms (Enterobacteriacea) at significant counts [12, 75]. Many standard identification schemes for *Bacteroides* spp. are designated for potentially pathogenic intestinal types and may misidentify isolates of oral origin [73].

Furthermore, similar glucose hydrogen breath tests in the elderly with and without omeprazole [76] and normal ^{14}C-*d*-xylose breath test in healthy old people with acquired gastric hypochlorhydria (pH > 6) [32] counterindicate that H_2 blockers induce colonization with strict anaerobes of intestinal types (colonic flora) in the upper gut.

An important novel finding in these studies was the detection of bile acid metabolism during acid suppression in healthy volunteers [66, 74], presumably caused by gastric bacteria, in particular when gastric pH exceeds 4 [66, 74, 77]. In vitro experiments showed that most of the bacteria recovered, mainly of oropharyngeal origin, were able to metabolize ox bile [66, 74]. In contrast, the ^{14}C glycocholic breath test was unchanged 6 weeks after omeprazole 40 mg and 26 weeks after 20 mg [78], and more studies of acid inhibition and microbial metabolism in the upper gut are thus needed.

The consequence of bacterial bile acid metabolism [66, 74, 77] is hardly clinically significant malabsorption [6] in otherwise healthy individuals [32, 79], but in predisposed individuals this may be different. Accordingly, omeprazole interferes with the absorption of vitamin B_{12} [80–83] and protein assimilation [84]. The mechanism for altered vitamin B_{12} absorption is prevention of its cleavage from dietary protein [83], for which the importance of the concurrent bacterial overgrowth has not yet been ruled out.

Shindo et al. [66, 74, 77] explain the presence of *Bacteroides* spp., presumably of the intestinal type, by migration from the ileum due to the change of pH in the small bowel. With a pH between 5 and 6 in the physiological state allowing bacterial colonization, the minor shift induced by cimetidine is unlikely to change significantly the microbial ecology of the small bowel. Accordingly, gastric pH did not correlate to Gram-negative colonization in jejunal aspirate [85].

Retrograde colonization is less likely in the absence of a widespread motility disorder or fistula [12, 75, 86]. When judged by defecatory intervals and stool form score, omeprazole was found to speed intestinal transit [87], which is comparable to experimental data showing that the predominant effect of commensal intestinal bacteria on physiological small bowel motility is the stimulation of myoelectric activity and transit [88, 89]. Elevated gastric pH will increase the load of bacteria that enter small intestine (fig. 3). Accordingly, in a recent thesis the combination of 40 mg of omeprazole twice daily and 300 mg of H_2 blocker at bedtime induced intestinal contractile activity during the fasting state by increasing phase II activity at the expense of phase I of migrating motor complex [90] (fig. 4).

In conclusion, total bacterial counts in the duodenum and the most proximal part of the jejunum of healthy subjects increase by about 2 log during standard proton pump inhibition with omeprazole 20 mg daily [87]. The bacterial species encountered are mainly of the URT flora. Gram-negative bacilli are occasionally recovered at low counts, the origin of which may be ingested food or oral carriage. There is disagreement concerning gastrointestinal bacterial metabolism during acid inhibition. Most studies have been negative [32, 76, 78, 87], but recent data [66, 72, 74, 77, 91] may indicate otherwise, at least for bile acids. Gastric overgrowth by URT flora, the ultimate result of elevated gastric pH, may thus not be as harmless as currently thought [52, 81, 83, 84]. Further studies are required [92] to clarify this important issue regarding the safety of pharmacological acid suppression in clinical practice.

Age-Associated *H. pylori*-Induced Hypochlorhydria

Healthy old people with fasting gastric hypochlorhydria and preserved intestinal motility [79] had normal ^{14}C-*d*-xylose breath test, corresponding with gastric culture showing predominantly URT flora in >90% of the individuals [32]. Overgrowth with Gram-negative bacilli in the upper gut is thus not a consequence of failure of the gastric acid barrier per se [32]. This corresponds to the absence of Gram-negative bacilli in the upper gut of patients with normal migrating motor complex in proximal small bowel [12], and malnourished children during recovery when hypochlorhydria is still present [55].

Intestinal Microflora in Patients with Gastric Hypochlorhydria

Cregan et al. [93] showed that neither gastric hypochlorhydria nor the presence of a profuse gastric microflora necessarily lead to the development of a resident flora in the mid-small bowel: 'an antibacterial mechanism, distinct from that in the stomach, must operate in small intestine'. Accordingly, Frederiksen et al. [85] could not find any relationship between gastric secretory capacity and Gram-negative bacilli in jejunal aspirate in a large series of patients.

Of 41 patients with chronic abdominal complaints after previous successful abdominal radiotherapy for pelvic malignancy, 29 patients had preserved intestinal peristalsis and clearance evidenced by normal migrating motor complex activity during prolonged ambulatory intestinal manometry, and normal anatomy by small bowel follow-through [12] (fig. 5). Five of these 29 (18%) had gastric hypochlorhydria. Dense gastric bacterial colonization was found in all, consisting of only URT flora in 4 of 5 (80%). *E. coli* was recovered in only 1 patient and strict anaerobic bacteria of colonic origin were not detected. Despite dense colonization of the stomach, the duodenum was only moderately colonized [12] by principally the same bacterial species. This corresponds to the findings of Sherwood et al. [75], sampling from five sites along the small bowel. They showed that intestinal anaerobic overgrowth occurred in relation to local or general stasis in the small bowel. In their study group with previous partial gastrectomy, intestinal anaerobes were not recovered from any site of the small bowel, despite marked gastric hypochlorhydria and complementary gastric bacterial overgrowth [75].

A correspondence between gastric and duodenal microflora when the gastric acid barrier fails has also been shown in patients with pernicious anemia [17].

Summary of Failure of the Gastric Acid Barrier: Intestinal Bacterial Overgrowth

When the gastric acid barrier fails the bacterial counts in the most proximal part of small bowel increase. Standard proton pump inhibition by omeprazole 20 mg daily will increase bacterial density by about 2 log, because bacteria are continuously emptied from the colonized gastric reservoir. In the duodenum the species will be quite similar to those cultured from the stomach. Unless there are concurrent factors or conditions predisposing to colonization with intestinal Gram-negative bacilli, URT flora will predominate. Recent data suggest that this URT flora may cause bacterial metabolism of bile acids and alter the assimilation and proteins and vitamin B_{12}, the significance of which remains to be clarified. In patients with a failure of other defense mechanisms predisposing to colonization

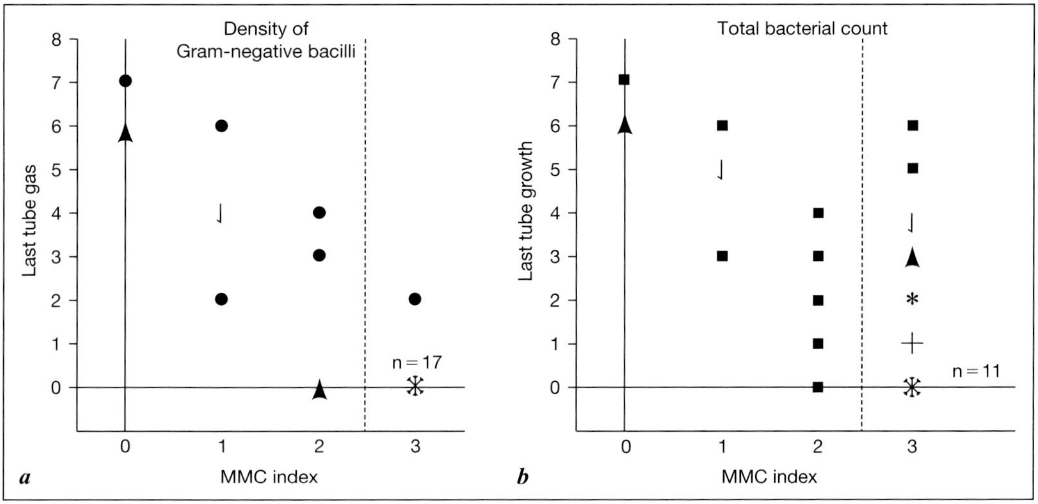

Fig. 5. Relationship between fasting intestinal motility [x-axis: migrating motor complex (MMC) index] and bacterial colonization of small bowel in 41 patients with late radiation enteropathy (LRE) is shown by two plots. Relationship to Gram-negative bacilli (***a***) and to total bacterial count (***b***) in the duodenum is shown. Note that no significant Gram-negative colonization was found in patients with normal MMC (index = 3). The vertical dotted lines show the normal limit for MMC index. Increased bacterial counts due to URT flora were found in some patients with normal MMC (***b***). Tied observations are indicated as follows: n = 1: ●, ■; n = 2: ↓; n = 3: ▲; n = 4: +; n = 6: ✱. For n > 6 number is given (with permission from Husebye et al. [12]). For total bacterial count 'last tube growth' indicates $\log_{10}$ for CFU/ml. For 'last tube gas' see [12].

by Gram-negative bacilli, proton pump inhibition will augment this type of bacterial overgrowth, which may be clinically harmful.

When intestinal peristalsis and clearance are intact, the bacteria are rapidly transported aborally, and in the mid jejunum bacterial counts are in general low (normal) despite dense gastric colonization. Considerable evidence indicates that bacteria recovered from small bowel under such conditions are transient rather than resident.

Intestinal Clearance

Defining Intestinal Clearance

Intestinal clearance is henceforth defined as the ability of the small bowel to clear its lumen of bacteria. The known conditions of major clinical importance for intact intestinal clearance are (1) normal gastrointestinal anatomy, including the absence of intestinal diverticula and fistula, and (2) normal intestinal motility.

Secretion and the immune system also contribute to luminal clearance of bacteria, but dysfunction and abnormalities of clinical relevance for the development of bacterial overgrowth have so far been associated with the factors outlined above. Moreover, normal intestinal motility, tested by manometry, also indicates that the enteric neuroendocrine control of motility, secretion, absorption and circulation is intact [24, 25, 94]. To the extent that gastrointestinal secretion has been studied, failure does not seem to result in bacterial overgrowth [95–98]. Studies on the immune system are briefly discussed later. The failure to recognize the clinical importance of these factors in the present context may, however, also reflect current methodological and scientific limitations. Although a failure of the gastric acid barrier increases the bacterial load to the small intestine from the gastric reservoir, evidence does not indicate that this defense mechanism contributes significantly to intestinal clearance of bacteria.

Intestinal Motor Activity and Clearance of Bacteria

Rolly and Liebermeister [95] showed that bacteria introduced into the small bowel disappeared rapidly, without bile, pancreatic, and intestinal juices having antibacterial properties alone or mixed. Later studies, of which those by Dack and Petran [96], Dixon [99] and Dixon and Paulley [100] are of particular importance, provided considerable further evidence that intestinal peristalsis is the main line of defense against bacterial colonization of the small bowel. This was also concluded by Donaldson [101–103] when he reviewed host defense mechanisms in 1964. At that time, however, the insights into small bowel motility were confined to the reflex-mediated peristaltic behavior.

Bayliss and Starling [104] described the peristaltic reflex of small intestine in 1899. This enterically controlled reflex elicits a contraction oral to and a relaxation distal to a segmental distension, resulting in the movement of contents in the aboral direction [104]. The peristaltic reflex is fundamental for understanding the behavior of the small bowel during nutrient stimulation, and there is a revived interest in the control mechanisms involved [105].

Reflex behavior, however, does not fully explain intestinal motor activity. During the fasting state, the small bowel moves at intervals, apparently spontaneously, in the absence of nutrients. The enteric nervous system intermittently inhibits the intestinal smooth muscle cells, which would otherwise spontaneously contract at a regular rate, like the cardiac muscle, due to the intrinsic pacemaker properties [106, 107]. The fasting state thus shows periods of both silence and contractile activity, depending on the degree of enteric inhibitory control with a maximum contractile rate of 11/min in the duodenum, decreasing to 7–8/min in the ileum. Regular contractions at this frequency occur for time periods of about 5 min at intervals ranging from 20 min to hours in healthy individuals [21, 23]. This band of regular propagating contractions, called phase III of the migrating motor complex, migrates in the aboral direction (fig. 4). C.F. Code named the migrating motor complex the gastrointestinal housekeeper, due to its propulsive properties capable of clearing the lumen of contents during the fasting state [22].

Intestinal mechanical clearance thus consists of both reflex-mediated contractions (peristalsis) elicited by the stimulatory effect of luminal contents and of periods of spontaneous contractile activity (e.g. the migrating motor complex). During fasting about 50% of intestinal transit has been attributed to phase III of the migrating motor complex, the remaining mostly to the propulsive contractions and motor patterns during phase II [108]. Luminal flow can also occur in the absence of propagating contractions of the circular muscle layer, so far considered the motor event mainly responsible for flow in the small intestine.

The motility of the small bowel has been studied in great detail in experimental, physiological and clinical research [21, 71, 106, 107, 109], and the patterns are well defined in man [21, 23, 110]. Although a standard test of intestinal motor activity with regard to the efficiency of mechanical luminal clearance is not yet established for clinical use, means to evaluate this function have been proposed.

Testing Intestinal Clearance

Microbial Culture of Intestinal Contents

The absence of Gram-negative bacilli in the small bowel is a reliable indicator of preserved intestinal clearance [12, 75, 111]. Although significant colonization of Gram-negative bacilli results from failure of intestinal clearance [12, 75, 111], oral carriage due to malnutrition [55], illness and reduced health [56], and other structural and functional changes [36, 39, 67] can also be the cause. The presence of Gram-negative bacilli in small bowel is therefore an indication, but no proof of failing intestinal clearance. The denser the colonization, however, the more likely there is a failure of clearance. When strict anaerobic bacteria of the intestinal type are present, advanced failure with stagnation is indicated [12, 75], unless there is a blind loop or a fistula [7].

Reference to the normal oropharyngeal microflora is required to distinguish the URT flora [112], for which α-hemolytic streptococci are predominant and the candidate marker. Among the Gram-negative bacilli of the intestinal type, Enterobacteriacea are easy to recover by culture because they are facultative and their prevalence in bacterial overgrowth is high. *E. coli* is the predominant species, and therefore the candidate marker. The limit of 10^5 CFU/ml serves to distinguish transient Gram-negative bacilli that may be recovered in health [7]. When strict anaerobic species of the colonic type are recovered this limit may be too high, but this depends largely on the culturing technique. Standardization of culture for bacterial overgrowth is required to establish more specific quantitative limits at the species level. Microbiological expertise and control data are, therefore, required for an appropriate interpretation of cultures for the diagnosis of bacterial overgrowth. This also concerns the occasionally difficult distinction between strict anaerobic bacteria of oral and colonic types [73].

Testing the Intestinal Mechanical Clearance (Intestinal Motor Activity)

If anatomical abnormalities have been ruled out, testing of the small bowel motor activity is useful to elucidate the pathogenesis of bacterial overgrowth with Gram-negative bacilli (table 1). This choice is encouraged by the correlation between clinical disorders associated with bacterial overgrowth and disorders associated with dysmotility of the small bowel [113].

Manometry remains the gold standard test, because phasic contractions are generally lumen occlusive in small bowel and thus reliably detected by intraluminal pressure measurements. Transit tests are more convenient; nevertheless, they are time-consuming and do not provide the same detailed information about contractile activity [114, 115]. These methods are briefly discussed.

Small Bowel Manometry

Data on small bowel motility disorders have been obtained by using both stationary techniques [21, 71, 114, 116, 117] with external transducers and water-perfused catheters [117] and by the use of ambulatory techniques [21, 118]. The establishment [110] and further implementation [119–121] of ambulatory techniques allow prolonged recording throughout the day and night at home [118]. Testing of both the response to nutrient challenge and the fasting motility is required in the present context, which implies prolonged recordings. This favors the use of ambulatory techniques.

Stanghellini et al. [122] have carefully defined the most common abnormalities of phase III activity and other abnormal motility patterns that occur in patients with chronic intestinal pseudoobstruction, who often suffer from bacterial overgrowth [113]. This concerns phase III with abnormal migration (stationary or retrograde) and with abnormal isotonic component, abnormal burst activity, and a failure of the postprandial pattern.

Phase III of the migrating motor complex serves as a marker of intestinal motility for several reasons. When phase III fails, concurrent abnormalities of postprandial motility patterns and other propulsive patterns during fasting are common [12, 21, 71, 117, 122–124]. Normal occurrence of the migrating motor complex and absence of strictly abnormal motor patterns during prolonged recording, including both the fed and fasting states, are valid and reliable indicators of preserved intestinal mechanical clearance [21]. In a large series comparing prolonged ambulatory small bowel manometry and culture, failure of the migrating motor complex predicted colonization by Gram-negative bacilli in the small bowel [12]. A semiquantitative migrating motor complex index was, therefore, proposed [12]. Schemes to analyze and evaluate a small bowel manometric record have been proposed [21, 125] (fig. 5), and international consensus is pending.

Small Bowel Transit

A small bowel transit study can be used to evaluate intestinal propulsion and clearance, and the presence of Enterobacteriacea (Gram-negative bacilli) in the small bowel indicates delayed transit [111]. The wide normal variability, however, makes transit tests rather insensitive, and thus less useful clinically [126, 127]. It is also a problem that accelerated and delayed transit may coexist in neuropathies and confuse the interpretation. Finally, as nutrients are mostly absorbed in the proximal small bowel, and the rate and pattern of transit vary along the intestine, segmental failure of transit is easily missed by global transit measurements. Although easier to perform, the clinical utility is often limited unless the dysfunction is severe [127]. The most commonly used transit tests available are briefly discussed with reference to the current study.

Scintigraphy

Single- and dual-isotope techniques have been applied [126] with labeling of the liquid and solid phase by ^{99m}Tc, ^{111}In or ^{113}In, or ^{67}Ga. The difference between the half-emptying time of the stomach and the half-filling time of the cecum has usually been estimated. The more accurate approach, however, is to use the technique of deconvolving the profiles for gastric emptying and colonic filling to obtain a spectrum of transit times, and then to calculate the mean value [126]. By this technique there was no discrimination between transit of liquids and solids [126]. Transit time ranged from 1.5 to 6 h in healthy subjects after a mixed meal [126], reflecting the limitations for clinical use. Only marked acceleration or delay can be detected, which apply mainly to patients with intestinal pseudoobstruction. Modified and simplified scintigraphic tests have been developed [114, 128], the use of which should be encouraged if a transit test is chosen to evaluate intestinal peristalsis in the presence of bacterial overgrowth.

Breath Tests

Studies of small bowel transit time have demonstrated a great variability both within and between individuals. When the hydrogen breath test was performed under fasting conditions, using 10 ml of lactulose, the coefficient of variation amounted to 18%. Di Lorenzo et al. [129] showed that variations under fasting conditions are partly accounted for by the phase of the migrating motor complex at the intake of test solution. Moreover, when a lactose-containing meal was used, the coefficient of variation was reduced to 4% [130].

The main limitation of breath tests in this setting is the bias induced by the intestinal overgrowth flora, generating a breath signal that can be difficult to distinguish from the arrival of the substrate in the cecum. This is further hampered by the intermittent passage of the head of a meal into the colon, which may, also under normal conditions, generate multiple signal peaks before a more sustained signal is obtained.

Breath tests are, therefore, less useful for testing of intestinal transit in the presence of bacterial overgrowth.

Failure of Intestinal Clearance

Causes of Failing Intestinal Clearance

Abnormal Intestinal Anatomy

Anatomical changes can alter luminal flow into a surgically prepared blind loop, a diverticulum, or through a fistula. These anatomical abnormalities of relevance for the development of bacterial overgrowth have been carefully defined in previous literature [2, 7, 98].

When significant Gram-negative overgrowth is detected, anatomical abnormalities should be considered prior to studies of intestinal mechanical clearance. The anatomy is revealed by X-ray using small bowel follow-through, optionally supplied by new modalities of ultrasound, computer tomography and magnetic resonance imaging.

Failure of Intestinal Mechanical Clearance (Intestinal Motility)

Although hereditary neuropathies and myopathies affecting small intestinal motility are rare, the entire spectrum of diseases that can interfere with motility is wide, including for example diabetes mellitus, Crohn's disease, scleroderma, and postoperative and radiation sequelae [21, 71, 116, 123, 131].

Failure of intestinal motility can be severe leading to frank intestinal pseudoobstruction [122, 132] or mild to moderate depending on the underlying disease, its severity, and the degree of intestinal involvement.

In some patients believed to suffer from the irritable bowel syndrome, an underlying enteric neuromuscular disorder has later been identified [133]. The bridge to infectious diseases is also of interest, with several enterotropic viruses in focus, and reports of lymphocytic infiltration of enteric neural structures in patients with unexplained intestinal dysmotility require further studies.

Neuromuscular Diseases

Enteric Neuropathies. Different kinds of familial visceral neuropathies have been described: the dominant type 1 [134], the recessive type 2 [135] and a recessive form with calcified basal ganglia [134]. Furthermore, aganglionosis of the small bowel (Hirschsprung's disease) [136], hyperganglionosis (neurofibromatosis) [137], neuronal intestinal dysplasia [138] and Parkinson's disease [139] are neuropathies to consider. The recognition of the pacemaker cells of the small bowel, the interstitial cells of Cajal, has prompted studies to detect abnormalities of these cells, another possible cause of pseudoobstruction [140].

Extrinsic Neuropathies. Autonomic dysfunction [141], pandysautonomia [142, 143], Shy-Drager syndrome [144] and sympathetic dysfunction are conditions associated with intestinal dysmotility.

Vagal neuropathy in diabetes mellitus [145, 146] and truncal vagotomy [147] may markedly change intestinal motility, as do heart-lung transplantation [148]. Spinal cord lesions also alter gut function, but the outlet obstruction due to failure of the striated muscles involved in defecation is more important than the enteric smooth muscle effects [149].

Enteric Myopathies. The familial types include the dominant type 1 [150], the recessive type 2 with ophthalmoplegia [151] and the recessive type 3 [116]. The sporadic types include muscular dystrophies [152] including myotonic dystrophy [153] and Duchenne's dystrophy. Dysmotility has been associated with all these diseases.

Diseases and Injury of the Gut Wall

Radiation Injury. Late radiation enteropathy is associated with alterations of small intestinal motility [154], intestinal pseudoobstruction [154, 155] and Gram-negative colonization of the small bowel in patients with impaired small bowel motility [12]. In patients with severe injury, alterations in the motility and microflora are of main importance for the clinical symptoms [154].

Inflammation. Chronic inflammatory bowel disease affecting the small bowel can lead to disturbances of intestinal motility [146]. Potential mechanisms are previous surgery, development of fibrosis and strictures, malabsorption, and 'cross-talk' between inflammatory and enteric nerves [156, 157]. Patients with Crohn's disease are often included in aggregate studies of bacterial overgrowth [23, 75, 158], reflecting this link.

Connective Tissue Diseases. Scleroderma is the connective tissue disease most frequently associated with intestinal dysmotility and bacterial overgrowth [159, 160]. Although the motility of the esophagus is most frequently affected, and a prerequisite for the label CREST syndrome, small bowel involvement is seen in a proportion of these patients. When present, intestinal clearance is usually impaired because of shallow contractions resulting in ineffective peristalsis and clearance. This can lead to overgrowth with Gram-negative bacilli, in part responsible for the malabsorption [161].

The neuromuscular compartment of the bowel wall is also affected in certain types of the Ehler-Danlos syndrome [162], maybe in amyloidosis [163], and in the presence of diffuse lymphocytic infiltration [164].

Infectious Diseases

Chagas disease affects enteric ganglionic cells. This leads to altered motility with a reduced rate of migration for the migrating motor complex [165], a change associated with colonization with Gram-negative bacilli [12].

Dysmotility has been reported in Lyme disease [166] and in postviral syndromes associated with cytomegalovirus and herpes simplex virus [167]. Altered intestinal motility can also be part of infectious mononucleosis [168].

Metabolic and Endocrine Disorders

Thyroid Disease. Hypothyroidism (myxedema) [169] and hyperthyroidism [170] alter small bowel motility. Although today these diseases are usually recognized before such symptoms develop, thyroid function must be examined in unexplained intestinal pseudoobstruction.

Diabetes Mellitus. Diabetes mellitus interferes with gastrointestinal motility through different mechanisms including blood sugar oscillations, extrinsic vagal neuropathy, vascular changes and enteric neural injury. Intestinal dysmotility [145, 146] is seen in a proportion of the diabetics, and intestinal pseudoobstruction associated with bacterial overgrowth can develop. When abdominal complaints are chronic and disabling, studies of intestinal microflora and clearance should be considered, in particular if nutritional problems occur.

Paraneoplastic Syndromes

Intestinal pseudoobstruction is also part of paraneoplastic syndromes. The anti-*hu* antibodies are useful to indicate this condition, as shown in bronchial small cell carcinoma [171]. In pheochromocytoma [172] and carcinoid [173] neuromediators affecting small bowel motility are produced by the tumor cells. Intestinal pseudoobstruction has also been reported in neuroblastoma [174].

Hepatic Disease

Patients with advances liver cirrhosis often suffer from bacterial overgrowth [175]. Chang et al. [176] reported a reduced frequency and rate of migration for migrating motor complexes in patients with liver cirrhosis, alterations that predispose to colonization of the small bowel by Gram-negative bacilli [12].

Drug-Induced Dysmotility

The perhaps most important and easily ignored cause of secondary dysmotility is the drug-induced toxic type. Pharmaceuticals are important to consider, in particular those with anticholinergic and/or opioid properties [177]. In individuals with reduced reserve capacity of the gut, either due to concomitant disease or age, such drugs may elicit pseudoobstruction. Although aging does not lead to clinically significant dysmotility, the reduction in the rate of migration for migrating motor complexes and increased prevalence of clustered contractions indicate reduced reserve capacity [21, 79].

Surgery

Although the gastrointestinal tract has great adaptive and reserve capacities, surgery can directly or indirectly through generation of fibrosis, adhesions and strictures interfere with small intestinal motility [178, 179]. Vagal injury will be of importance in particular for the motor response to feeding, whereas direct injury or modifications of intestinal loops are usually present if pseudoobstruction results. The Billroth type II resection of the stomach and the Roux-en-Y anastomosis result in chronic dysmotility, likely to be of importance when postoperative abdominal complaints occur [178].

Consequences for the Gastric Microflora

Gastric emptying is delayed in patients with intestinal pseudoobstruction [180]. Intestinogastric reflexes including the duodenal and ileal brakes are candidate mechanisms for this effect. Recent data indicate that delayed gastric emptying per se does not interfere significantly with gastric microflora, when the gastric acid barrier is maintained [181].

A certain proportion of short-reaching retroperistaltic waves at the gastroduodenal junction is physiological [182], but in severe functional dyspepsia both segmental spread and the contribution of retroperistalsis in the duodenum was increased [183]. Paradoxical gastric colonization by Gram-negative bacilli despite the presence of a normal gastric acid barrier has been reported in some patients with severe late radiation enteropathy associated with marked intestinal dysmotility [12]. Giant retrogradely migrating contractions, observed in these patients, may also reflux intestinal contents into the gastric lumen.

In conclusion, gastric microflora is altered in patients with severe forms of intestinal pseudoobstruction due to frequent duodenogastric reflux episodes caused by abnormal retrogradely propagating contractions.

Consequences for the Intestinal Microflora

Pharmacological suppression of intestinal peristalsis in experimental animals leads to bacterial colonization of small bowel by all types of bacteria present in the gut, including Gram-negative bacilli [100, 184, 185]. Similar studies cannot be performed in man, but patients taking opioids regularly show changes of intestinal motor activity with a slowing of peristalsis and transit resulting in constipation.

Intestinal Microflora in Patients with Failure of Intestinal Peristalsis

Vantrappen et al. [23] for the first time showed the relevance of phase III of the migrating motor complex in the current context, when reporting its absence in 5 of 12 patients with bacterial overgrowth detected by the bile acid breath test and response to antibiotics.

The consequences of altered intestinal motility patterns for the microflora of the small bowel have later been addressed in detail [12]. Forty-one patients with varying degrees of dysmotility due to previous successful abdominal radiotherapy for malignancy were studied. Impaired phase III of the migrating motor complex was invariably associated with intestinal colonization by Gram-negative bacilli, whereas normal phase III reliably predicted the absence of such microflora [12, 21] (fig. 5). Significant URT flora was detected in the small bowel of patients with normal motility patterns and failure of the gastric acid barrier [12]. The underlying pathophysiology could thus be established, considering the type of overgrowth flora [12].

Further analyses showed that not only the presence of phase III, but also its migration velocity determined clearance. Slow migration velocity was independently associated with Gram-negative bacilli colonization [12]. The migration velocity, the duration of each phase III activity, and the overall occurrence of phase III during prolonged recording in the fasting state were summarized by a migrating motor complex index. It was then possible to predict semiquantitatively the failure of intestinal clearance, as evidenced by Gram-negative bacilli in the small bowel, with a high sensitivity, superior to the qualitative evaluation of the presence or absence of phase III of the migrating motor complex [12, 21] (fig. 4, 5). The sensitivity and specificity of MMC index for the detection of Gram-negative bacilli in the duodenum were 91% and 90%, respectively [12].

There are also distinctly abnormal patterns of motility [21] that are independently associated with Gram-negative bacilli overgrowth, such as prolonged isolated irregular bursts and giant migrating contractions [12]. Accordingly, in enteric neuropathies uncoordinated contractile activity can cause temporal stagnation and even retropulsion [122–124].

Moreover, certain enteropathogenic microorganisms [186, 187] and commensal bacteria colonizing the small bowel in experimental bacterial overgrowth [188] induce giant migrating contractions that do not occur in healthy subjects [21]. Giant migrating contractions cause rapid intestinal clearance [189], and have been reported in patients with severe Gram-negative bacilli overgrowth with strict anaerobic bacteria of the intestinal type [12].

These data on the motility patterns of the small bowel and clearance concur with a recent study showing that Gram-negative bacilli (Enterobacteriacea) in the small bowel are associated with delayed small bowel transit [111], and the early pioneer study on bacterial overgrowth showing the association between local stasis and Gram-negative colonization including strict anaerobes [75]. Moreover, the absence of phase III in a subset of patients with bacterial overgrowth has been reconfirmed [190].

Summary of Consequences for Intestinal Microflora

Failure of intestinal clearance caused by impaired motor activity or local stagnation for anatomical reasons results in Gram-negative colonization of the small bowel. Small bowel aspirate, mucosal brush, or biopsies are optional samples for culture, which is still the gold standard for detecting this type of overgrowth.

The absence of Gram-negative bacilli is a reliable and valid indication of preserved intestinal clearance, which precludes a significant failure of intestinal motility and anatomical abnormalities inducing stasis or recycling of contents from the lower gastrointestinal tract.

The presence of Gram-negative bacilli, however, can also be due to alterations in oral and gastric microflora, or to the general effects of illness and malnutrition. Further diagnostic workup to elucidate the pathogenesis is thus encouraged when bacterial overgrowth of Gram-negative bacilli is found in patients with clinically significant gastrointestinal symptoms to detect anatomical abnormalities or intestinal dysmotility.

The Significance of Changes in Local Mucosal and Systemic Immunity

Systemic Immunity

Humoral Immunity

Blood donors with selective IgA deficiency have a normal gastrointestinal microflora without evidence of bacterial overgrowth [191]. In patients with complex immunodeficiency increased bacterial colonization is seen in the upper gut, predominantly by URT flora, which may be related to concurrent gastric hypo- or achlorhydria [54, 191]. Similar findings have been made in a limited study of jejunal flora in children [192].

Cellular Immunity

Patients with HIV display different degrees of failure of cell-mediated immunity. The prevalence of URT flora in the upper gut was in line with what was expected, and did not change with the clinical severity of the disease [193]. Colonization by Gram-negative bacilli was frequently found in HIV patients with diarrhea, regardless of its cause, but not in those with normal stools [193]. The cause and the consequences of Gram-negative bacilli in the upper gut of HIV patients remain unclear, but the degree of malnutrition [55] and illness [56] are likely to contribute. Children with a T cell defect have URT flora in the upper gut, but the prevalence is hardly significantly increased [192]. Duodenal microflora was examined in 32 patients with HIV infection [193]. Those with and without increased density of bacteria in the small bowel ($>10^5$ CFU/ml) had gastric pH 4.0 and 2.8 (nonsignificant), respectively. Gastric pH values for patients with and without Gram-negative bacilli flora in the duodenum were 3.3 and 3.2, respectively. This study could not establish a link between HIV infection and bacterial overgrowth, and provided further evidence that factors other than gastric hypochlorhydria explain the presence of Gram-negative bacilli in the small bowel.

Intestinal Mucosal Immunity

An identified specific defect of local mucosal immunity that results in bacterial overgrowth with URT flora or Gram-negative bacilli has not yet been detected, but there is evidence indicating that the mucosal immune system responds to a resident overgrowth flora with Gram-negative bacilli in the small intestine. The number of IgA2 immunocytes was increased in the jejunum, whereas the number of IgM immunocytes was reduced [194]. The increase in IgA2 may enhance mucosal protection and probably reflects immunomodulation caused by lipopolysaccharides of Gram-negative bacilli [194]. Accordingly, stimulated production of luminal IgA was recently reported in elderly patients with bacterial overgrowth with Gram-negative bacilli [195].

Moreover, bacterial overgrowth flora with Gram-negative bacilli, but not with URT flora, is associated with an increase in intraepithelial lymphocytes, reflecting an immune response in the small intestine [196]. These findings emphasize corresponding differences in the pathophysiology for the two types of bacterial overgrowth defined by pathogenesis.

From Pathogenesis to Clinical Management

Knowing the cause of the problem can facilitate and improve clinical management. In table 3 a clinical algorithm for dealing with each type of bacterial overgrowth is proposed based on the insight of the pathogenesis as discussed in the present review.

Failure of the gastric acid barrier and URT overgrowth are 'benign' alterations of gut function, as opposed to bacterial overgrowth with Gram-negative bacilli associated with a wide spectrum of potential clinical problems. This difference should not be attributed solely to the bacteria, but rather to the underlying defect of the host. Failure of intestinal motility, for example, can lead to problems of digestion and transport independent of the Gram-negative bacilli in the lumen. The overgrowth flora reflects microbial adaptation that may produce additional clinical symptoms, depending on density and composition.

The clear distinctions in the pathogenesis, microbial flora and pathophysiology of bacterial overgrowth with URT flora and Gram-negative bacilli, respectively, encourage a classification based on the pathogenesis (table 1). As shown in table 3, corresponding distinctions can be made in the diagnostic workup and further clinical management.

Findings and Insights of Particular Interest

Suppression of the Gastric Acid Barrier

Reduced protein and vitamin B_{12} assimilation, in particular in the elderly, is a recently recognized risk. Malabsorption due to acid deficiency, microbial metabolism of bile acids by the URT flora, and reduced reserve capacity of the gut in the elderly are candidate mechanisms, confined or combined. The increased risk of gastrointestinal infections is well established and more relevant nowadays with the marked increase in traveling between continents. This also involves elderly people, more often suffering from a failure of the gastric acid

Table 3. Algorithm for clinical management of bacterial overgrowth based on stratification by pathogenesis

<table>
<tr><th colspan="2">GNB overgrowth</th><th rowspan="2">URT overgrowth no further diagnostic measures</th></tr>
<tr><th>Anatomical disorder possible</th><th>Anatomical disorder ruled out or unsuitable for surgery</th></tr>
<tr><td>Diagnostic workup
Search for fistula, large or multiple small intestinal diverticula, and an enlarged surgical blind loop (X-ray) or confined segment of intestine</td><td>Diagnostic workup
Consider the presence of diseases and conditions associated with impairment of small bowel motility

If present and clinical symptoms are significant, test small bowel motility[a]</td><td>If patients are on PPI and nutritional deficiencies occur, the indication and further prescription should be reconsidered, in particular in the elderly</td></tr>
<tr><td>Management
If significant abnormality is detected, consider surgical correction</td><td>Management
If significantly abnormal, avoid drugs interfering with small bowel motility and/or intestinal microflora; give dietary advice to avoid nutrients requiring major grinding and mixing, and provide vitamin D, calcium, iron, and vitamin B_{12} as indicated; optimize treatment of underlying disorder, and provide drugs promoting small bowel motility</td><td></td></tr>
<tr><td colspan="3">If none of the above measures are relevant or sufficiently effective
Provide antibiotics, by preference poorly absorbed types, efficient against Enterobacteriacea and strict anaerobic bacteria; give intermittent trials and cycle different antibiotics to reduce the risk of resistance.
Avoid drugs suppressing gastric acid secretion.
Monitor effects by symptomatic improvement, gain of body weight and improved blood tests as indicated: hemoglobin, calcium, albumin, iron, B_{12} and folic acid.</td></tr>
</table>

GNB = Gram-negative bacilli; PPI = proton pump inhibitors.

[a]See text for testing of small bowel motility. If testing is not available, the management advice can be followed provided that significant colonization by Gram-negative bacilli is present in small bowel (see text for testing of bacterial overgrowth).

barrier due to *H. pylori*-induced gastritis or using proton pump inhibitors. Although no clear link exists between URT overgrowth in the upper gut and cancer, this issue has not been fully explored. Furthermore, precipitation or aggravation of bacterial overgrowth with Gram-negative bacilli in predisposed individuals has been demonstrated, and may be a problem with the more liberal use of long-term proton pump inhibitor treatment beyond study audit. Clinical data are still too sparse to justify management guidelines for these issues, prompting clinical awareness and further research.

Failure of Intestinal Clearance

By recognizing significant anatomical abnormalities and intestinal dysmotility, attempts to restore the causal problems are encouraged. This is important, because the Gram-negative bacilli can be innocent bystanders, a clinically silent consequence of the underlying problem rather than the cause of the symptoms. Attempts to modulate the abnormal microflora by anti-, pre-, or probiotics are justified when treatment of the underlying problem is impossible or ineffective. This will often be the case, and antibiotics usually have temporary effect. Studies comparing antibiotics are now emerging [197, 198]. Drugs with effects on intestinal anaerobic and facultative bacteria are in general effective, and poorly absorbed antibiotics, like rifaximin [198], are good candidates because of limited systemic effects and antimicrobial action along the entire length of the small intestine. This rifamycin derivative indeed proved to be one of the most effective antimicrobials in the treatment of bacterial overgrowth [199].

References

1 Drasar BS, Shiner M, Mcloed GM: Studies on the intestinal flora. The bacterial flora of the gastrointestinal tract in healthy and achlorhydric persons. Gastroenterology 1969;56:71–79.
2 Simon GL, Gorbach SL: Intestinal flora in health and disease. Gastroenterology 1984;86:174–193.
3 Savage DC: Microbial ecology of the gastrointestinal tract. Annu Rev Microbiol 1977;31:107–133.
4 Dickman MD, Chappelka AR, Schaedler RW: The microbial ecology of the upper small bowel. Am J Gastroenterol 1976;65:57–62.
5 Liljemark WF, Bloomquist CG: Normal microbial flora of the human body; in Newman MG, Nisengard R (eds): Oral Microbiology and Immunology. Philadelphia, Saunders, 1988, pp 140–142.
6 Saltzman JR, Kowdley KV, Pedrosa MC, Sepe T, Golner B, Perrone G, et al: Bacterial overgrowth without clinical malabsorption in elderly hypochlorhydric subjects. Gastroenterology 1994;106: 615–623.
7 King CE, Toskes PP: Small intestine bacterial overgrowth. Gastroenterology 1979;76:1035–1055.
8 Clarke RTJ, Beauchop T: Methods for studying gut microbes; in Clarke RTJ, Beauchop T (eds): Microbial Ecology of the Gut. London, Academic Press, 1977, pp 1–33.
9 Riordan SM, McIver CJ, Walker BM, Duncombe VM, Bolin TD, Thomas MC: The lactulose breath hydrogen test and small intestinal bacterial overgrowth. Am J Gastroenterol 1996;91:1795–1803.
10 Rumessen JJ, Gudmand-Hoyer E, Bachmann E, Justesen T: Diagnosis of bacterial overgrowth of the small intestine. Comparison of the ^{14}C-*D*-xylose breath test and jejunal cultures in 60 patients. Scand J Gastroenterol 1985;20:1267–1275.

11 Valdovinos MA, Camilleri M, Thomforde GM, Frie C: Reduced accuracy of ^{14}C-*D*-xylose breath test for detection of bacterial overgrowth in gastrointestinal motility disorders. Scand J Gastroenterol 1993;28:963–968.
12 Husebye E, Skar V, Hoverstad T, Iversen T, Melby K: Abnormal intestinal motor patterns explain enteric colonisation with Gram-negative bacilli in late radiation enteropathy. Gastroenterology 1995;109:1078–1089.
13 Riordan SM, McIver CJ, Duncombe VM, Thomas MC, Bolin TD: Evaluation of the rice breath hydrogen test for small intestinal bacterial overgrowth. Am J Gastroenterol 2000;95:2858–2864.
14 Giannella RA, Broitman SA, Zamcheck N: Gastric acid barrier to ingested microorganisms in man: Studies in vivo and in vitro. Gut 1972;13:251–256.
15 Hill M: Normal and pathological microbial flora of the upper gastrointestinal tract. Scand J Gastroenterol Suppl 1985;111:1–6.
16 Allan JD, Shiner M: Influence of gastric pH on gastric and jejunal flora. Gut 1967;8:574–581.
17 Stockbruegger RW, Cotton PB, Menon GG, Beilby JOW, Bartholomew BA, Hill MJ, et al: Pernicious anaemia, intragastric bacterial overgrowth, and possible consequences. Scand J Gastroenterol 1984;19:355–364.
18 Feldman M, Barnett C: Fasting gastric pH and its relationship to true hypochlorhydria in humans. Dig Dis Sci 1991;36:866–869.
19 Reback JF: Studies of Intestinal Flora of White Rat; thesis University of Notre Dame, Indiana, USA, 1942.
20 Mayer EA: The physiology of gastric storage and emptying; in Johnson LR, Alpers DH, Christensen J, Jacobson ED, Walsh JH (eds): Physiology of the Gastrointestinal Tract. New York, Raven Press, 1994, pp 929–976.
21 Husebye E: The patterns of small bowel motility: Physiology and implications in organic disease and functional disorders. Neurogastroenterol Motil 1999;11:141–161.
22 Code CF, Schlegel JF: The gastrointestinal housekeeper. Motor correlates of the interdigestive myoelectric complex of the dog. Proceedings from the 4th International Symposium on Gastro-Intestinal Motility. Vancouver, Mitchell Press, 1974, pp 631–634.
23 Vantrappen G, Janssens J, Hellemans J, Ghoos Y: The interdigestive motor complex of normal subjects and patients with bacterial overgrowth of the small intestine. J Clin Invest 1977;59:1158–1166.
24 Dalenback J, Mellander A, Olbe L, Sjovall H: Motility-related cyclic fluctuations of interdigestive gastric acid and bicarbonate secretion in man. A source of substantial variability in gastric secretion studies. Scand J Gastroenterol 1993;28:943–948.
25 Vantrappen G, Peeters TL, Janssens J: The secretory component of the interdigestive migrating motor complex in man. Scand J Gastroenterol 1979;14:663–667.
26 Verdu EF, Fraser R, Murphy GM, Blum AL, Armstrong D: The origin of nocturnal intragastric pH rises in healthy subjects. Scand J Gastroenterol 1995;30:935–943.
27 Bhaskar KR, Garik P, Turner BS, Bradley JD, Bansil R, Stanley HE, et al: Viscous fingering of HCl through gastric mucin. Nature 1992;360:458–461.
28 Mahalanabis D, Rahman MM, Sarker SA, Bardhan PK, Hildebrand P, Beglinger C, et al: *Helicobacter pylori* infection in the young in Bangladesh: Prevalence, socioeconomic and nutritional aspects. Int J Epidemiol 1996;25:894–898.
29 Lindkvist P, Asrat D, Nilsson I, Tsega E, Olsson GL, Wretlind B, et al: Age at acquisition of *Helicobacter pylori* infection: Comparison of a high and a low prevalence country. Scand J Infect Dis 1996;28:181–184.
30 van Herwaarden MA, Samsom M, Smout AJ: 24-hour recording of intragastric pH: Technical aspects and clinical relevance. Scand J Gastroenterol 1999;230(suppl):9–16.
31 Peterson WL, Barnett C, Feldman M, Richardson CT: Reduction of twenty-four-hour gastric acidity with combination of drug therapy in patients with duodenal ulcer. Gastroenterology 1979;77:1015–1020.
32 Husebye E, Skar V, Hoverstad T, Melby K: Fasting hypochlorhydria with gram positive gastric flora is highly prevalent in healthy old people. Gut 1992;33:1331–1337.
33 Fimmel CJ, Etienne A, Cilluffo T, Ritter C, Gasser T, Rey JP, et al: Long-term ambulatory gastric pH monitoring: Validation of a new method and effect of H2-antagonists. Gastroenterology 1985; 88:1842–1851.

34 Milton-Thompson GJ, Lightfoot NF, Ahmet Z, Hunt RH, Barnard J, Brimblecombe RW, et al: Intragastric acidity, bacteria, nitrite, and N-nitroso compounds before, during, and after cimetidine treatment. Lancet 1982;i:1091–1095.
35 Ruddel WWJ, Axon ATR, Findlay JM, Bartholomew BA, Hill MJ: Effect of cimetidine on the gastric bacterial flora. Lancet 1980;i:672–674.
36 Brummer RJ, Stockbruegger RW: Effect of nizatidine 300 mg at night and omeprazole 20 mg in the morning on 24-hour intragastric pH and bacterial overgrowth in patients with acute duodenal ulcer. Dig Dis Sci 1996;41:2048–2054.
37 Nwokolo CU, Smith JT, Gavey C, Sawyerr A, Pounder RE: Tolerance during 29 days of conventional dosing with cimetidine, nizatidine, famotidine or ranitidine. Aliment Pharmacol Ther 1990; 4(suppl 1):29–45.
38 Thorens J, Froehlich F, Schwizer W, Saraga E, Bille J, Gyr K, et al: Bacterial overgrowth during treatment with omeprazole compared with cimetidine: A prospective randomised double blind study. Gut 1996;39:54–59.
39 Stockbruegger RW, Cotton PB, Eugenides N, Bartholomew BA, Hill MJ, Walters CL: Intragastric nitrites, nitroamines, and bacterial overgrowth during cimetidine treatment. Gut 1982;23: 1048–1054.
40 Snepar R, Poporad GA, Romano JM, Kobasa WD, Kaye D: Effect of cimetidine and antacid on gastric microbial flora. Infect Immun 1982;36:518–524.
41 McColl KE, el-Omar E, Gillen D: *Helicobacter pylori* gastritis and gastric physiology. Gastroenterol Clin North Am 2000;29:687–703, viii.
42 Verdu EF, Armstrong D, Fraser R, Viani F, Idstrom JP, Cederberg C, et al: Effect of *Helicobacter pylori* status on intragastric pH during treatment with omeprazole. Gut 1995;36:539–543.
43 Verdu EF, Fraser R, Armstrong D, Blum AL: Effects of omeprazole and lansoprazole on 24-hour intragastric pH in *Helicobacter pylori*-positive volunteers. Scand J Gastroenterol 1994;29: 1065–1069.
44 Sharma BK, Santana IA, Wood EC, Walt RP, Pereira M, Noone P, et al: Intragastric bacterial activity and nitrosation before, during, and after treatment with omeprazole. Br Med J 1984;289: 717–719.
45 Calam J: *Helicobacter pylori* modulation of gastric acid. Yale J Biol Med 1999;72:195–202.
46 Morihara M, Aoyagi N, Kaniwa N, Kojima S, Ogata H: Assessment of gastric acidity of Japanese subjects over the last 15 years. Biol Pharm Bull 2001;24:313–315.
47 Kawaguchi H, Haruma K, Komoto K, Yoshihara M, Sumii K, Kajiyama G: *Helicobacter pylori* infection is the major risk factor for atrophic gastritis. Am J Gastroenterol 1996;91:959–962.
48 Feldman M, Cryer B, McArthur KE, Huet BA, Lee E: Effects of aging and gastritis on gastric acid and pepsin secretion in humans: A prospective study. Gastroenterology 1996;110:1043–1052.
49 Christiansen PM: The incidence of achlorhydria and hypochlorhydria in healthy subjects and patients with gastrointestinal diseases. Scand J Gastroenterol 1968;3:497–508.
50 Bird T, Hall MRP, Schade ROK: Gastric histology and its relation to anaemia in the elderly. Gerontology 1977;23:309–321.
51 Haruma K, Kamada T, Kawaguchi H, Okamoto S, Yoshihara M, Sumii K, et al: Effect of age and *Helicobacter pylori* infection on gastric acid secretion. J Gastroenterol Hepatol 2000;15: 277–283.
52 McCloy RF, Arnold R, Bardhan KD, Cattan D, Klinkenberg-Knol E, Maton PN, et al: Pathophysiological effects of long-term acid suppression in man. Dig Dis Sci 1995;40:96S–120S.
53 Marks IN, Louw JA, Young GO: Acid secretion, 1932–92: Advances, adaptations, and paradoxes. Scand J Gastroenterol Suppl 1992;193:7–13.
54 Dolby JM, Webster ADB, Borriello SP, Barclay FE, Bartholomew BA, Hill MJ: Bacterial colonization and nitrite concentration in the achlorhydric stomachs of patients with primary hypogammaglobulinaemia or classic pernecious anaemia. Scand J Gastroenterol 1984;19:105–110.
55 Gilman RH, Partanen R, Brown KH, Spira WM, Khanam S, Greenberg B, et al: Decreased gastric acid secretion and bacterial colonization of the stomach in severely malnourished Bangladeshi children. Gastroenterology 1988;94:1308–1314.
56 Johanson WG, Pierce AK, Sanford JP: Changing pharyngeal bacterial flora of hospitalized patients. N Engl J Med 1969;281:1137–1140.

57 Muscroft TJ, Deane SA, Young D, Burdon DW, Keighley MRB: The microflora of the postoperative stomach. Br J Surg 1981;68:560–564.
58 Greenlee HB, Vivit R, Paez J, Dietz A: Bacterial flora of the jejunum following peptic ulcer surgery. Arch Surg 1971;102:260–265.
59 Greenlee HB, Gelbart SM, DeOrio AJ, Francescatti DS, Paez J, Reinhardt GF: The influence of gastric surgery on the intestinal flora. Am J Clin Nutr 1977;30:1826–1833.
60 Browning GG, Buchan KA, Mackay C: The effect of vagotomy and drainage on the small bowel flora. Gut 1974;15:139–142.
61 Gorbach LS, Plaut AG, Nahas L, Weinstein L: Studies of intestinal microflora. Microorganisms of the small intestine and their relations to oral and fecal flora. Gastroenterology 1967;53:856–867.
62 Savage DC: Gastrointestinal microflora in mammalian nutrition. Annu Rev Nutr 1986;6:155–178.
63 Gorbach SL: Bengt E. Gustafsson memorial lecture. Function of the normal human microflora. Scand J Infect Dis Suppl 1986;49:17–30.
64 Di Lorenzo C, Flores AF, Buie T, Hyman PE: Intestinal motility and jejunal feeding in children with chronic intestinal pseudo-obstruction. Gastroenterology 1995;108:1379–1385.
65 Yeomans ND, Brimblecombe RW, Elder J, Heatley RV, Misiewicz JJ, Northfield TC, et al: Effects of acid suppression on microbial flora of upper gut. Dig Dis Sci 1995;40:81S–95S.
66 Shindo K, Machida M, Fukumura M, Koide K, Yamazaki R: Omeprazole induces altered bile acid metabolism. Gut 1998;42:266–271.
67 Fried M, Pignata C, Frei R, Froehlich F, Duroux P, Thorens J, et al: Duodenal bacterial overgrowth during treatment in outpatients with omeprazole. Gut 1994;35:23–26.
68 Kerrigan DD, Taylor ME, Read NW, Johnson AG: Acid, motility, and ulcers: A comparison of cisapride with placebo in the prevention of duodenal ulcer relapse. Gut 1993;34:1042–1046.
69 McCallum RW, Berkowitz DM, Lerner E: Gastric emptying in patients with gastroesophageal reflux. Gastroenterology 1981;80:285–291.
70 Smout AJPM: Gastroesophageal reflux disease: Pathogenesis and diagnosis; in Champion MC, Orr WC (eds): Gastrointestinal Motility. Oxford, Blackwell Science, 2001, pp 46–63.
71 Quigley EMM: Gastric and small intestinal motility in health and disease; in Camilleri M (ed): Gastrointestinal Motility in Clinical Practice. Philadelphia, Saunders, 1996, pp 113–147.
72 Shindo K, Machida M, Koide K, Fukumura M, Yamazaki R: Deconjugation ability of bacteria isolated from the jejunal fluid of patients with progressive systemic sclerosis and its gastric pH. Hepatogastroenterology 1998;45:1643–1650.
73 Kornman K: Bacteroides; in Newman MG, Nisengard R (eds): Oral Microbiology and Immunology. Philadelphia, Saunders, 1988, pp 243–250.
74 Shindo K, Yamazaki R, Koide K, Fukumura M, Hirai Y: Alteration of bile acid metabolism by cimetidine in healthy humans. J Investig Med 1996;44:462–469.
75 Sherwood L, Gorbach SL, Tabaqchali S: Bacteria, bila, and the small bowel. Gut 1969;10:963–972.
76 Hutchinson S, Logan R: The effect of long-term omeprazole on the glucose-hydrogen breath test in elderly patients. Age Ageing 1997;26:87–89.
77 Shindo K, Fukumura M: Effect of H_2-receptor antagonists on bile acid metabolism. J Investig Med 1995;43:170–177.
78 Nelis GF, Engelage AH, Samson G: Does long-term inhibition of gastric acid secretion with omeprazole lead to small intestinal bacterial overgrowth? Neth J Med 1994;45:93–100.
79 Husebye E, Engedal K: The patterns of motility are maintained in the human small intestine throughout the process of aging. Scand J Gastroenterol 1992;27:397–404.
80 Saltzman JR, Kemp JA, Golner BB, Pedrosa MC, Dallal GE, Russell RM: Effect of hypochlorhydria due to omeprazole treatment or atrophic gastritis on protein-bound vitamin B_{12} absorption. J Am Coll Nutr 1994;13:584–591.
81 Marcuard SP, Albernaz L, Khazanie PG: Omeprazole therapy causes malabsorption of cyanocobalamin (vitamin B_{12}). Ann Intern Med 1994;120:211–215.
82 Bellou A, Aimone-Gastin I, De Korwin JD, Bronowicki JP, Moneret-Vautrin A, Nicolas JP, et al: Cobalamin deficiency with megaloblastic anaemia in one patient under long-term omeprazole therapy. J Intern Med 1996;240:161–164.
83 Bradford GS, Taylor CT: Omeprazole and vitamin B_{12} deficiency. Ann Pharmacother 1999; 33:641–643.

84 Evenepoel P, Claus D, Geypens B, Maes B, Hiele M, Rutgeerts P, et al: Evidence for impaired assimilation and increased colonic fermentation of protein, related to gastric acid suppression therapy. Aliment Pharmacol Ther 1998;12:1011–1019.
85 Frederiksen W, Bruusgaard A, Hess Thaysen E: Assessment of the relationship between gastric secretory capacity and jejunal bacteriology. Scand J Gastroenterol 1973;8:353–359.
86 Bishop RF, Andersson CM: The bacterial flora of the stomach and small intestine in children with intestinal obstruction. Arch Dis Child 1960;35:487–491.
87 Lewis SJ, Franco S, Young G, O'Keefe SJ: Altered bowel function and duodenal bacterial overgrowth in patients treated with omeprazole. Aliment Pharmacol Ther 1996;10:557–561.
88 Husebye E, Hellström PM, Midtvedt T: The intestinal microflora stimulates myoelectric activity of rat small intestine by promoting cyclic initiation and aboral propagation of the migrating myoelectric complex. Dig Dis Sci 1994;39:946–956.
89 Husebye E, Hellström PM, Sundler F, Chen J, Midtvedt T: Influence of microbial species on small intestinal myoelectric activity and transit in germ-free rats. Am J Physiol Gastrointest Liver Physiol 2001;280:G368–G380.
90 van Felius LD: The Role of the Small Intestine in Acute Pancreatitis; Dissertation University of Utrecht, 2002, pp 101–115.
91 Shindo K, Machida M, Miyakawa K, Fukumura M: A syndrome of cirrhosis, achlorhydria, small intestinal bacterial overgrowth, and fat malabsorption. Am J Gastroenterol 1993;88:2084–2091.
92 Murphy GM: Depressing acid, deconjugating bile. Gut 1998;42:154–155.
93 Cregan J, Dunlop EE, Hayward NJ: The bacterial content of human small intestine in disease of the stomach. Br Med J 1953;5:1248–1251.
94 Sjövall H, Hagman I, Abrahamsson H: Relationship between interdigestive duodenal motility and fluid transport in humans. Am J Physiol 1990;259:G348–G354.
95 Rolly, Liebermeister G: Experimentelle Untersuchungen über die Ursachen der Abtötung von Bacterien im Dünndarm. Dtsch Arch Klin Med 1905;83:413–451.
96 Dack GM, Petran E: Bacterial activity in different levels of the intestine. J Infect Dis 1934;54:204–220.
97 Anderson CM, Langford RF: Bacterial content of small intestine of children in health, in coeliac disease, and in fibrocystic disease of pancreas. Br Med J 1958;i:803–806.
98 Toskes PP, Donaldson RM: Enteric bacterial flora and bacterial overgrowth syndrome; in Sleisenger MH, Fordtran JS (eds): Gastrointestinal Disease. Philadelphia, Saunders, 1993, pp 1106–1125.
99 Dixon JMS: The fate of bacteria in the small intestine. J Pathol Bacteriol 1960;79:131–140.
100 Dixon JMS, Paulley JW: Bacteriological and histological studies of the small intestine of rats treated with mecamylamine. Gut 1963;4:169–173.
101 Donaldson RM: Normal bacterial populations of the intestine and their relation to intestinal function (continued). N Engl J Med 1964;270:994–1001.
102 Donaldson RM: Normal bacterial populations of the intestine and their relation to intestinal function. N Engl J Med 1964;270:938–945.
103 Donaldson RM: Normal bacterial populations of the intestine and their relation to intestinal function (concluded). N Engl J Med 1964;270:1050–1056.
104 Bayliss WM, Starling EH: The movements and innervation of the small intestine. J Physiol 1899;24:99–143.
105 Spencer NJ, Smith TK: Simultaneous intracellular recordings from longitudinal and circular muscle during the peristaltic reflex in guinea-pig distal colon. J Physiol 2001;533:787–799.
106 Weisbrodt NW: Intestinal motility; in Johnson LR (ed): Physiology of the Gastrointestinal Tract. New York, Raven Press, 1987, pp 631–663.
107 Makhlouf G: Neuromuscular function of the small intestine; in Johnson LR (ed): Physiology of the Gastrointestinal Tract. New York, Raven Press, 1994, pp 977–990.
108 Kerlin P, Zinsmeister A, Phillips S: Relationship of motility to flow of contents in the human small intestine. Gastroenterology 1982;82:701–706.
109 Van Eldere J, Robben J, Caenepeel PH, Eyssen H: Influence of a cecal volume-reducing intestinal microflora on the excretion and entero-hepatic circulation of steroids and bile acids. J Steroid Biochem 1988;29:33–39.

110 Thompson DG, Wingate DL, Archer L, Benson MJ, Green WJ, Hardy RJ: Normal patterns of human upper small bowel motor activity recorded by prolonged radiotelemetry. Gut 1980;21: 500–506.
111 Riordan SM, McIver CJ, Walker BM, Duncombe VM, Bolin TD, Thomas MC: Bacteriological method for detecting small intestinal motility. Am J Gastroenterol 1996;91:2399–2405.
112 Newman MG, Nisengard R: Oral Microbiology and Immunology. Philadelphia, Saunders, 1988.
113 Husebye E: Gastrointestinal motility disorders and bacterial overgrowth. J Intern Med 1995;237: 419–427.
114 Camilleri M, Hasler WL, Parkman HP, Quigley EM, Soffer E: Measurement of gastrointestinal motility in the GI laboratory. Gastroenterology 1998;115:747–762.
115 Clements JA, Heading RC, Nimmo WS, Prescott LF: Kinetics of acetaminophen absorption and gastric emptying in man. Clin Pharmacol Ther 1978;24:420–431.
116 Anuras S: Motility Disorders of the Gastrointestinal Tract. New York, Raven Press, 1992.
117 Camilleri M: Study of human gastroduodenojejunal motility. Dig Dis Sci 1993;38:785–794.
118 Soffer EE, Summers RW: Ambulant manometry; in Kumar D, Wingate DL (eds): An Illustrated Guide to Gastrointestinal Motility. Edinburgh, Churchill Livingstone, 1993, pp 200–210.
119 Gill RC, Kellow JE, Browning C, Wingate DL: The use of intraluminal strain gauges for recording ambulant small bowel motility. Am J Physiol 1990;258:G610–G615.
120 Husebye E, Skar V, Aalen OO, Osnes M: Digital ambulatory manometry of the small intestine in healthy adults: Estimates of the variation within and between individuals and statistical management of incomplete MMC periods. Dig Dis Sci 1990;35:1057–1065.
121 Lindberg G, Iwarzon M, Stål P, Seensalu R: Digital ambulatory monitoring of small-bowel motility. Scand J Gastroenterol 1990;25:216–224.
122 Stanghellini V, Camilleri M, Malagelada JR: Chronic idiopathic intestinal pseudo-obstruction: Clinical and intestinal manometric findings. Gut 1987;28:5–12.
123 Malagelada JR, Camilleri M, Stanghellini V: Manometric Diagnosis of Gastrointestinal Motility Disorders. New York, Thieme, 1986.
124 Malagelada JR, Stanghellini V: Manometric evaluation of functional upper gut symptoms. Gastroenterology 1985;88:1223–1231.
125 Quigley EM, Deprez PH, Hellstrom P, Husebye E, Soffer EE, Stanghellini V, et al: Ambulatory intestinal manometry: A consensus report on its clinical role. Dig Dis Sci 1997;42:2395–2400.
126 Malagelada J-R, Robertson JS, Brown ML, Remmington M, Duven JA, Thomford GM, et al: Intestinal transit of solid and liquid components of a meal in health. Gastroenterology 1984;87: 1255–1263.
127 der Ohe MR, Camilleri M: Measurement of small bowel and colonic transit: Indications and methods. Mayo Clin Proc 1992;67:1169–1179.
128 Charles F, Camilleri M, Phillips SF: Scintigraphy of the whole gut: Clinical evaluation of transit disorders. Mayo Clin Proc 1995;70:113.
129 Di Lorenzo C, Dooley CP, Valenzula JE: Role of fasting gastrointestinal motility in the variability of gastrointestinal transit time assessed by hydrogen breath test. Gut 1991;32:1127–1130.
130 Staniforth DH, Rose D: Statistical analysis of the lactulose/breath hydrogen test in the measurement of orocecal transit: Its variability and predictive value in assessing drug action. Gut 1989;30: 171–175.
131 Kumar D, Wingate D: An Illustrated Guide to Gastrointestinal Motility. Edinburgh, Churchill Livingstone, 1993.
132 Summers RW, Anuras S, Green J: Jejunal manometry patterns in health, partial intestinal obstruction, and pseudoobstruction. Gastroenterology 1983;85:1290–1300.
133 Camilleri M, Fealey RD: Idiopathic autonomic denervation in eight patients presenting with functional gastrointestinal disease. Dig Dis Sci 1990;35:609–616.
134 Roy AD, Bharucha H, Nevin NC, Odling-Smee GW, Cockel R, Hill EE, et al: Idiopathic intestinal pseudo-obstruction: A familial visceral neuropathy. Clin Genet 1980;18:291–297.
135 Schuffler MD, Bird TD, Sumi M, Cook A: A familial neuronal disease presenting as intestinal pseudoobstruction. Gastroenterology 1978;75:889–898.
136 Careskey JM, Weber TR, Grosfeld JL: Total colonic aganglionosis. Analysis of 16 cases. Am J Surg 1982;143:160–168.

137 Riccardi VM: Von Recklinghausen neurofibromatosis. N Engl J Med 1981;305:1617–1627.
138 Milla PJ, Smith VV: Intestinal neuronal dysplasia. J Pediatr Gastroenterol Nutr 1993;17:356–357.
139 Boseman T, Anuras S, Hutton E, Ghandour E, Mikeska C: Abnormal motility of the upper gastrointestinal tract in Parkinson's disease. Am J Gastroenterol 1990;85:1264A.
140 Kenny SE, Vanderwinden JM, Rintala RJ, Connell MG, Lloyd DA, Vanderhaegen JJ, et al: Delayed maturation of the interstitial cells of Cajal: A new diagnosis for transient neonatal pseudoobstruction. Report of two cases. J Pediatr Surg 1998;33:94–98.
141 Cohen J, Low P, Fealey R, Sheps S, Jiang NS: Somatic and autonomic function in progressive autonomic failure, a multiple system atrophy. Ann Neurol 1987;22:692–699.
142 Low PA, Dyck PJ, Lambert EH, Brimijoin WS, Trautmann JC, Malagelada JR, et al: Acute panautonomic neuropathy. Ann Neurol 1983;13:412–417.
143 Bharucha AE, Camilleri M, Low PA, Zinsmeister AR: Autonomic dysfunction in gastrointestinal motility disorders. Gut 1993;34:397–401.
144 Camilleri M, Malagelada JR, Stanghellini V, Fealey RD, Sheps SG: Gastrointestinal motility disturbances in patients with orthostatic hypotension. Gastroenterology 1985;88:1852–1859.
145 Malagelada JR, Rees WD, Mazzotta LJ, Go VL: Gastric motor abnormalities in diabetic and postvagotomy gastroparesis: Effect of metoclopramide and bethanechol. Gastroenterology 1980;78: 286–293.
146 Annese V, Bassotti G, Caruso N, De Cosmo S, Gabbrielli A, Modoni S, et al: Gastrointestinal motor dysfunction, symptoms, and neuropathy in noninsulin-dependent (type 2) diabetes mellitus. J Clin Gastroenterol 1999;29:171–177.
147 Thompson DG, Ritchie HD, Wingate DL: Pattern of small intestine motility in duodenal ulcer patients before and after vagotomy. Gut 1982;23:517–523.
148 Mathias JR, Baskin GS, Reeves-Darby VG, Clench MH, Smith LL, Calhoon JH: Chronic intestinal pseudoobstruction in a patient with heart-lung transplant. Dig Dis Sci 1992;37:1761–1768.
149 Fealey RD, Szurszewski JH, Merritt JL, Di-Magno EP: Effect of traumatic spinal cord transection on human upper gastrointestinal motility and gastric emptying. Gastroenterology 1984;87:69–75.
150 Schuffler MD, Lowe MC, Bill AH: Studies of idiopathic intestinal pseudoobstruction. I. Hereditary hollow visceral myopathy: Clinical and pathological studies. Gastroenterology 1977;73:327–338.
151 Anuras S, Mitros FA, Nowak TV, Ionasescu VV, Gurll NJ, Christensen J, Green JB: A familial visceral myopathy with external ophthalmoplegia and autosomal recessive transmission. Gastroenterology 1983;84:346–353.
152 Novak TV, Ionasescu VV, Anuras S: Gastrointestinal manifestations of the muscular dystrophies. Gastroenterology 1982;82:800–810.
153 Nowak TV, Anuras S, Brown BP, Ionasescu V, Green JB: Small intestinal motility in myotonic dystrophy patients. Gastroenterology 1984;86:808–813.
154 Husebye E, Hauer-Jensen M, Kjorstad K, Skar V: Severe late radiation enteropathy is characterised by impaired motility of proximal small intestine. Dig Dis Sci 1994;39:2341–2349.
155 Conklin JL, Anuras S: Radiation-induced recurrent intestinal pseudoobstruction. Am J Gastroenterol 1981;75:440–444.
156 de Jonge WJ, van den Wijngaard RM, The FO, ter Beek ML, Bennink RJ, Tytgat GN, et al: Postoperative ileus is maintained by intestinal immune infiltrates that activate inhibitory neural pathways in mice. Gastroenterology 2003;125:1137–1147.
157 Spiller RC: Role of nerves in enteric infection. Gut 2002;51:759–762.
158 Tabaqchali S: The pathophysiological role of small intestinal bacterial flora. Scand J Gastroenterol Suppl 1970;6:139–163.
159 Rees WDW, Leigh RJ, Christofides ND, Bloom SR, Turnberg LA: Interdigestive motor activity in patients with systemic sclerosis. Gastroenterology 1982;83:575–580.
160 Soudah HC, Hasler WL, Owyang C: Effect of octreotide on intestinal motility and bacterial overgrowth in scleroderma. N Engl J Med 1991;325:1461–1467.
161 Kahn IJ, Jeffries GH, Sleisenger MH: Malabsorption in intestinal scleroderma. Correction by antibiotics. N Engl J Med 1993;274:1339–1344.
162 Ryan JC, Sleisenger MH: Effects of systemic and extraintestinal diseases on the gut; in Sleisenger MH, Fordtran JS (eds): Gastrointestinal Disease: Pathophysiology/Diagnosis/Management. Philadelphia, Saunders, 1993, pp 193–224.

163 Wald A, Kichler J, Mendelow H: Amyloidosis and chronic intestinal pseudoobstruction. Dig Dis Sci 1981;26:462–465.
164 Krishnamurthy S, Schuffler MD: Pathology of neuromuscular disorders of the small intestine and colon. Gastroenterology 1987;93:610–639.
165 Oliveira RB, Menghelli UG, De Godoy RA, Dantas RO, Padovan W: Abnormalities of interdigestive motility of the small intestine in patients with Chagas disease. Dig Dis Sci 1983;28/4: 294–299.
166 Chatila R, Kapadia CR: Intestinal pseudoobstruction in acute Lyme disease: A case report. Am J Gastroenterol 1998;93:1179–1180.
167 Sonsino E, Mouy R, Foucaud P, Cezard JP, Aigrain Y, Bocquet L, et al: Intestinal pseudoobstruction related to cytomegalovirus infection of myenteric plexus. N Engl J Med 1984;311:196–197.
168 Vassallo M, Camilleri M, Caron BL, Low PA: Gastrointestinal motor dysfunction in acquired selective cholinergic dysautonomia associated with infectious mononucleosis. Gastroenterology 1991;100:252–258.
169 Abbasi AA, Douglass RC, Bissell GW, Chen Y: Myxedema ileus: A form of intestinal pseudo-obstruction. JAMA 1975;234:181–183.
170 Christensen J, Schedl HP, Clifton JA: The basic electrical rhythm of the duodenum in normal human subjects and in patients with thyroid disease. J Clin Invest 1964;43:1659–1667.
171 Gerl A, Storck M, Schalhorn A, Müller-Hörker J, Jauch KW, Schildberg FW, et al: Paraneoplastic chronic intestinal pseudoobstruction as a rare complication of bronchial carcinoid. Gut 1992;33:1000–1003.
172 Khafagi FA, Lloyd HM, Gough IR: Intestinal pseudo-obstruction in pheochromocytoma. Aust NZ J Med 1987;17:246–248.
173 der Ohe MR, Camilleri M, Kvols LK, Thomforde GM: Motor dysfunction of the small bowel and colon in patients with the carcinoid syndrome and diarrhea. N Engl J Med 1993;329:1073–1078.
174 Schobinger-Clement S, Gerber HA, Stallmach T: Autoaggressive inflammation of the myenteric plexus resulting in intestinal pseudoobstruction. Am J Surg Pathol 1999;23:602–606.
175 Morencos FC, las Heras CG, Martin RL, Lopez Arias MJ, Ledesma F, Pons RF: Small bowel bacterial overgrowth in patients with alcoholic cirrhosis. Dig Dis Sci 1995;40:1252–1256.
176 Chang CS, Chen GH, Lien HC, Yeh HZ: Small intestine dysmotility and bacterial overgrowth in cirrhotic patients with spontaneous bacterial peritonitis. Hepatology 1998;28:1187–1190.
177 Christensen J, Dent J, Malagelada JR, Wingate DL: Pseudo-obstruction. Gastroenterology 1990; 3/3:107–119.
178 Moody FG, Weisbrodt NW: Post-surgical motility disorders; in Kumar D, Wingate D (eds): An Illustrated Guide to Gastrointestinal Motility. Edinburgh, Churchill Livingstone, 1993, pp 673–690.
179 Quigley EMM: The effects of resection, restorative procedures and transplantation on intestinal motility; in Kumar D, Wingate D (eds): An Illustrated Guide to Gastrointestinal Motility. Edinburgh, Churchill Livingstone, 1993, pp 691–716.
180 Camilleri M, Brown ML, Malagelada JR: Relationship between impaired gastric emptying and abnormal gastrointestinal motility. Gastroenterology 1986;91:94–99.
181 Vilbergsson S, Melby K, Keirung G, Petlund K, Husebye E: The influence of significant delay of gastric emptying on the gastric microflora. Gastroenterology 2002;122/4(suppl 1):T1300.
182 Dalenback J, Abrahamson H, Bjornson E, Fandriks L, Mattsson A, Olbe L, et al: Human duodenogastric reflux, retroperistalsis, and MMC. Am J Physiol 1998;275:R762–R769.
183 Bjornsson ES, Abrahamsson H: Contractile patterns in patients with severe chronic dyspepsia. Am J Gastroenterol 1999;94:54–64.
184 Scott LD, Cahall DL: Influence of the interdigestive myoelectric complex on enteric flora in the rat. Gastroenterology 1982;82:737–745.
185 Nieuwenhuijs VB, Verheem A, van Duijvenbode-Beumer H, Visser MR, Verhoef J, Gooszen HG, et al: The role of interdigestive small bowel motility in the regulation of gut microflora, bacterial overgrowth, and bacterial translocation in rats. Ann Surg 1998;228:188–193.
186 Cowles VE, Sarna SK: Effect of *T. spiralis* infection on intestinal motor activity in the fasted state. Am J Physiol 1990;259:G693–G701.
187 Cowles VE, Sarna SK: *Trichinella spiralis* infection alters small bowel motor activity in the fed state. Gastroenterology 1991;101:664–669.

188 Justus PG, Fernandez A, Martin JL, King CE, Toskes PP, Mathias JR: Altered myoelectric activity in the experimental blind loop syndrome. J Clin Invest 1983;72:1064–1071.
189 Sarna SK: Giant migrating contractions and their myoelectric correlates in the small intestine. Am J Physiol 1987;253:G697–G705.
190 Stotzer PO, Björnsson ES, Abrahamsson H: Interdigestive and postprandial motility in small intestinal bacterial overgrowth. Scand J Gastroenterol 1996;31:875–880.
191 McLoughlin GA, Hede JE, Temple JG, Bradley J, Capman DM, McFarland J: The role of IgA in the prevention of bacterial colonization of the jejunum in the vagotomized subject. Br J Surg 1978;65:435–437.
192 Pignata C, Budillon G, Monaco G, Nani E, Cuomo R, Pamilli G, et al: Jejunal bacterial overgrowth and intestinal permeability in children with immunodeficiency syndromes. Gut 1990;31:879–882.
193 Wilcox CM, Waites KB, Smith PD: No relationship between gastric pH, small bowel bacterial colonisation, and diarrhoea in HIV-1-infected patients. Gut 1999;44:101–105.
194 Kett K, Baklien K, Bakken A, Kral JG, Fausa O, Brandtzaeg P: Intestinal B-cell isotype response in relation to local bacterial load: Evidence for immunoglobulin A subclass adaptation. Gastroenterology 1995;109:819–825.
195 Riordan SM, McIver CJ, Wakefield D, Bolin TD, Duncombe VM, Thomas MC: Small intestinal bacterial overgrowth in the symptomatic elderly. Am J Gastroenterol 1997;92:47–51.
196 Riordan SM, McIver CJ, Wakefield D, Duncombe VM, Thomas MC, Bolin TD: Small intestinal mucosal immunity and morphometry in luminal overgrowth of indigenous gut flora. Am J Gastroenterol 2001;96:494–500.
197 Attar A, Flourie B, Rambaud JC, Franchisseur C, Ruszniewski P, Bouhnik Y: Antibiotic efficacy in small intestinal bacterial overgrowth-related chronic diarrhea: A crossover, randomized trial. Gastroenterology 1999;117:794–797.
198 Scarpignato C, Pelosini I: Rifaximin, a poorly absorbed antibiotic: Pharmacology and clinical potential. Chemotherapy 2005;51(suppl 1):36–66.
199 Di Stefano M, Corazza GR: Treatment of small intestine bacterial overgrowth and related symptoms by rifaximin. Chemotherapy 2005;51(suppl 1):103–109.

Note Added in Proof

After submission of this paper I came across the interesting review by Singh and Toskes [1] where the pathophysiology of bacterial overgrowth is carefully presented. In the most recent article by Lin [2] the possible role of bacterial overgrowth in the pathogenesis of irritable bowel syndrome is discussed, paying particular attention to the high prevalence of bloating in this syndrome.

The high prevalence of bacterial overgrowth in patients with chronic renal failure is a novel finding [3], and a condition to add to the list in the current review. Interestingly, concurrent abnormalities of small bowel motility were detected, of which increased prevalence of retrograde pressure waves in duodenum is of particular relevance in the present context [12, 183]. Castiglione et al. [4] further indicate the usefulness of both metronidazole and cipro-floxacin in the treatment of bacterial overgrowth associated with Crohn's disease. Indeed both clinical improvement and normalization of the lactose and glucose breath tests occurred after antibiotic treatment. The symbiotic modulation of the gut flora [5] is an interesting new approach for the management of minimal hepatic encephalopathy, emphasizing the importance of understanding the role of changes in gut flora.

References

1 Castiglione F, Rispo A, Di Girolamo E, Cozzolino A, Manguso F, Grassia R, et al: Antibiotic treatment of small bowel bacterial overgrowth in patients with Crohn's disease. Aliment Pharmacol Ther 2003;18:1107–1112.

2 Lin HC: Small intestinal bacterial overgrowth: A framework for understanding irritable bowel syndrome. JAMA 2004;292:852–858.

3 Liu Q, Duan ZP, Ha DK, Bengmark S, Kurtovic J, Riordan SM: Symbiotic modulation of gut flora: Effect on minimal hepatic encephalopathy in patients with cirrhosis. Hepatololy 2004;39:1441–1449.

4 Singh VV, Toskes PP: Small bowel bacterial overgrowth: Presentation, diagnosis, and treatment. Curr Gastroenterol Rep 2003;5:365–372.

5 Strid H, Simren M, Stotzer PO, Ringstrom G, Abrahamsson H, Bjornsson ES: Patients with chronic renal failure have abnormal small intestinal motility and a high prevalence of small intestinal bacterial overgrowth. Digestion 2003;67:129–137.

Einar Husebye, MD, PhD
Department of Medicine
Clinic of Medicine
NO–3004 Drammen (Norway)
Tel. +47 328 03410, Fax +47 671 47958, E-Mail einarhu@ioks.uio.no

This chapter should be cited as follows:

Husebye E: The Pathogenesis of Gastrointestinal Bacterial Overgrowth. Chemotherapy 2005; 51(suppl 1):1–22.

Scarpignato C (ed): Rifaximin: A Poorly Absorbed Antibiotic.
Pharmacology and Clinical Use.

Pathophysiology and Impact of Enteric Bacterial and Protozoal Infections: New Approaches to Therapy

Gerly A.C. Brito[a,b], *Cirle Alcantara*[a,c], *Benedito A. Carneiro-Filho*[a], *Richard L. Guerrant*[a]

[a]Division of Geographic Medicine, Department of Internal Medicine, School of Medicine, University of Virginia, Charlottesville, Va., USA; [b]Department of Morphology, School of Medicine, Federal University of Ceará, Fortaleza, Brazil; [c]National Institutes of Health, University of the Philippines, Manila, Philippines

Abstract

Despite numerous scientific advances in the past few years regarding the pathogenesis, diagnostic tools and treatment of infectious enteritis, enteric infections remain a serious threat to health worldwide. With globalization of the food supply, the increase in travel, mass food processing and antibiotic resistance, infectious diarrhea has become a critical concern for both developing and developed countries. Oral rehydration therapy has been cited as the most important medical discovery of the century due to the millions of lives that have been saved. However, statistics concerning diarrhea-induced mortality and the highly underestimated morbidity continue to demonstrate the severity of the problem. A more complete understanding of the pathogenesis of infectious diarrhea and potential new vaccines and effective treatments are badly needed. In addition, public health preventive actions, such as early detection of outbreaks, care with food, water and sanitation and, where relevant, immunization, should be considered a priority. This article provides an overview of the epidemiological impact, pathogenesis and new approaches to the management of enteric infections.

Introduction

Enteric infections are among the leading causes of mortality worldwide. They are estimated to cause 2.5 million deaths per year, which translates to over 6,800 children who die each day from diarrheal diseases, and the huge morbidity from diarrhea has not been reduced but may actually be increasing [1]. Even more impressive is the long-term developmental impact of repeated childhood diarrheal disease [2]. Diarrhea further aggravates malnutrition, especially in developing countries. Studies done in Brazil show that diarrhea in the first 2 years of life is associated with an approximate 4% decrement in physical fitness, a growth shortfall of 3.6 cm and impaired cognition and school performance at 6–9 years of age [3–6]. In addition to acute morbidity and mortality, some causes of infectious diarrheal disease result in serious long-term sequelae such as hemolytic-uremic syndrome with renal failure following enterohemorrhagic *Escherichia coli* (EHEC) infection (a risk that may be increased by treatment with certain antimicrobial agents such as sulfa-trimethoprim or quinolones). Other examples include Guillain-Barré syndrome following *Campylobacter jejuni* infection and malnutrition with or without diarrhea following infection with enteroaggregative *E. coli* (EAggEC), *Cryptosporidium* species or other enteric infections [7–10].

With the globalization of our food supply and increasing international travel, enteric infection is now also a serious threat to industrialized countries, as demonstrated in recent years by diarrheal outbreaks in North America due to *Cyclospora* following ingestion of imported Guatemalan raspberries [11]. Other examples include water-borne outbreaks caused by *Cryptosporidium* and food-borne outbreaks caused by EHEC. The economic cost of infectious diarrheal diseases is also considerable. In the United States, an estimated USD 6 billion each year is spent on medical care and loss of productivity due to food-borne diseases, most of which cause diarrhea [12, 13]. The exploding developing world's population, the disparity between the rich and the poor, and emerging antibiotic-resistant infections make enteric infections a critical global health concern.

This article provides an overview of the epidemiological impact, pathogenesis and new approaches to the management of enteric infections. Although several enteric viruses are important causes of diarrhea in both developed and developing country, we will focus this overview on bacterial and selected parasitic pathogens.

Epidemiology

EHEC, *Salmonella*, *Shigella*, *Vibrio cholerae*, *Cyclospora*, *Cryptosporidium*, *Giardia*, *C. jejuni*, *Clostridium difficile*, caliciviruses and other viruses such as rotavirus, astrovirus and torovirus are the main causes of diarrhea worldwide, and cause more than 211–375 million cases of diarrheal illnesses in the United States each year [14, 15]. In addition, in the last 2 or 3 decades, other enteric pathogens have been recognized as emerging causes of enteric infections. There are now several types of *E. coli* enteropathogens in addition to the classical enteropathogenic *E. coli* (EPEC), including enterotoxigenic *E. coli* (ETEC), which produces a cholera-like heat-labile toxin (LT) or heat-stable toxins STa or STb, EHEC, which produces a Shiga-like toxin (SLT), enteroinvasive *E. coli* (EIEC) and EAggEC, which is associated with persistent diarrhea in developing and developed countries. Among the parasitic protozoa, microsporidia can also be included as emerging infectious pathogens especially in immunocompromised hosts, as well as *Cyclospora* and *Cryptosporidium* [16, 17].

Many of these organisms are easily transmitted through food and water or by human contact. Thus, prevention by avoiding the ingestion of raw or undercooked meat, seafood or unpasteurized milk products, and the selective use of available vaccines are the key to the control of infectious diarrhea.

In the United States alone, episodes of diarrheal illness result in 73 million physician consultations, 1.8 million hospitalizations and 3,100 deaths each year. Food-borne illnesses alone account for 76 million illnesses and 350,000 hospitalizations each year [15, 18, 19].

Traveler's diarrhea is a common problem that occurs in 20–50% of the 35 million people who cross international borders from the developed to tropical or semitropical developing countries every year, resulting in more than 7 million cases [20–23]. The etiological agents of traveler's diarrhea depend on the geographical location, standards of food, hygiene, sanitation, water supply and season. The most common causes of traveler's diarrhea in adults in developed countries include *E. coli*, specially ETEC, *Shigella* spp., *Salmonella* spp., *Campylobacter* spp., *Vibrio parahaemolyticus* (in Asia), rotavirus (in Latin America) and protozoa (*Giardia*, *Cryptosporidium* and *Cyclospora* spp., and *Entamoeba histolytica*) [24, 25].

Pathogenesis

There are several mechanisms by which enteric pathogens can cause diarrhea (table 1). Recent progress in understanding of the pathogenesis at the molecular level opens new perspectives on the treatment of infectious diarrhea. Furthermore, different microorganisms often share common pathogenic pathways. Microbes must first adhere to the mucosa in order to elicit disease. Thereafter, some microorganisms such as *V. cholerae* or ETEC produce toxins that can subvert ion transport across the intestinal epithelium. Other microorganisms such as *Shigella* and *Salmonella* species can invade the mucosa causing inflammation. In extreme cases, microorganisms can also invade the bloodstream [26].

Table 1. Clinical, epidemiological and pathogenic features of enteric infections

Pathogenic agent	Epidemiology	Incubation period	Diarrhea	Virulence determinant/mechanism
V. cholerae	All ages in developing world/related to poor sanitation	18–40 h but can be as short as 12 h or as long as 72 h	Profuse watery diarrhea causing severe dehydration	**Cholera toxin** → G_s protein → adenylate cyclase → secretion → prostaglandin → secretion → enteroendocrine cells → endogenous secretagogues → secretion
ETEC	Young children > adults in developing world/travelers to tropics	10–72 h	Acute watery	**CFA-I-IV** → colonization **LT-I** and **-II** → adenylate cyclase → secretion **STa** → guanylate cyclase → secretion **STb** → cyclic nucleotide-independent HCO_3^- secretion
EPEC	Infants in developing world	As short as 9–12 h	Acute→ persistent watery	Not fully understood, possibilities are increase in mucosal permeability and loss of microvilli leading to malabsorption
EHEC	All ages/primarily in US, Canada, Europe, South America and Japan	12–60 h	Acute bloody (hemorrhagic colitis in 31–61%); occasionally nonbloody diarrhea	**SLT-I** and **-II** → bloodstream → inhibition of protein synthesis → endothelial cell damage → microvascular thrombosis → hemolytic-uremic syndrome
EAggEC	Children in the developing world	20–48 h	Persistent	**FliC** → inflammation **EAST-1** → guanylate cyclase → secretion **Heat-labile toxin** → Ca^{2+}-dependent actin phosphorylation; cytoskeletal damage **Pet** → histopathologic effects on human intestinal mucosa

EIEC	All ages/primarily in the developing regions; occasional outbreaks in industrialized countries	As short as 10–18 h	Acute watery diarrhea followed by dysentery	Cell invasion → spread → inflammation
C. difficile	History of antibiotic use, advanced age, underlying illness	5–10 days of anti-bacteria treatment (range 1st day to 10 weeks of antibiotics)	Mild to severe inflammatory diarrhea	**Toxins A** and **B** → monoglucosylation of Rho protein → disruption of actin cytoskeleton → mucosal disruption → COX-2 → prostaglandin E_2 → synthesis of inflammatory cytokines
Cryptosporidium	All ages/children in developing areas/ immunocompromised adults/outbreaks in developed areas	7–10 days (range 5–28 days)	Intermittent and scant to continuous and watery	Prostaglandins → cAMP-mediated apical chloride secretion and inhibition of electroneutral sodium chloride and water absorption release of IL-1, IL-8 and TNF-α
Salmonella	All ages/travelers to tropics	6–48 h	Moderate volume, and usually without blood	Mucosal invasion via M cells or enterocytes → macrophages and lymphocytes in Peyer's patches and other lymphoid tissue → bloodstream
Shigella	Incidence highest in children 1–5 years of age	24–72 h	Watery at the onset and may evolve to bloody diarrhea or dysentery	Invasion and destruction of the distal ileal and colonic mucosa → release of cytokines → PMN mucosal infiltration

FliC = Flagellin sequence in EAggEC responsible for IL-8 induction [64].

Other organisms such as *C. difficile* produce enterocytotoxin, which causes intense disruption of the intestinal mucosa [27].

Aside from the features of the microorganisms cited above, the host defenses also play an important role in the acquisition of enteric infection. Host defenses include normal gastric acidity, intestinal mucus, cellular and humoral immunity, motility and intestinal microbial flora.

A bacterial enteric infection may manifest as diarrhea or may also remain asymptomatic. Recently, it was recognized that even asymptomatic enteric infections by *Cryptosporidium*, EAggEC and *Giardia lamblia* may be associated with nutritional shortfalls, even in the absence of overt diarrheal illness [17].

Intestinal infections that cause persistent diarrhea normally result in histopathological changes to the intestine including villus blunting, crypt hypertrophy and inflammatory infiltrate in the lamina propria. These histopathological disarrangements are seen in *Cryptosporidium*, *Cyclospora* and microsporidial infections [28]. Furthermore, it has been documented that there are substantial disruptions of intestinal barrier function as measured by lactulose:mannitol permeability ratios in patients with AIDS and in children with diarrhea in northeast Brazil [29, 30].

Among functional alterations in patients with infectious diarrhea are increased secretion, failure of barrier function and reduction of absorptive function causing dehydration and nutritional deficiency. An understanding of the molecular pathogenesis with regard to each enteric pathogen will likely lead to a quicker diagnosis, more effective treatment and prevention of enteric infections.

Vibrio cholerae

V. cholerae (01 and 0139) pathogenesis has been extensively studied. This pathogen causes a devastating diarrhea characterized by severe dehydration without mucosal disruption or invasion. The microbe interacts with the host cell mainly in the proximal small intestine where the motile vibrios penetrate the mucus and bind to the enterocytes via toxin-coregulated pili, producing several toxins including cholera toxin [31]. Cholera toxin binds to the membrane of enterocytes and is subsequently internalized, thus causing activation of the catalytic unit of the stimulatory G protein (GS). The activation of GS protein results in uncontrolled production of cyclic AMP (cAMP), which inhibits sodium absorption and induces chloride secretion [32–34]. For decades, this was the only mechanism that explained the large loss of liquid associated with cholera-induced diarrhea. However, there is now evidence that prostaglandins are also involved in the secretion induced by cholera toxin [35]. Additionally, it has been shown that cholera toxin interacts with enteroendocrine cells, stimulating the release of endogenous secretagogues. Cholera toxin also interacts with the enteric nervous system, altering electrolyte transport and motility [36].

Escherichia coli

Several types of *E. coli* have been recognized, each with its own pathogenesis. ETEC is a major cause of dehydrating infant diarrhea in the developing world. It is also the most common cause of travelers' diarrhea [31, 37]. Like *V. cholerae*, ETEC causes an acute, watery diarrhea following the ingestion of contaminated water or food. The incubation period has been found to be 10–72 h. The organism attaches via the fimbrial colonization factor antigens (CFAs), multiplies in the proximal small intestine and produces one or more enterotoxins [38, 39]. Of the four known enterotoxins (LT-I, LT-II, STa, STb) produced by ETEC, LT-I and STa are well established in the literature as important human secretagogues. LT-I is similar to cholera toxin with respect to structure and mechanism. After binding to a GM_1 ganglioside receptor, LT-I activates adenylate cyclase, resulting in an increase of the intracellular levels of cAMP, which ultimately stimulates chloride secretion and inhibits sodium absorption [40, 41]. The ST toxin family bears significant homology to the endogenous intestinal peptide guanylin. STa binds to an extracellular domain of particulate guanylate cyclase, resulting in increased intracellular levels of cyclic guanosine monophosphate (cGMP), which leads to decreased absorption of sodium and increased chloride secretion [42]. Protective immunity to ETEC appears to be mediated by secretory IgA antibodies directed against fimbrae and LT. One of the most promising vaccine candidates, now in a phase III clinical trial, is an oral ETEC vaccine containing recombinant cholera B subunit in combination with five different formalin-inactivated *E. coli* strains expressing common fimbrial CFA-I and coli surface antigen 1–6 [31].

EPEC causes a degeneration of the microvillus brush border, with 'cupping and pedestal' formation of the plasma membrane at the sites of bacterial attachment and reorganization of cytoskeletal proteins [43, 44]. Invasion has been observed in some clinical specimens, but the mechanism of how this bacteria produces diarrhea is not fully understood. Some possibilities include an increase in permeability and loss in microvilli leading to malabsorption.

With mass food processing and fast food practices, EHEC, also called Shiga toxin-producing *E. coli*, has emerged as an important bacterial pathogen in industrialized countries [45]. Like EPEC, EHEC causes filamentous actin accumulation at the site of attachment in association with 'cup and pedestal' formation [46]. The toxins of EHEC bear both structural and functional similarity with Shiga toxin and are named SLTs or verotoxins, reflecting their cytotoxic effect in Vero cells. There are at least two immunologically different forms of SLT (SLT-I and SLT-II). These toxins are capable of inducing secretion and mucosal injury in animal models [47]. In severe disease, especially when bloody diarrhea is present, it is thought that these toxins gain access to the bloodstream and are involved in the pathogenesis of hemolytic-uremic syndrome. It is proposed that SLT binds to receptors on host cells named Gb_3

(glycolipid globotriaosylceramide) [48]. The variability in surface expression of this receptor determines the cell susceptibility to damage induced by these toxins. In addition, the proliferation rate and tissue origin of endothelial cells influence their susceptibility to the cytotoxicity of these toxins [49, 50]. For example, human renal and intestinal endothelial cells are very sensitive to SLTs [48, 51, 52], whereas human brain endothelial cells and endothelial cells derived from large vessels such as saphenous vein or human umbilical vein are relatively resistant [50, 53, 54]. Evidence shows that coincubation of endothelial cell culture with proinflammatory cytokines, such as interleukin (IL)-1 and tumor necrosis factor (TNF)-α, stimulates the expression of Gb_3 and markedly increases the cytotoxicity of the toxins towards endothelial cells [50, 53]. The damage of endothelial cells stimulates the expression of adhesion molecules, leading to leukocyte recruitment [55]. Activation of adherent leukocytes would result in the release of leukocyte products, such as reactive oxygen metabolites and proteases which exacerbate the endothelial damage. The detachment of endothelial cells as a result of direct and indirect effects of SLTs expose the basement membrane and underlying matrix, initiating the coagulation characteristic of hemolytic-uremic syndrome [56–58].

EAggEC include a heterogeneous group of organisms, some strains exhibiting no virulence. The characteristic HEp-2 adherence occurs via a flexible bundle-forming fimbrial structure, aggregative adherence fimbriae I [59, 60]. EAggEC also secretes an enterotoxin named EAST-1, which bears homology to domains of guanylin and ST, sharing with them the capacity to increase cGMP and induce secretion [61]. However, the role of EAST-1 in EAggEC-induced diarrhea is questionable given the lack of diarrhea in volunteers challenged with EAST-1-producing EAggEC strains that colonized the intestine at high levels [62]. EAggEC is also able to produce a heat-labile toxin which increases the intracellular level of calcium and stimulates calcium-dependent phosphorylation [63], but no in vivo effect of this protein has been shown. It was also shown that a product from EAggEC induces secretion of IL-8 by intestinal epithelial cells in vitro [8], and this could contribute to the intestinal inflammation detected in children with EAggEC infection [8]. This IL-8-releasing factor from EAggEC has been cloned, sequenced and expressed as a unique flagellin [64]. In addition, a 104-kD protein termed Pet (plasmid-encoded toxin), secreted by some strains of EAggEC, has been cloned and sequenced and bears homology to a class of serine protease auto-transporter proteins from *E. coli* and *Shigella* spp. [65]. Pet raises the transepithelial short-circuit current, decreases the electrical resistance of rat jejunum mounted in an Ussing chamber, causes contraction of cytoskeleton and loss of actin stress fibers, and is required for the histopathologic effects of EAggEC on human intestinal mucosa [65–67]. A definitive role of these virulent factors in the pathogenesis of EAggEC diarrhea remains to be established.

EIEC invades and multiples within colonic epithelial cells, causing cell death and inducing inflammation. This inflammatory response, along with necrosis and ulceration of the large bowel, leads to a bloody and mucoid diarrhea. Among the virulence factors, a 140-MD plasmid has been described to encode the genes responsible for outer membrane proteins important for invasion [68]. In addition, some strains produce enterotoxins capable of inducing secretion in Ussing chambers that might play a role in the watery diarrhea seen after an incubation period as short as 10–18 h [69, 70].

Clostridium difficile

C. difficile colonization and infection occur in the setting of altered intestinal microflora, usually precipitated by antibiotic exposure. Colitis and diarrhea are mediated by large exotoxins, *C. difficile* toxin A and toxin B. These toxins are produced intraluminally, bind to specific epithelial surface receptors and are internalized [71, 72]. Once in an intracellular location, both toxins monoglucosylate small GTP-binding proteins. Modification and inactivation of small GTPases (Rho, Rac, Cdc42) cause disruption of the actin cytoskeleton [73, 74]. This leads to loosening of tight junctions and eventually mucosal disruption. Interestingly, toxin A also appears to alter the morphology of neutrophils and adversely affect nondirected and direct migration induced by FMLP (f-met-leu-phe) through inactivation of Rho [75]. Toxin A-negative/toxin B-positive strains have been documented to cause disease, even nosocomial outbreaks [76]. Although both toxins can cause clinical disease, many of the secretory and inflammatory effects of *C. difficile* infection are attributed to toxin A, while the cytopathic effect is more prominent with toxin B. Toxin A has been demonstrated to cause the release of proinflammatory cytokines in an animal model [77]. Indeed, upregulation of IL-8 transcription [78] and generation of prostaglandin E_2 by inducing cyclooxygenase-2 (COX-2) expression have been recently reported along with blockade of toxin A-induced secretion and inflammatory damage by COX-2 inhibition [79]. Chemotaxis of polymorphonuclear cells and monocytes and recruitment of mast cells further contribute to the intense inflammatory reaction [80, 81]. Activation of the enteric nervous system as evidenced by increased substance P in intestinal macrophages and dorsal root ganglia in toxin A-induced enteritis in rats has also been demonstrated [82]. Disruption of the epithelial barrier, release of proinflammatory cytokines and recruitment of immune and inflammatory cells all contribute to fluid accumulation and mucosal injury.

Cryptosporidium

The *Cryptosporidium* parasite attaches to the host's intestinal epithelium, becomes intracellular but remains extracytoplasmic. In vitro studies suggest that attachment is mediated by a *Cryptosporidium parvum* sporozoite ligand and an intestinal epithelial cell surface protein interaction [83, 84].

Although infection with *C. parvum* is considered predominantly secretory, histopathologic studies have revealed varying degrees of villous atrophy and infiltration of inflammatory cells beneath the epithelial mucosa [85, 86]. Prostaglandins, which are known to induce cAMP-mediated apical chloride secretion and inhibit electroneutral sodium chloride and water absorption in enterocytes, have been demonstrated to be elevated in a porcine model of cryptosporidiosis [87]. Inflammatory cytokines such as IL-1, IL-8 and TNF-α are induced in intestinal epithelial cell lines infected with *Cryptosporidium* and in animal models of cryptosporidiosis and have been postulated to play a role in pathogenesis [88, 89]. Expression of TNF-α and IL-1 mRNA in the majority of jejunal biopsies of adult volunteers after experimental infection were also observed, although this did not correlate with the enteric symptoms [90].

Lactoferrin, a protein found in secondary granules of polymorphonuclear cells, was observed to be mildly to moderately elevated in the stools of children with endemic cryptosporidiosis [91] and healthy adult volunteers with experimental infection [92]. Indeed, in another study of malnourished children in Haiti, cryptosporidiosis was noted to stimulate an inflammatory response, as evidenced by elevated IL-8, TNF-α, lactoferrin, IL-13 and IL-10 [93]. Further studies are needed to elucidate the role of inflammatory mediators in the development of prolonged diarrhea, malabsorption and malnutrition in immunocompromised hosts and children in endemic areas.

Shigella

Shigella is the most common etiological agent of dysentery. Initially, this pathogen produces a watery diarrhea, followed by the onset of dysentery that is characterized by scanty stools of blood and mucus. The pathogen invades the mucosa of the distal ileum and colon via the M cells overlying the gut-associated lymphoid tissue [94, 95]. Invasion plasmid antigens, which are secreted by the bacteria on contact with M cells or epithelial cells, lead to reorganization of the cytoskeleton through activation of small GTPases of the Rho family and recruitment of the protooncogene *c-src*, resulting in internalization of the bacterium by macropinocytosis [95–97]. The internalized bacterium lyses its phagocytotic vacuole and initiates intracytoplasmic movement, resulting from polar assembly of actin filaments caused by a bacterial surface protein, VirG (also called IcsA), which binds and activates neuronal Wiskoff-Aldrich syndrome protein, thus inducing actin nucleation [98–101]. Actin-driven motility promotes efficient colonization of the host cell cytoplasm and rapid cell-to-cell spread via protrusions that are engulfed by adjacent cells in a cadherin-dependent process [102]. Bacterial invasion causes an intense proinflammatory response from invaded cells through activation of nuclear factor-κB [103]. A major consequence is IL-8 production, which attracts polymorphonuclear leukocytes (PMN) [104]. On transmigration, PMN disrupt the permeability of this epithelium and promote its invasion by *Shigella*, leading to mucosal ulceration and microabscess formation [31]. Subsequent apoptotic killing of macrophages in a caspase 1-dependent process causes the release of IL-1β and IL-18, which accounts for the initial steps of inflammation [105–107]. There are four species or groups of *Shigella*: *S. dysenteriae*, *S. flexneri*, *S. boydii* and *S. sonnei.* All include multiple serotypes, complicating vaccine development strategies. One approach that is being followed is to prepare conjugate vaccines for parenteral administration by covalently linking O polysaccharides of the most prevalent *Shigella* serotypes to carrier proteins [108]. Another approach that has been studied is that of attenuated strains. Investigators have attempted to apply tools of biotechnology to develop modern attenuated strains *of Shigella* that can serve as live oral vaccines. One of these prototype vaccines contain a strain that harbors a mutation in a plasmid virulence gene *ics*A (i.e. *vir*G) that limits the intra- and intercellular spread of the bacteria, combining with other mutations. Proteosomes are outer-membrane proteins of meningococci that are highly hydrophobic and assemble into membranous vesicles and can combine with antigens to form a competent antigen delivery system. One of the most successful uses of proteosomes has been to prepare complexes with the lipopolysaccharides of *S. sonnei* and *S. flexneri* [31, 109]. Clinical trials of these candidate vaccines are currently under way.

Salmonella

Salmonella species are a major source of food-borne disease throughout the developing and the developed countries [110]. This pathogen invades the mucosa through the M cells or through enterocytes, resulting in the extrusion of infected epithelial cells into the intestinal lumen with consequent villus blunting and loss of absorptive surfaces. *Salmonella* also elicit a PMN influx into infected mucosa and induce watery diarrhea, which may contain blood [111]. Wallis and Galyov [111] reviewed and proposed a sequence of events occurring during the pathogenesis of *Salmonella*-induced enteritis: (1) *Salmonella* interacts with enterocytes and delivers *Salmonella* outer proteins (Sops) into the cell cytoplasm via a TTSS-1 (TTSS are secreted virulence-associated effector proteins) and *Salmonella* invasion protein (Sip)-dependent pathway. (2) Sips, SopE and possibly other Sops induce enterocyte membrane ruffling promoting bacterial invasion. (3) Intracellular bacteria reside within membrane-bound vesicles and possibly continue translocation of TTSS-1 secreted effectors. The replication of *Salmonella* within the vesicles is promoted by TTSS-2. (4) The intracellular SopB protein affects inositol phosphate signaling events, causing a transient increase in the concentration of Ins(1,4,5,6)P_1, which in turn can antagonize the closure of chloride channels, influencing net electrolyte transport and thus fluid secretion. (5) *Salmonella-infected* epithelial cells secrete chemokines and prostaglandins that act to recruit inflammatory cells to foci of infection. The release of at least some chemokines and prostaglandins is probably affected by the intracellular activity of Sops. (6) *Salmonella* interacts with inflammatory cells and stimulates the release of proinflammatory cytokines that enhance the inflammatory response. *Salmonella*-infected epithelial cells release pathogen-elicited epithelial chemoattractant across the apical membrane, which stimulates PMN trans-epithelial migration between the enterocytes. (8) Infiltrating inflammatory cells phagocytose *Salmonella.* (9) *Salmonella*-infected enterocytes become extruded from the villus surface, leading to shedding of infected cells into the intestinal lumen and resulting in villus blunting and loss of absorptive surfaces. (10) Some of the infected cells migrate to the draining lymphatics, carrying *Salmonella* to systemic sites.

Campylobacter

Although not reviewed in detail here, *C. jejuni* and *C. coli* are another major cause of inflammatory colitis that may be complicated by Guillain-Barré syndrome or reactive arthritis. In addition, their resistance to antimicrobials (particularly to quinolones) is increasing. In the United States, fluoroquinolone resistance of *C. jejuni* rose from 13% in 1997 to 18% in 1999 [112].

Management of Enteric Infections

Because the most common risks of diarrhea are dehydration and malnutrition, the critical initial treatment must be rehydration. Thus, the first approach to patients with enteritis should be the evaluation of their hydration status by checking mucosal hydration, skin turgor and orthostatic changes in pulse and blood pressure. Oral or intravenous rehydration therapy should precede any search for etiological diagnosis. Although both methods are life-saving procedures, oral rehydration is better tolerated, safer and more inexpensive than intravenous fluid administration. Some patients with mild diarrhea can compensate for water loss in the stool by ingesting more dietary liquids such as soups, juices, etc. However, patients with severe diarrhea may need additional rehydration. Rehydration can be accomplished by providing the patient with an oral solution containing electrolytes and glucose. The concentrations recommended by the World Health Organization are as follows: glucose 111 m*M*, Na 90 m*M*, K 20 m*M*, Cl 80 m*M* and HCO_3 30 m*M* [113]. The principle behind the use of this solution is that nutrients such as glucose and amino acids are transported across the apical membrane of the enterocyte by a carrier that cotransports sodium [114]. Unlike apical sodium-hydrogen exchange, nutrient-sodium cotransport is not impeded by elevated intracellular cAMP levels [115]. Recently, it has been shown that glutamine and especially its stable derivative alanyl-glutamine may not only increase sodium absorption but also improve the repair of intestinal epithelium after damage [116–120]. Alanyl-glutamine is more advantageous than glutamine due to its much greater solubility and its stability in solution and in acidic conditions such as the stomach. Other advantages include its ability to be heat sterilized and capacity for long term storage (US patent No. 5,561,111).

The second step in the management of the patient with enteritis is the collection of a detailed clinical history including the epidemiological features. Relevant clinical information includes symptomatic onset, stool characteristics (watery, bloody, mucous, purulent, greasy, etc.), frequency of bowel movements, quantity of stool produced, presence of dysenteric symptoms (fever, tenesmus, blood and/or pus in the stool), symptoms of volume depletion (thirst, tachycardia, orthostasis, decreased urination, lethargy, decreased skin turgor) and associated symptoms (nausea, vomiting, abdominal pain, cramps, headache, myalgias, altered sensorium). In addition, all patients must be asked about potential epidemiological risks such as travel to endemic areas, day care center attendance or employment, consumption of unsafe foods (raw meats, seafood, unpasteurized milk or juices), contact with pets with diarrhea, use of antibiotics and underlying medical conditions (AIDS, immunosuppressive medication, etc.).

Physical examination is essential for evaluation of signs of hydration status. In addition, it is important to screen for the presence of fever, and to evaluate diagnostic findings that may indicate another etiology.

Combining clinical and epidemiological features with fecal analysis gives important clues to the etiological diagnosis. For example, any patients with diarrheal illness lasting more than 1 day, accompanied by fever, bloody stools, systemic illness, signs of serious dehydration and recent use of antibiotics, day care attendance and hospitalization should have a fecal sample specimen sent for evaluation. Additional laboratory exams may be necessary for selected cases. The Infectious Diseases Society of America Practice Guidelines for the Management of Infectious Diarrhea recommend a selective approach such as that shown in figure 1 [113].

With the increasing appearance of antibiotic-resistant infections, the side effects of antibiotics and superinfection as a consequence of the disturbance of the intestinal microflora, the immediate decision to use antibiotics should be reconsidered. Although most forms of traveler's diarrhea can be managed effectively with symptomatic treatment alone, with agents such as loperamide or bismuth preparations, empirical antibiotics are commonly recommended.

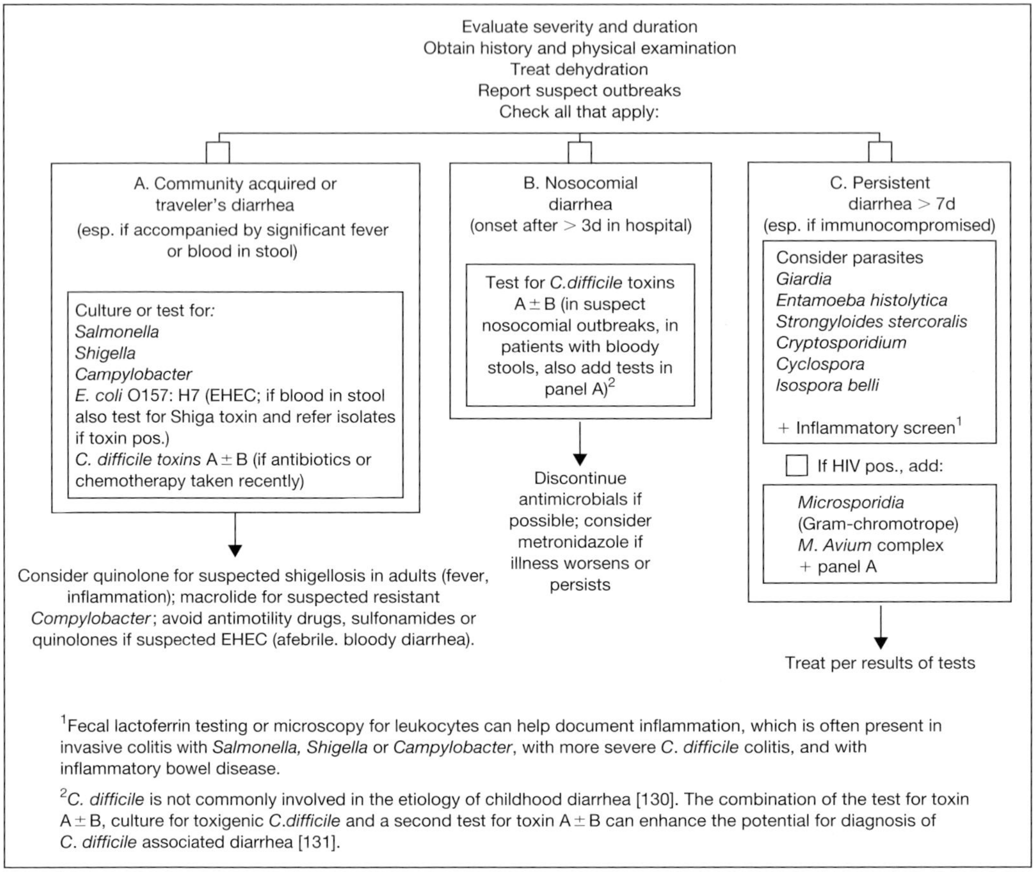

Fig. 1. Recommendations for the diagnosis and management of enteric infections. Adapted from Guerrant et al. [113], Infectious Diseases Society of America Practice Guidelines for the Management of Infectious Diarrhea.

Treatment with fluoroquinolone or, in children, trimethoprim-sulfamethoxazole (TMP-SMZ) can reduce the duration of the diarrhea from 3–5 days to less than 1–2 days [24, 113]. Some also consider empirical treatment of diarrhea that lasts longer than 10–14 days for suspected giardiasis, if other evaluations are negative and, especially, if the patient's history of travel or water exposure is suggestive [113]. For patients with febrile diarrheal illnesses, especially those believed to have moderate to severe invasive disease, empirical treatment should be considered after a fecal specimen is obtained for performance of the studies noted in figure 1. This empirical treatment can be with an agent such as a quinolone antibiotic or, for children, TMP-SMZ [113]. The increasing worldwide resistance to TMP-SMZ and the more recently reported resistance to fluoroquinolones [122, 123] is a driving force for the development of new antimicrobial agents, such as rifaximin and azithromycin. Rifaximin (a rifamycin derivative) is poorly absorbed when administered orally, but it has been shown to be safe and effective in comparison with TMP-SMX and ciprofloxacin [122, 123]. A study performed with adult students from United States in Mexico or international tourists in Jamaica showed that treatment for 3 days with rifaximin (400 mg twice a day) was as effective as ciprofloxacin (500 mg twice a day) with regard to the duration of disease, clinical improvement and microbiological cure. The incidence of adverse events was low and similar in each group [123]. Another study suggested that rifaximin (600 mg, 3 times a day, for 14 days) may improve clinical symptoms and clearing of protozoan infections in HIV-1-infected patients with CD4 $\geq 200/\text{mm}^3$ who presented with *Cryptosporidium* or *Blastocystis* associated with bacteria [124]. Additionally, the effect of rifaximin was compared with neomycin plus bacitracin in children with bacterial diarrhea in which the etiologic agents were *Salmonella* spp. and EPEC. Rifaximin yielded bacteriological cure in 12 out of 14 children, the reference drug in 13 of 17. With both drugs, the stool number per day fell after 1 day; within 2 days, stool consistency shifted to normal [125].

Because the development of antibiotic resistance will continue to be a problem, the development of effective alternative treatments is imperative. Immunization, probiotics, antisecretory agents, improved oral rehydration and nutrition therapy and nonabsorbable antibiotics are being considered by clinicians and researchers. Novel therapeutic agents, other than antimicrobials, include the 5-hydroxytryptamine-2 and -3 receptor antagonists [126, 127], calcium-calmodulin antagonists, zaldaride maleate and σ-receptor agonist igmesine [126]. An enkephalinase inhibitor named racecadotril has also been developed, based on the antisecretory role of the neurotransmitter enkephalin, and it has been reported to have good efficacy and tolerability in clinical trials [128].

Prevention

Education, simple rules of personal hygiene and safe food preparation can prevent many diarrheal diseases. Hand washing with soap is an effective step in preventing spread of illness. Human feces must always be considered potentially hazardous. Immunocompromised persons, alcoholics, persons with chronic liver disease and pregnant women may require additional attention, and health care providers can play an important role in providing information about food safety. These populations should avoid undercooked meat, raw shellfish, raw dairy products, French-style cheeses and unheated deli meats [114].

Several bacterial pathogens have been targeted as a priority for the development of new or improved vaccines, such as *V. cholerae*, *Shigella*, *E. coli* and *Salmonella.* Substantial progress in molecular biology, bacterial pathogenesis, and immunology make possible the development of new candidate vaccines, but the evaluation of these candidates is a long and expensive process [31, 129]. In the developing countries, where the incidence of diarrhea is greater, financial resources are scarce and few countries have incorporated immunization for enteric pathogens into their immunization program. In the USA, only cholera and typhoid fever vaccines are commercially available. Immunization is recommended for typhoid fever (types Vi, Ty21a or the heat-phenol-inactivated vaccine for those under 2 years of age) in individuals living in or traveling to high-risk areas. Two modern oral cholera vaccines have been licensed by regulatory authorities in a number of countries. One is a nonliving vaccine consisting of inactivated *V. cholerae* O1 administered in combination with the B subunit of cholera toxin, so-called B subunit whole-cell cholera vaccine. The other vaccine is a genetically engineered attenuated strain of *V. cholerae* O1, CVD 103-HgR, which is used as a single-dose live oral vaccine [31]. Older cholera vaccines are not recommended in the US because of their limited efficacy and the low risk of cholera to the traveler [114].

Conclusion

Emerging infectious pathogens, increasing antimicrobial resistance, recognition of the long-term impact of diarrheal diseases and the appearance of diseases that decrease the host defense have heightened the necessity to develop new and more specific treatments and further clarify the pathogenesis of diarrheal illnesses. New antibiotics, vaccines and micronutrients that improve mucosal recovery and host defenses are currently being tested. Additionally, it is critical to prevent enteric infections by increasing vaccination and improving sanitary conditions and the availability of safe drinking water.

References

1 Kosek M, Bern C, Guerrant RL: The global burden of diarrhoeal disease, as estimated from studies published between 1992 and 2000. Bull World Health Organ 2003;81:197–204.

2 Guerrant RL, Kosek M, Lima AA, Lorntz B, Guyatt HL: Updating the DALYs for diarrhoeal disease. Trends Parasitol 2002;18:191–193.

3 Guerrant DI, Moore SR, Lima AA, Patrick PD, Schorling JB, Guerrant RL: Association of early childhood diarrhea and cryptosporidiosis with impaired physical fitness and cognitive function four to seven years later in a poor urban community in northeast Brazil. Am J Trop Med Hyg 1999; 61:707–713.

4 Moore SR, Lima AA, Conaway MR, Schorling JB, Soares AM, Guerrant RL: Early childhood diarrhoea and helminthiases associate with long-term linear growth faltering. Int J Epidemiol 2001;30:1457–1464.

5 Lorntz B, Lima AA, Silva R, Chen P, Kosek M, Moore S, Guerrant RL: Diarrhea in first two years of life is associated with increase age for grade and age at starting school five to nine years later. 49th Annual Meeting of the American Society of Tropical Medicine and Hygiene, Houston, Tex., 2000.

6 Niehaus MD, Moore SR, Patrick PD, Derr LL, Lorntz B, Lima AA, Guerrant RL: Early childhood diarrhea is associated with diminished cognitive function 4 to 7 years later in children in a northeast Brazilian shantytown. Am J Trop Med Hyg 2002;66:590–593.

7 Nachamkin I, Allos BM, Ho T: Campylobacter species and Guillain-Barre syndrome. Clin Microbiol Rev 1998;11:555–567.

8 Steiner TS, Lima AAM, Nataro JP, Guerrant RL: Enteroaggregative *Escherichia coli* produce intestinal inflammation and growth impairment and cause interleukin-8 release from intestinal epithelial cells. J Infect Dis 1998;177:88–96.

9 Checkley W, Gilman RH, Epstein LD, Suarez M, Diaz JF, Cabrera L, Black RE, Sterling CR: Asymptomatic and symptomatic cryptosporidiosis: Their acute effect on weight gain in Peruvian children. Am J Epidemiol 1997;145:156–163.

10 Checkley W, Epstein LD, Gilman RH, Black RE, Cabrera L, Sterling CR: Effects of *Cryptosporidium parvum* infection in Peruvian children: Growth faltering and subsequent catchup growth. Am J Epidemiol 1998;148:497–506.

11 Herwaldt BL, Beach MJ: The return of Cyclospora in 1997: Another outbreak of cyclosporiasis in North America associated with imported raspberries. Cyclospora Working Group (see comments). Ann Intern Med 1999;130:210–220.

12 Buzby JC, Roberts T, Jordan Lin C-T, MacDonald JM: Bacterial foodborne disease: Medical costs and productivity losses. Agricultural Economic Report. Economic Research Service, USDA, 1996.

13 NIAID Foodborne Diseases Fact Sheet. http://www.niaid.nih.gov/factsheets/foodborne-dis.htm. Bethesda, NIH, 1999.

14 LeDuc JW, Hughes JM: Surveillance for emerging infectious diseases; in Guerrant RL, Walker DH, Weller PF (eds): Tropical Infectious Diseases: Principles, Pathogens, and Practice. Philadelphia, Churchill Livingstone, 1999, pp 251–260.

15 Mead PS, Slutsker L, Dietz V, McCaig LF, Bresee JS, Shapiro C, Griffin PM, Tauxe RV: Food-related illness and death in the United States. Emerg Infect Dis 1999;5:607–625.

16 Thielman NM, Guerrant RL: Enteric *Escherichia coli* infections; in Guerrant RL, Walker DH, Weller PF (eds): Tropical Infectious Diseases: Principles, Pathogens, and Practice. Philadelphia, Churchill Livingstone, 1999, pp 261–276.

17 Guerrant RL, Lima AA, Barboza M, Young S, Silva T, Barrett L, Bao Y, Fox J, Moore S: Mechanisms and impact of enteric infections. Adv Exp Med Biol 1999;473:103–112.

18 Heriskstadt H, Vergia D, Hadler J, et al: Population-based estimate of the burden of diarrheal illnesses; FoodNet 1996–1997. 1st International Conference on Emerging Infectious Diseases, Atlanta, Ga., 1998.

19 LeClere FB, Moss AJ, Everhart JE, Roth HP: Prevalence of major digestive disorders and bowel symptoms, 1989. Adv Data 1992;(212):1–15.

20 Adachi JA, Ostrosky-Zeichner L, DuPont HL, Ericsson CD: Empirical antimicrobial therapy for traveler's diarrhea. Clin Infect Dis 2000;31:1079–1083.

21 DuPont HL, Ericsson CD: Prevention and treatment of traveler's diarrhea. N Engl J Med 1993; 328:1821–1827.

22 Ericsson CD: Travelers' diarrhea. Epidemiology, prevention, and self-treatment. Infect Dis Clin North Am 1998;12:285–303.

23 Gorbach SL, Edelman R: Traveler's diarrhea: National Institutes of Health Consensus Conference. JAMA 1985;253:2700–2704.

24 Lima AA: Tropical diarrhoea: New developments in traveller's diarrhoea. Curr Opin Infect Dis 2001;14:547–552.

25 Keystone J, Kozarsky PE: Health advice for international travel; in Guerrant RL, Walker DH, Weller PF (eds): Essentials of Tropical Infectious Diseases. New York, Churchill Livingstone, 2001, pp 128–140.

26 Schiller LR: Secretory diarrhea. Curr Gastroenterol Rep 1999;1:389–397.
27 Lima AA, Innes DJ Jr, Chadee K, Lyerly DM, Wilkins TD, Guerrant RL: *Clostridium difficile* toxin A. Interactions with mucus and early sequential histopathologic effects in rabbit small intestine. Lab Invest 1989;61:419–425.
28 Thielman NM, Guerrant RL: Persistent diarrhea in the returned traveler. Infect Dis Clin North Am 1998;12:489–501.
29 Bao YD, Silva TJ, Guerrant RL, Lima AM, Fox JW: Direct analysis of mannitol, lactulose and glucose in urine samples by high-performance anion-exchange chromatography with pulse amperometric detection – clinical evaluation of intestinal permeability in human immunodeficiency virus infection. J Chromatogr 1996;685:105–112.
30 Lima AAM, Silva TJ, Gifoni AMR, Barrett LJ, McAuliffe IT, Bao Y, Fox JW, Fedorko DP, Guerrant RL: Mucosal injury and disruption of intestinal barrier function in HIV-infected individuals with and without diarrhea and cryptosporidiosis in Northeast Brazil. Am J Gastroenterol 1997;92:1861–1866.
31 Levine MM: Immunization against bacterial diseases of the intestine. J Pediatr Gastroenterol Nutr 2000;31:336–355.
32 Moss J, Vaughan M: Activation of adenylate cyclase by choleragen. Annu Rev Biochem 1979;48: 581–600.
33 Guerrant RL, Brunton LL, Schnaitman RC, Rebhun LI, Gilman AG: Cyclic adenosine monophosphate and alteration of Chinese hamster ovary cell morphology: A rapid, sensitive in vitro assay for the entertoxins of *Vibrio cholerae* and *Escherichia coli*. Infect Immun 1974;10:320–327.
34 Field M: Ion transport in rabbit ileal mucosa. II. Effects of cyclic 3′,5′-AMP. Am J Physiol 1971;255:781–786.
35 Peterson JW, Ochoa LG: Role of prostaglandins and cAMP in the secretory effects of cholera toxin. Science 1989;245:857–859.
36 Lundgren O: 5-Hydroxytryptamine, enterotoxins, and intestinal fluid secretion. Gastroenterology 1998;115:1009–1012.
37 Black RE, Brown KH, Becker S, Yunus M: Longitudinal studies of infectious diseases and physical growth of children in rural Bangladesh. II. Incidence of diarrhea and association with known pathogens. Am J Epidemiol 1982;115:315–324.
38 Oyofo BA, el Etr SH, Wasfy MO, Peruski L, Kay B, Mansour M, Campbell JR, Svennerholm AM, Churilla AM, Murphy JR: Colonization factors of enterotoxigenic *E. coli* (ETEC) from residents of northern Egypt. Microbiol Res 1995;150:429–436.
39 Knutton S, Lloyd DR, McNeish AS: Identification of a new fimbrial structure in enterotoxigenic *Escherichia coli* (ETEC) serotype O148: H28 which adheres to human intestinal mucosa: A potentially new human ETEC colonization factor. Infect Immun 1987;55:86–92.
40 Dallas WS, Falkow S: Amino acid sequence homology between cholera toxin and *Escherichia coli* heat-labile toxin. Nature 1980;288:499–501.
41 Lockman H, Kaper JB: Nucleotide sequence analysis of the A2 and B subunits of *Vibrio cholerae* enterotoxin. J Biol Chem 1983;258:13722–13726.
42 Forte LR, Eber SL, Turner JT, Freeman RH, Fok KF, Currie MG: Guanylin stimulation of Cl–secretion in human intestinal T84 cells via cyclic guanosine monophosphate. J Clin Invest 1993;91:2423–2428.
43 Rothbaum R, McAdams AJ, Giannella R, Partin JC: A clinicopathologic study of enterocyteadherent *Escherichia coli:* A cause of protracted diarrhea in children. Gastroenterology 1982;83: 441–454.
44 Kenny B, DeVinney R, Stein M, Reinscheid DJ, Frey EA, Finlay BB: Enteropathogenic *E. coli* (EPEC) transfers its receptor for intimate adherence into mammalian cells. Cell 1997;91: 511–520.
45 Griffin PM, Tauxe RV: The epidemiology of infections caused by *Escherichia coli* O157:H7, other enterohemorrhagic *E. coli*, and the associated hemolytic uremic syndrome. Epidemiol Rev 1991; 13:60–98.
46 Knutton S, Baldwin T, Williams PH, McNeish AS: Actin accumulation at sites of bacterial adhesion to tissue culture cells: Basis of a new diagnostic test for enteropathogenic and enterohemorrhagic *Escherichia coli*. Infect Immun 1989;57:1290–1298.

47 Tzipori S, Karch H, Wachsmuth KI, Robins-Browne RM, O'Brien AD, Lior H, Cohen ML, Smithers J, Levine MM: Role of a 60-megadalton plasmid and Shiga-like toxins in the pathogenesis of infection caused by enterohemorrhagic *Escherichia coli* O157: H7 in gnotobiotic piglets. Infect Immun 1987;55:3117–3125.

48 Obrig TG, Louise CB, Lingwood CA, Boyd B, Barley-Maloney L, Daniel TO: Endothelial heterogeneity in Shiga toxin receptors and responses. J Biol Chem 1993;268:15484–15488.

49 Obrig TG, Del Vecchio PJ, Brown JE, Moran TP, Rowland BM, Judge TK, Rothman SW: Direct cytotoxic action of Shiga toxin on human vascular endothelial cells. Infect Immun 1988;56:2373–2378.

50 Louise CB, Obrig TG: Shiga toxin-associated hemolytic-uremic syndrome: Combined cytotoxic effects of Shiga toxin, interleukin-1 beta, and tumor necrosis factor alpha on human vascular endothelial cells in vitro. Infect Immun 1991;59:4173–4179.

51 Louise CB, Obrig TG: Specific interaction of *Escherichia coli* O157: H7-derived Shiga-like toxin II with human renal endothelial cells. J Infect Dis 1995;172:1397–1401.

52 Jacewicz MS, Acheson DW, Binion DG, West GA, Lincicome LL, Fiocchi C, Keusch GT: Responses of human intestinal microvascular endothelial cells to Shiga toxins 1 and 2 and pathogenesis of hemorrhagic colitis. Infect Immun 1999;67:1439–1444.

53 Kaye SA, Louise CB, Boyd B, Lingwood CA, Obrig TG: Shiga toxin-associated hemolytic uremic syndrome: Interleukin-1 beta enhancement of Shiga toxin cytotoxicity toward human vascular endothelial cells in vitro. Infect Immun 1993;61:3886–3891.

54 Ramegowda B, Samuel JE, Tesh VL: Interaction of Shiga toxins with human brain microvascular endothelial cells: Cytokines as sensitizing agents. J Infect Dis 1999;180:1205–1213.

55 Morigi M, Micheletti G, Figliuzzi M, Imberti B, Karmali MA, Remuzzi A, Remuzzi G, Zoja C: Verotoxin-1 promotes leukocyte adhesion to cultured endothelial cells under physiologic flow conditions. Blood 1995;86:4553–4558.

56 O'Brien AD, Holmes RK: Shiga and Shiga-like toxins. Microbiol Rev 1987;51:206–220.

57 O'Loughlin EV, Robins-Browne RM: Effect of Shiga toxin and Shiga-like toxins on eukaryotic cells. Microbes Infect 2001;3:493–507.

58 Su C, Brandt LJ: *Escherichia coli* O157: H7 infection in humans. Ann Intern Med 1995;123: 698–714.

59 Nataro JP, Deng Y, Maneval DR, German AL, Martin WC, Levine MM: Aggregative adherence fimbriae I of enteroaggregative *Escherichia coli* mediate adherence to HEp-2 cells and hemagglutination of human erythrocytes. Infect Immun 1992;60:2297–2304.

60 Nataro JP, Yikang D, Giron JA, Savarino SJ, Kothary MH, Hall R: Aggregative adherence fimbria I expression in enteroaggregative *Escherichia coli* requires two unlinked plasmid regions. Infect Immun 1993;61:1126–1131.

61 Savarino SJ, Fasano A, Watson J, Martin BM, Levine MM, Guandalini S, Guerry P: Enteroaggregative *Escherichia coli* heat-stable enterotoxin 1 represents another subfamily of *E. coli* heat-stable toxin. Proc Natl Acad Sci USA 1993;90:3093–3097.

62 Nataro JP, Deng Y, Cookson S, Cravioto A, Savarino SJ, Guers LD, Levine MM, Tacket CO: Heterogeneity of enteroaggregative *Escherichia coli* virulence demonstrated in volunteers. J Infect Dis 1995;171:465–468.

63 Baldwin TJ, Knutton S, Sellers L, Hernandez HA, Aitken A, Williams PH: Enteroaggregative *Escherichia coli* strains secrete a heat-labile toxin antigenically related to *E. coli* hemolysin. Infect Immun 1992;60:2092–2095.

64 Steiner TS, Nataro JP, Poteet-Smith CE, Smith JA, Guerrant RL: Enteroaggregative *Escherichia coli* expresses a novel flagellin that causes IL-8 release from intestinal epithelial cells. J Clin Invest 2000;105:1769–1777.

65 Henderson IR, Navarro-Garcia F, Nataro JP: The great escape: Structure and function of the autotransporter proteins. Trends Microbiol 1998;6:370–378.

66 Navarro-Garcia F, Eslava C, Villaseca JM, Lopez-Revilla R, Czeczulin JR, Srinivas S, Nataro JP, Cravioto A: In vitro effects of a high-molecular-weight heat-labile enterotoxin from enteroaggregative *Escherichia coli*. Infect Immun 1998;66:3149–3154.

67 Navarro-Garcia F, Canizalez-Roman A, Luna J, Sears C, Nataro JP: Plasmid-encoded toxin of enteroaggregative *Escherichia coli* is internalized by epithelial cells. Infect Immun 2001;69: 1053–1060.

68 Sansonetti PJ, d'Hauteville H, Ecobichon C, Pourcel C: Molecular comparison of virulence plasmids in *Shigella* and enteroinvasive *Escherichia coli*. Ann Microbiol (Paris) 1983;134A: 295–318.

69 Fasano A, Kay BA, Russell RG, Maneval DR Jr, Levin MM: Enterotoxin and cytotoxin production by enteroinvasive *Escherichia coli*. Infect Immun 1990;58:3717–3723.

70 Nataro JP, Seriwatana J, Fasano A, Maneval DR, Guers LD, Noriega F, Dubovsky F, Levine MM, Morris JG Jr: Identification and cloning of a novel plasmid-encoded enterotoxin of enteroinvasive *Escherichia coli* and *Shigella* strains. Infect Immun 1995;63:4721–4728.

71 Eichel-Streiber C, Warfolomeow I, Knautz D, Sauerborn M, Hadding U: Morphological changes in adherent cells induced by *Clostridium difficile* toxins. Biochem Soc Trans 1991;19:1154–1160.

72 Krivan HC, Clark GF, Smith DF, Wilkins TD: Cell surface binding site for *Clostridium difficile* enterotoxin: Evidence for a glycoconjugate containing the sequence Gal alpha 1–3Gal beta 1–4GlcNAc. Infect Immun 1986;53:573–581.

73 Just I, Wilm M, Selzer J, Rex G, von Eichel-Streiber C, Mann M, Aktories K: The enterotoxin from *Clostridium difficile* (ToxA) monoglucosylates the Rho proteins. J Biol Chem 1995;270: 13932–13936.

74 Just I, Selzer J, Wilm M, von Eichel-Streiber C, Mann M, Aktories K: Glucosylation of Rho proteins by *Clostridium difficile* toxin B. Nature 1995;375:500–503.

75 Brito GA, Sullivan GW, Ciesla WP Jr, Carper HT, Mandell GL, Guerrant RL: *Clostridium difficile* toxin A alters in vitro-adherent neutrophil morphology and function. J Infect Dis 2002;185: 1297–1306.

76 Alfa MJ, Kabani A, Lyerly D, Moncrief S, Neville LM, Al Barrak A, Harding GK, Dyck B, Olekson K, Embil JM: Characterization of a toxin A-negative, toxin B-positive strain of *Clostridium difficile* responsible for a nosocomial outbreak of *Clostridium difficile*-associated diarrhea. J Clin Microbiol 2000;38:2706–2714.

77 Flegel WA, Muller F, Daubener W, Fischer HG, Hadding U, Northoff H: Cytokine response by human monocytes to *Clostridium difficile* toxin A and toxin B. Infect Immun 1991;59:3659–3666.

78 Jefferson KK, Smith MF Jr, Bobak DA: Roles of intracellular calcium and NF-kappa B in the *Clostridium difficile* toxin A-induced up-regulation and secretion of IL-8 from human monocytes. J Immunol 1999;163:5183–5191.

79 Alcantara C, Stenson WF, Steiner TS, Guerrant RL: Role of inducible cyclooxygenase and prostaglandins in *Clostridium difficile* toxin A-induced secretion and inflammation in an animal model. J Infect Dis 2001;184:648–652.

80 Pothoulakis C, Sullivan R, Malnick DA, Triadafilopoulos G, Gadenne AS, Meshulam T, La-Mont JT: *Clostridium difficile* toxin A stimulates intracellular calcium release and chemotactic response in human granulocytes. J Clin Invest 1988;81:1741–1745.

81 Wershil BK, Castagliuolo I, Pothoulakis C: Direct evidence of mast cell involvement in *Clostridium difficile* toxin A-induced enteritis in mice. Gastroenterology 1998;114:956–964.

82 Castagliuolo I, Keates AC, Qiu B, Kelly CP, Nikulasson S, Leeman SE, Pothoulakis C: Increased substance P responses in dorsal root ganglia and intestinal macrophages during *Clostridium difficile* toxin A enteritis in rats. Proc Natl Acad Sci USA 1997;94:4788–4793.

83 Langer RC, Riggs MW: *Cryptosporidium parvum* apical complex glycoprotein CSL contains a sporozoite ligand for intestinal epithelial cells. Infect Immun 1999;67:5282–5291.

84 Langer RC, Schaefer DA, Riggs MW: Characterization of an intestinal epithelial cell receptor recognized by the *Cryptosporidium parvum* sporozoite ligand CSL. Infect Immun 2001;69: 1661–1670.

85 Godwin TA: Cryptosporidiosis in the acquired immunodeficiency syndrome: A study of 15 autopsy cases. Hum Pathol 1991;22:1215–1224.

86 Genta RM, Chappell CL, White AC Jr, Kimball KT, Goodgame RW: Duodenal morphology and intensity of infection in AIDS-related intestinal cryptosporidiosis. Gastroenterology 1993;105: 1769–1775.

87 Argenzio RA, Lecce J, Powell DW: Prostanoids inhibit intestinal NaCl absorption in experimental porcine cryptosporidiosis. Gastroenterology 1993;104:440–447.

88 Laurent F, Eckmann L, Savidge TC, Morgan G, Theodos C, Naciri M, Kagnoff MF: *Cryptosporidium parvum* infection of human intestinal epithelial cells induces the polarized secretion of C-X-C chemokines. Infect Immun 1997;65:5067–5073.
89 Seydel KB, Zhang T, Champion GA, Fichtenbaum C, Swanson PE, Tzipori S, Griffiths JK, Stanley SL Jr: *Cryptosporidium parvum* infection of human intestinal xenografts in SCID mice induces production of human tumor necrosis factor alpha and interleukin-8. Infect Immun 1998; 66:2379–2382.
90 Robinson P, Okhuysen PC, Chappell CL, Lewis DE, Shahab I, Janecki A, White AC Jr: Expression of tumor necrosis factor alpha and interleukin 1 beta in jejuna of volunteers after experimental challenge with *Cryptosporidium parvum* correlates with exposure but not with symptoms. Infect Immun 2001;69:1172–1174.
91 Newman RD, Sears CL, Moore SR, Nataro JP, Wuhib T, Agnew DA, Guerrant RL, Lima AAM: Longitudinal study of *Cryptosporidium* infection in children in northeastern Brazil. J Infect Dis 1999;180:167–175.
92 Alcantara CS, Yang CH, Steiner TS, Barrett LJ, Lima AAM, Chappell CL, Okhuysen PC, White AC, Guerrant RL: Interleukin-8, tumor necrosis factor-α and lactoferrin in immunocompetent hosts with experimental and Brazilian children with acquired cryptosporidiosis. Am J Trop Med Hyg 2003;68:325–328.
93 Kirkpatrick BD, Daniels MM, Jean SS, Pape JW, Karp C, Littenberg B, Fitzgerald DW, Lederman HM, Nataro JP, Sears CL: Cryptosporidiosis stimulates an inflammatory intestinal response in malnourished Haitian children. J Infect Dis 2002;186:94–101.
94 Phalipon A, Sansonetti PJ: Microbial-host interactions at mucosal sites. Host response to pathogenic bacteria at mucosal sites. Curr Top Microbiol Immunol 1999;236:163–189.
95 Sansonetti PJ, Phalipon A: M cells as ports of entry for enteroinvasive pathogens: Mechanisms of interaction, consequences for the disease process. Semin Immunol 1999;11:193–203.
96 Dehio C, Prevost MC, Sansonetti PJ: Invasion of epithelial cells by *Shigella flexneri* induces tyrosine phosphorylation of cortactin by a pp60c-src-mediated signalling pathway. EMBO J 1995; 14:2471–2482.
97 Hall A: Rho GTPases and the actin cytoskeleton. Science 1998;279:509–514.
98 Egile C, Loisel TP, Laurent V, Li R, Pantaloni D, Sansonetti PJ, Carlier MF: Activation of the CDC42 effector N-WASP by the *Shigella flexneri* IcsA protein promotes actin nucleation by Arp2/3 complex and bacterial actin-based motility. J Cell Biol 1999;146:1319–1332.
99 Lett MC, Sasakawa C, Okada N, Sakai T, Makino S, Yamada M, Komatsu K, Yoshikawa M: virG, a plasmid-coded virulence gene of *Shigella flexneri*: Identification of the virG protein and determination of the complete coding sequence. J Bacteriol 1989;171:353–359.
100 Makino S, Sasakawa C, Kamata K, Kurata T, Yoshikawa M: A genetic determinant required for continuous reinfection of adjacent cells on large plasmid in *S. flexneri* 2a. Cell 1986;46: 551–555.
101 Suzuki T, Miki H, Takenawa T, Sasakawa C: Neural Wiskott-Aldrich syndrome protein is implicated in the actin-based motility of *Shigella flexneri*. EMBO J 1998;17:2767–2776.
102 Sansonetti PJ, Mounier J, Prevost MC, Mege RM: Cadherin expression is required for the spread of *Shigella flexneri* between epithelial cells. Cell 1994;76:829–839.
103 Philpott DJ, Yamaoka S, Israel A, Sansonetti PJ: Invasive *Shigella flexneri* activates NF-kappa B through a lipopolysaccharide-dependent innate intracellular response and leads to IL-8 expression in epithelial cells. J Immunol 2000;165:903–914.
104 Jung HC, Eckmann L, Yang SK, Panja A, Fierer J, Morzycka-Wroblewska E, Kagnoff MF: A distinct array of proinflammatory cytokines is expressed in human colon epithelial cells in response to bacterial invasion. J Clin Invest 1995;95:55–65.
105 Chen Y, Smith MR, Thirumalai K, Zychlinsky A: A bacterial invasin induces macrophage apoptosis by binding directly to ICE. EMBO J 1996;15:3853–3860.
106 Whyte M: ICE/CED-3 proteases in apoptosis. Trends Cell Biol 1996;6:245–248.
107 Sansonetti PJ: Microbes and microbial toxins: Paradigms for microbial-mucosal interactions. III. Shigellosis: From symptoms to molecular pathogenesis. Am J Physiol Gastrointest Liver Physiol 2001;280:G319–G323.

108 Robbins JB, Schneerson R: Polysaccharide-protein conjugates: A new generation of vaccines. J Infect Dis 1990;161:821–832.
109 Orr N, Robin G, Cohen D, Arnon R, Lowell GH: Immunogenicity and efficacy of oral or intranasal *Shigella flexneri* 2a and *Shigellasonnei* proteosome-lipopolysaccharide vaccines in animal models. Infect Immun 1993;61:2390–2395.
110 Baird-Parker AC: Foodborne salmonellosis. Lancet 1990;336:1231–1235.
111 Wallis TS, Galyov EE: Molecular basis of *Salmonella*-induced enteritis. Mol Microbiol 2000;36:997–1005.
112 Swartz MN: Human diseases caused by food-borne pathogens of animal origin. Clin Infect Dis 2002;34(suppl 3):S111–S122.
113 Guerrant RL, Van Gilder T, Steiner TS, Thielman NM, Slutsker L, Tauxe RV, Hennessy T, Griffin PM, DuPont H, Sack RB, Tarr P, Neill M, Nachamkin I, Reller LB, Osterholm MT, Bennish ML, Pickering LK: Practice guidelines for the management of infectious diarrhea. Clin Infect Dis 2001;32:331–351.
114 Farthing MJ: Oral rehydration therapy. Pharmacol Ther 1994;64:477–492.
115 Schiller LR, Santa Ana CA, Porter J, Fordtran JS: Glucose-stimulated sodium transport by the human intestine during experimental cholera. Gastroenterology 1997;112:1529–1535.
116 Carneiro-Filho BA, Bushen OY, Brito GA, Lima AA, Guerrant RL: Glutamine analogues as adjunctive therapy for infectious diarrhea. Curr Infect Dis Rep 2003;5:114–119.
117 Argenzio RA, Rhoads JM, Armstrong M, Gomez G: Glutamine stimulates prostaglandin-sensitive Na(+)-H+ exchange in experimental porcine cryptosporidiosis. Gastroenterology 1994; 106:1418–1428.
118 Lima AA, Carvalho GH, Figueiredo AA, Gifoni AR, Soares AM, Silva EA, Guerrant RL: Effects of an alanyl-glutamine-based oral rehydration and nutrition therapy solution on electrolyte and water absorption in a rat model of secretory diarrhea induced by choleratoxin. Nutrition 2002; 18:458–462.
119 Daniele B, Perrone F, Gallo C, Pignata S, DeMartino S, De Vivo R, Barletta E, Tambaro R, Abbiati R, D'Agostino L: Oral glutamine in the prevention of fluorouracil induced intestinal toxicity: A double blind, placebo controlled, randomised trial. Gut 2001;48:28–33.
120 Brito GAC, Alcantara C, Guerrant RL: Effect of glutamine an alanyl-glutamine on apoptosis induced by *C. difficile* toxin A on intestinal epithelial cells. Am J Trop Med Hyg 2001; 65(suppl):293.
121 Vila J, Vargas M, Ruiz J, Corachan M, Jimenez De Anta MT, Gascon J: Quinolone resistance in enterotoxigenic *Escherichia coli* causing diarrhea in travelers to India in comparison with other geographical areas. Antimicrob Agents Chemother 2000;44:1731–1733.
122 DuPont HL, Ericsson CD, Mathewson JJ, Palazzini E, DuPont MW, Jiang ZD, Mosavi A, de la Cabada FJ: Rifaximin: A nonabsorbed antimicrobial in the therapy of travelers' diarrhea. Digestion 1998;59:708–714.
123 DuPont HL, Jiang ZD, Ericsson CD, Adachi JA, Mathewson JJ, DuPont MW, Palazzini E, Riopel LM, Ashley D, Martinez-Sandoval F: Rifaximin versus ciprofloxacin for the treatment of traveler's diarrhea: A randomized, double-blind clinical trial. Clin Infect Dis 2001;33:1807–1815.
124 Amenta M, Dalle Nogare ER, Colomba C, Prestileo TS, Di Lorenzo F, Fundaro S, Colomba A, Ferrieri A: Intestinal protozoa in HIV-infected patients: Effect of rifaximin in *Cryptosporidium parvum* and *Blastocystis hominis* infections. J Chemother 1999;11:391–395.
125 Beseghi U, De'Angelis GL: Comparison of two non-absorbable antibiotics for treatment of bacterial enteritis in children. Eur Rev Med Pharmacol Sci 1998;2:131–136.
126 Farthing MJ: Diarrhoea: A significant world wide problem. Int J Antimicrob Agents 2000;14: 65–69.
127 Turvill JL, Farthing MJ: Effect of granisetron on cholera toxin-induced enteric secretion. Lancet 1997;349:1293.
128 Roge J, Baumer P, Berard H, Schwartz JC, Lecomte JM: The enkephalinase inhibitor, acetorphan, in acute diarrhoea. A double-blind, controlled clinical trial versus loperamide. Scand J Gastroenterol 1993;28:352–354.
129 Bass DM: Vaccines for bacterial enteritis: What is new and why it matters. J Pediatr Gastroenterol Nutr 2000;31:365–366.

130 Cerquetti M, Luzzi I, Caprioli A, Sebastianelli A, Mastrantonio P: Role of *Clostridium difficile* in childhood diarrhea. Pediatr Infect Dis J 1995;14:598–603.
131 Bouza E, Pelaez T, Alonso R, Catalan P, Munoz P, Creixems MR: 'Second-look' cytotoxicity: An evaluation of culture plus cytotoxin assay of *Clostridium difficile* isolates in the laboratory diagnosis of CDAD. J Hosp Infect 2001;48:233–237.

Richard L. Guerrant MD, FACP
Center for Global Health, School of Medicine, University of Virginia
MR4, Lane Road, Room 3148, Charlottesville, VA 22908 (USA)
Tel. +1 804 924 5242, Fax +1 804 977 5323, E-Mail rlg9a@virginia.edu

This chapter should be cited as follows:

Brito GAC, Alcantara C, Carneiro-Filhoa BA, Guerrant RL: Pathophysiology and Impact of Enteric Bacterial and Protozoal Infections: New Approaches to Therapy. Chemotherapy 2005;51(suppl 1): 23–35.

Scarpignato C (ed): Rifaximin: A Poorly Absorbed Antibiotic.
Pharmacology and Clinical Use.

Rifaximin, a Poorly Absorbed Antibiotic: Pharmacology and Clinical Potential

Carmelo Scarpignato, Iva Pelosini

Laboratory of Clinical Pharmacology, Department of Human Anatomy, Pharmacology and Forensic Sciences, School of Medicine and Dentistry, University of Parma, Parma, Italy

Abstract

Rifaximin (4-deoxy-4′-methylpyrido[1′,2′-1,2]imidazo-[5,4-c]rifamycin SV) is a synthetic antibiotic designed to modify the parent compound, rifamycin, in order to achieve low gastrointestinal (GI) absorption while retaining good antibacterial activity. Both experimental and clinical pharmacology clearly show that this compound is a nonsystemic antibiotic with a broad spectrum of antibacterial action covering Gram-positive and Gram-negative organisms, both aerobes and anaerobes. Being virtually non-absorbed, its bioavailability within the GI tract is rather high with intraluminal and fecal drug concentrations that largely exceed the minimal inhibitory concentration values observed in vitro against a wide range of pathogenic organisms. The GI tract represents, therefore, the primary therapeutic target and GI infections the main indication. The appreciation of the pathogenic role of gut bacteria in several organic and functional GI diseases has increasingly broadened its clinical use, which is now extended to hepatic encephalopathy, small intestine bacterial overgrowth, inflammatory bowel disease and colonic diverticular disease. Potential indications include the irritable bowel syndrome and chronic constipation, *Clostridium difficile* infection and bowel preparation before colorectal surgery. Because of its antibacterial activity against the microorganism and the lack of strains with primary resistance, some preliminary studies have explored the rifaximin potential for *Helicobacter pylori* eradication. Oral administration of this drug, by getting rid of enteric bacteria, could also be employed to achieve selective bowel decontamination in acute pancreatitis, liver cirrhosis (thus preventing spontaneous bacterial peritonitis) and nonsteroidal anti-inflammatory drug (NSAID) use (lessening in that way NSAID enteropathy). This antibiotic has, therefore, little value outside the enteric area and this will minimize both antimicrobial resistance and systemic adverse events. Indeed, the drug proved to be safe in all patient populations, including young children. Although rifaximin has stood the test of time, it still attracts the attention of both basic scientists and clinicians. As a matter of fact, with the advancement of the knowledge on microbial-gut interactions in health and disease novel indications and new drug regimens are being explored. Besides widening the clinical use, the research on rifaximin is also focused on the synthesis of new derivatives and on the development of original formulations designed to expand the spectrum of its clinical use.

Introduction

Hundreds of bacterial species make up the human gut flora. The intestine has at least 400 different species of bacteria totaling over 1,012 organisms. Of these, 99% are anaerobic bacteria. Although anaerobes are part of the normal commensal flora, they can become opportunistic pathogens, causing serious, sometimes fatal infections if they escape from the colonic milieu. Most often, this escape occurs as a result of perforation, surgery, diverticulitis or cancer [1]. Pathogens range from highly virulent organisms, which infect people with well-functioning immune systems as well as people with poorly functioning immune systems, to opportunistic organisms, which infect only those with impaired immune systems (e.g. HIV-infected patients or transplant and oncology patients taking immunosuppressive drugs) [2]. In these subjects infection can be particularly severe, debilitating, and difficult to treat.

The host gastrointestinal (GI) tract is exposed to countless numbers of foreign antigens and has embedded a unique and complex network of immunological and non-immunological mechanisms, often termed the GI 'mucosal barrier', to protect the host from potentially harmful pathogens while at the same time 'tolerating' other resident microbes to allow absorption and utilization of nutrients. Of the many important roles of this barrier, it is the distinct responsibility of the mucosal immune system to sample and discriminate between harmful and beneficial antigens and to prevent entry of food-borne pathogens through the GI tract. This system comprises an immunological network termed the gut-associated lymphoid tissue (GALT) that consists of unique arrangements of B cells, T cells and phagocytes which sample luminal antigens through specialized epithelia termed the follicle-associated epithelia (FAE) and orchestrate coordinated molecular responses between immune cells and other components of the mucosal barrier [3].

Certain pathogens have developed ways to bypass and/or withstand defense by the mucosal immune system to establish disease in the host. Some 'opportunistic' pathogens (such as *Clostridium difficile*) take advantage of host or other factors (diet, stress, antibiotic use) which may alter or weaken the response of the immune system. Other pathogens have developed mechanisms for invading the GI epithelium and evading phagocytosis/destruction by immune system defenses [4]. Once cellular invasion occurs, host responses are activated to limit local mucosal damage and repel the foreign influence. Some pathogens (*Shigella* spp., parasites and viruses) primarily establish localized disease while others (*Salmonella*, *Yersinia*, *Listeria*) use the lymphatic system to enter organs or the bloodstream and cause more systemic illness. In some cases, pathogens (*Helicobacter pylori* and *Salmonella typhi*) colonize the GI tract or associated lymphoid structures for extended periods of time and these persistent pathogens may also be potential triggers for other chronic or inflammatory diseases, including inflammatory bowel disease (IBD) and malignancies [5]. The ability of certain pathogens to avoid or withstand the host's immune assault and/or utilize these host responses to their own advantage (i.e. enhance further colonization) will dictate the pathogen's success in promoting illness and furthering its own survival [4].

Emerging infectious pathogens, increasing antimicrobial resistance (mediated primarily through horizontal transfer of a plethora of mobile DNA transfer factors) and the appearance of diseases that decrease the host defense have increased the need for more effective and safe treatments [6]. Antibiotics have an important place in the management of GI diseases [7–9]. Antibiotic use in gastroenterology falls into three general settings [8]: (1) GI infections (e.g. bacterial diarrhea, cholangitis, diverticulitis), (2) GI diseases that may involve infectious agents but are not 'classic' infectious diseases (e.g. *H. pylori*-positive peptic ulcer, Whipple's disease, IBD), and (3) antibiotic prophylaxis for GI procedures.

The proliferation of antibacterial agents has made the choice of antibiotics increasingly complex. General considerations in selecting antibiotic therapy include (1) the identity and susceptibility pattern of the infecting organisms, (2) the anatomic localization of the infection, (3) the antimicrobial spectrum of the drug, and (4) its pharmacokinetic properties. Other important considerations include the possible selection of resistant organisms, interactions with other drugs, toxicity and cost [8].

The anatomic location of the GI infection influences the selection of the antimicrobial agent and the route of administration. For instance, oral administration of a poorly absorbable antibiotic may be used for the eradication of noninvasive enteric pathogens [10]. Although the importance of attaining high biliary concentrations of antimicrobial agents in treating patients with cholangitis is still debated, it has been suggested that agents undergoing biliary secretion have a higher efficacy in the treatment of these infections [11].

It is well known that the dynamic bacterial community lining the gut exerts many physiological functions [12, 13]. These include metabolic activities that result in the salvage of energy and absorbable nutrients, important trophic effects on intestinal epithelia and on immune structure and function, and protection of the colonized host against invasion by alien microbes [13]. Oral administration of antibiotics can cause 'ecological' disturbances in the normal

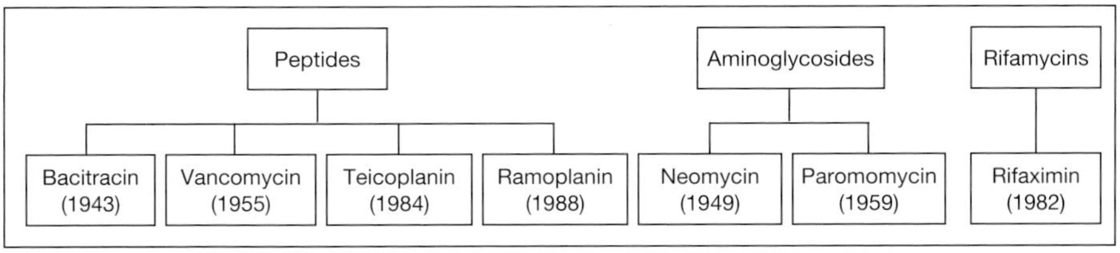

Fig. 1. Poorly absorbed antibiotics currently used in the treatment of GI infections. The date in parentheses refers to the first full description of the chemical synthesis of each compound.

intestinal microflora [12]. Suppression of the normal microflora may lead to reduced colonization resistance with subsequent overgrowth of preexisting, naturally resistant microorganisms, such as yeasts and *C. difficile.* Although the incidence varies among antibiotics, the occurrence of pseudomembranous colitis has been associated with virtually every antibiotic [14]. New colonization by resistant potential pathogens may also occur and may spread within the body or to other patients and cause severe infections.

Nonabsorbed oral antibiotic therapy, unlike systemically available antibiotics, allows localized enteric targeting of pathogens and is associated with a minimal risk of systemic toxicity or side effects [15]. Provided that nonabsorbed antibiotics are as effective as systemically absorbed drugs for the target illness, their safety and tolerability profiles may render them more appropriate for certain patient groups, such as young children, pregnant or lactating women, and the elderly, among whom side effects are a particular concern. The restricted use of nonabsorbed oral antibiotics only for enteric infections should also reduce the development of widespread resistance, a major limitation of current antibiotics for enteric infections [15].

Compared to systemic drugs, the number of poorly absorbed antimicrobials that would best target the GI tract is relatively small and almost completely limited to aminoglycosides (fig. 1). Indeed, oral vancomycin [16], teicoplanin [17], and bacitracin [18] are confined to the treatment of *C. difficile* infection [19–21]. Ramoplanin, a glycolipodepsipeptide antibiotic [22], is being developed for the treatment of *C. difficile*-associated diarrhea [23] and vancomycin-resistant enterococcal infection in high-risk patients [24]. Paromomycin and neomycin represent therefore the most widely used compounds [25, 26]. Neomycin is often associated with bacitracin, which is highly active against Gram-positive microorganisms, in order to extend its antibacterial activity. However, even poorly absorbed aminoglycosides are not completely devoid of untoward effects. Indeed, both ototoxicity [27–29] and nephrotoxicity [30] have been reported after oral neomycin especially in patients with renal dysfunction. Such patients can in fact accumulate toxic levels of the antimicrobial since the kidneys represent the major route of drug excretion [31]. Ototoxicity has actually been reported after ototopic (i.e. ear drops) aminoglycoside administration [32].

In order to overcome the limitations of the above drugs, a series of rifamycin derivatives with improved pharmacokinetic (i.e. virtually absence of GI absorption) and pharmacodynamic (i.e. with broad spectrum of antibacterial activity) properties have been synthesized at Alfa Wassermann laboratories [33]. Amongst the different molecules, the compound marked L-105 and later named rifaximin was selected for further development. The antibiotic was first marketed in Italy and subsequently introduced in other European countries. Rifaximin was also licensed in some Northern African and Asian areas as well as in Mexico. The compound has recently been approved by the US FDA for the treatment of infectious diarrhea in the traveler (TD) [34].

The aim of this review is to summarize the available pharmacology and safety data on this nonsystemic antibiotic as well to outline its current and potential clinical use.

Rifaximin: Structure and Physicochemical Properties

Rifamycin is a clinically useful macrolide antibiotic produced by the Gram-positive bacterium *Amycolatopsis mediterranei* (originally classified as *Streptomyces mediterranei*). Rifamycin B, the compound originally isolated, has no antibacterial activity, but it is oxidized to the very active derivative rifamycin S, which inhibits the growth of Gram-positive bacteria. This antibiotic is primarily used against *Mycobacterium tuberculosis* and *Mycobacterium leprae*, causative agents of tuberculosis and leprosy, respectively. In these bacteria, rifamycin treatment specifically inhibits the initiation of RNA synthesis by binding to the β subunit of RNA polymerase. Apart from its activity against the bacteria, rifamycin has also been reported to inhibit reverse transcriptase (RT) of certain RNA viruses. Rifamycin derivatives have also been discovered that are effective against *Mycobacterium avium*, which is associated with the AIDS complex. Consequently, the importance of and demand for rifamycin have increased tremendously worldwide [35]. The rifamycin antibiotics, namely rifampicin (called rifampin in the US), rifabutin and rifapentine, are uniquely potent in the treatment of tuberculosis and chronic staphylococcal infections. Intestinal absorption of these drugs does occur and it is affected by the presence of food [36].

Rifaximin (4-deoxy-4′-methylpyrido[1′,2′-1,2]imidazo-[5,4-c]rifamycin SV, fig. 2) is a synthetic product designed to modify the parent compound, rifamycin, in order to achieve low GI absorption while retaining good antibacterial

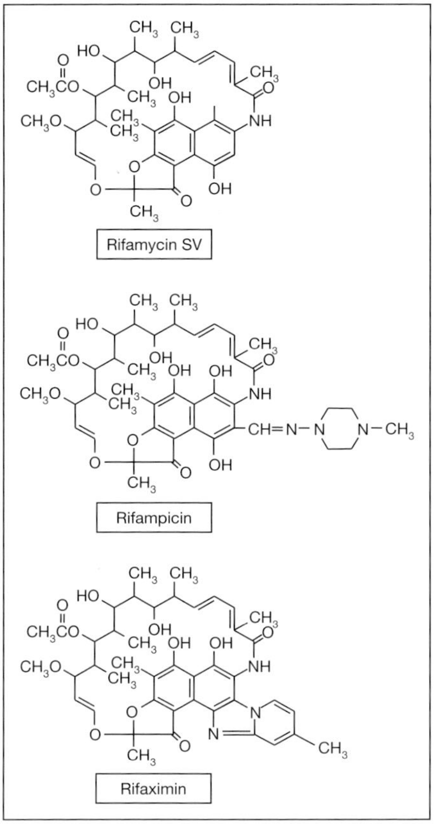

Fig. 2. Chemical structures of rifampicin and rifaximin as well as of their parent compound, rifamycin SV. The empirical formula of rifaximin is $C_{43}H_{51}N_3O_{11}$ and its molecular weight 785.9 daltons.

activity [37]. It is a rifamycin SV derivative, prepared by condensing 2-aminopyridine derivatives to 3-bromorifamycin S (fig. 3) [37–39]. This pyridoimidazo rifamycin SV derivative, which proved to be stable in gastric juice for 24 h, displays a zwitterionic nature at physiological pH [38].

A solid-state X-ray study [40] did confirm the structure proposed on the basis of ^{1}H-NMR studies in solution and showed that the compound is in a mesomeric betaine form, the pyrido nitrogen being positively charged and the imidazo nitrogen being negatively charged, a feature most likely responsible for the pharmacokinetic behavior of these new drugs. Indeed, since rifamycins are generally absorbed by passive diffusion, the presence of the two opposite charged nitrogens, together with the presence of the phenolic hydroxyls, leads to a molecule ionized at all the pH values encountered along the GI tract, which thus prevents its absorption. Rifaximin also displays a strong tendency to self-associate both in solution and in the solid state, and the increase in molecular size may also play a role in preventing its absorption [41].

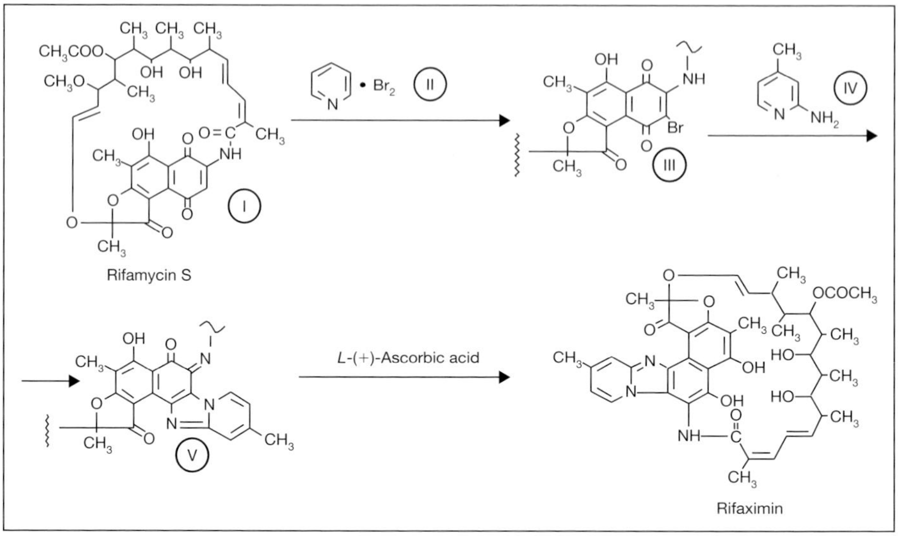

Fig. 3. Stepwise synthesis of rifaximin (from De Angelis [39]). The reaction of rifamycin S (I) with pyridine perbro-mide (II) in 2-propanol/chloroform (70/30) mixture at 0°C gives 3-bromorifamycin S (III), which is then condensed with 2-amino-4-methyl-pyridine (IV) at 10°C. The *o*-quinonimic compound (V) is then obtained. This compound is finally reduced with ascorbic acid to rifaximin.

Antimicrobial Activity

In vitro Activity

The in vitro antibacterial activity of rifaximin has been determined by using minimum inhibitory concentrations (MIC) against bacteria from clinical isolates or stock culture collections. It should be pointed out that – in the absence of known GI concentrations – the interpretation of MICs is difficult. It is likely, however, that the drug concentration achieved at the desired site of action, i.e. the GI tract, will largely exceed the reported MIC values. For instance, fecal levels after oral administration of the antibiotic range between 4,000 and 8,000 μg/g of stool, which is 160–250 times higher than the MIC_{90} for the various bacterial enteropathogens [42].

Several in vitro studies, summarized by Gillis and Brogden [33] and Jiang and DuPont [43], have shown that – like rifampicin – rifaximin displays an inhibitory activity against Gram-positive and Gram-negative, aerobic and anaerobic bacteria. Sharing the properties of the rifamycin family, the drug was shown to be active against the H37RV *M. tuberculosis* [44] as well as five *Mycobacterium* isolates from patients with tuberculosis [45]. In general,

Table 1. MICs (μg/ml) of rifaximin and other antimicrobials against 40 strains (39 clinical isolates and the NCTC 11638 strain) of *H. pylori* at pH 7.0 (from Holton et al. [53])

	MIC_{50}	MIC_{90}	Range
Rifaximin	4	8	4–6
Ampicillin	0.03	0.25	0.03–0.5
Metronidazole	0.5	4	0.12–4
Omeprazole	32	>128	32–>128

the activity of rifaximin proved to be greater against Gram-positive than Gram-negative bacteria. Amongst Gram-positive microorganisms, the susceptibility of oxacillin-resistant strains of *Staphylococcus aureus* [46, 47] and of *C. difficile* [47, 48] is particularly interesting. Of the Gram-negative rods, identified in patients with GI disease, those belonging to the Enterobacteriaceae family appear to be the most sensitive ones [49, 50]. Interestingly enough, rifaximin was found to inhibit the growth of *H. pylori* [51–54] with MIC values (table 1) intermediate between those of amoxicillin and colloidal bismuth subcitrate [55]. In contrast to metronidazole, no strain tested exhibited primary resistance [52, 53]. Furthermore, the activity of rifaximin was only slightly affected by lowering the pH of the medium, conversely from what is currently observed with other antibiotics [56]. Last but not least, rifaximin was shown to be active against clarithromycin-resistant strains [54].

Finally, a recent study [57] found rifaximin active against 408 clinical strains of *Vibrio cholerae* isolated from different geographical areas and with different antimicrobial resistance patterns, the MIC values ranging from 0.5 to 4 μg/ml for all strains. These findings, together with the pharmacokinetic properties of the drug, suggest that rifaximin could be an attractive antimicrobial agent for cholera.

Mechanism of Action

To establish whether rifaximin, like the other members of the rifamycin family [36, 58], specifically inhibits bacterial RNA synthesis the effect of this antibiotic as well as that of rifampicin and chloramphenicol on RNA (via-^{3}H-uridine incorporation), DNA (via ^{3}H-thymidine incorporation) and protein (via ^{35}S-methionine incorporation) synthesis was studied in growing cultures of *Escherichia coli* [59]. While chloramphenicol reduced protein synthesis, both rifaximin and rifampicin inhibited RNA synthesis in a concentration-dependent fashion. In contrast, none of them affected ^{3}H-thymidine incorporation into DNA. These data suggest that rifaximin, like rifampicin, inhibits RNA synthesis by binding the β subunit of the bacterial DNA-dependent RNA polymerase [60].

In vitro Antimicrobial Resistance

Despite much effort, antibiotic resistance continues to increase [61]. Looking back, it is clear that this was an inevitable consequence of antibiotic use [62]. Antibiotic resistance, which has been recognized to be an important clinical problem, varies in prevalence from one country to another and among the pathogens themselves. This has great clinical, economic, political and environmental implications worldwide [63]. Strict adherence to the ongoing measures of infection control, education and antibiotic policy should minimize antibiotic resistance [64].

Development of resistance to rifaximin may be similar to that of rifampicin, which is primarily due to a chromosomal single-step alteration in the drug target, the DNA-dependent RNA polymerase [65, 66]. This differs from the plasmid-mediated resistance commonly acquired by bacteria to aminoglycoside antibiotics, such as neomycin or bacitracin [67]. The spread of resistance due to the chromosomal mechanism is less frequent than that due to plasmid-mediated transfer [63, 66].

The development of resistance to rifaximin was studied in detail on several aerobic (Gram-negative and Gram-positive) and anaerobic strains using two different methods, i.e. the agar dilution and broth dilution methods [68, 69]. In the agar dilution method bacterial inocula were spread onto plates containing antibiotics at concentrations 2, 4 or 8 times the MIC value. After incubation under aerobic and anaerobic conditions for the appropriate species of bacteria, surviving colonies were counted, purified and the frequency of spontaneous resistant mutants was evaluated. Incubation in an anaerobic atmosphere was used to mimic the situation of the human GI tract environment (prevalently anaerobic). In the broth dilution method bacteria were inoculated in test tubes containing subinhibitory concentrations of the drug tested and incubated at 37°C. Aliquots of these cultures were transferred from tubes containing the highest drug concentration that permitted bacterial growth to another series of tubes containing 2-, 4-, 8- and 16-fold the concentration of the antimicrobial agent. The experiments were ended when the test bacteria were able to grow in media containing at least 100 μg/ml of the drug tested. Thanks to the well-known ability of suboptimal concentrations of antibiotics to promote this phenomenon [70] it is obviously easier to select resistant mutants with this second method, where exposure to subinhibitory concentrations of antimicrobials is allowed.

As expected [71], spontaneous selection of resistance was rare for the anaerobic bacteria; in fact, among these anaerobes only a few species showed spontaneous emergence of resistant mutants [46, 48].

The selection of rifaximin-resistant strains was also investigated on five different isolates of *H. pylori.* None of the strains exhibited primary resistance to rifaximin, but, after exposure to subinhibitory concentrations of the antibiotic, all five strains became resistant. The mutation frequency was similar to that observed with macrolides and quinolones, but was less frequent than that observed with metronidazole [52, 53].

Rifaximin selected resistant Gram-positive cocci mutants more easily under aerobic conditions than in an anaerobic atmosphere [46, 48]. In comparison with Gram-positive microorganisms, drug-resistant Gram-negative bacilli were rarely detected [46, 48].

Spontaneously resistant mutants were more easily selected after preincubation of the test bacteria with subinhibitory concentrations of rifaximin rather than after exposing the microorganisms to high levels of the antibiotic. Taking into account that rifaximin is poorly absorbed (see below) the high amounts of the drug available within the digestive lumen compare better with supra- rather than with subinhibitory concentrations of the drug. Furthermore, since the anaerobic atmosphere did hinder the selection of rifaximin-resistant enterobacteria, it is expected that – during antibiotic therapy with this drug – the selection of resistant mutants in the GI tract (a prevalently anaerobic environment) is very low. In summary, thanks to the high drug bioavailability in an oxygen-deficient milieu, the in vivo occurrence of bacterial resistance should with rifaximin be an infrequent phenomenon. The constant therapeutic efficacy of the antibiotic in the management of various GI infections [33, 71] clearly suggests that this is the case.

In vivo Activity

The antibacterial activity of rifaximin has been confirmed by in vivo studies performed in both laboratory animals and humans.

Two studies compared the effect of rifaximin to that of neomycin and/or of rifampicin [72, 73] on the fecal flora in rats. In the first study [72] the antibiotic (1, 10, 30 and 100 mg/kg orally for 7 days) did inhibit both aerobic (especially coliforms and cocci) and anaerobic bacterial growth. Its activity was similar to that of neomycin and stronger than that of rifampicin. In the second investigation [73] the antibiotic effect on aerobic microorganisms was specifically investigated. Oral rifaximin treatment (50 mg/kg for 3 days) caused a marked reduction in the number of total aerobic bacteria and salmonellae, while neomycin led only to a decrease in salmonella counts, but did not cause statistically significant changes in the total aerobic bacterial population.

The in vivo protective activity of rifaximin was studied in mice, infected experimentally by intraperitoneal inoculation of *S. aureus* Colliva and compared to that of rifampicin (a systemic rifamycin) and gentamicin (a poorly absorbed aminoglycoside) [74]. After oral administration, only rifampicin was

Table 2. Therapeutic activity of rifaximin and other antibiotics on experimentally induced infection in mice (from Venturini and Marchi [74])

Route of administration	ED_{50}, mg/kg		
	Rifaximin	Rifampicin	Gentamycin
Oral	>10	0.15	>10
Subcutaneous	0.46	ND	ND

Swiss mice were infected by intraperitoneal injection of 0.25 ml of *S. aureus* Colliva (clinical isolate). The bacterial suspension contained a sufficient number of organisms to kill all the animals within 72 h. Antibiotics were given orally or subcutaneously 1 h after bacterial inoculation. ND = Not determined.

Table 3. Effect of rifaximin and rifampicin on experimentally induced tubeculosis in guinea pigs (from Lucchesi et al. [76])

Treatment	Feldman's index	Pathological findings
Saline	54.11	Extensive tuberculosis
Rifaximin (60 mg/kg daily)	54.47	Extensive tuberculosis
Rifampicin (30 mg/kg daily)	11.00	Very limited infection

Albino male guinea pigs were infected by subcutaneous injection of 0.001 mg of bacterial (*M. tuberculosis*) coating and treated with rifamycins by oral route immediately after the infection. The antibiotic treatment lasted 4 months, after which the animals were sacrificed and inguinal lymph nodes, spleen, liver and lungs examined to quantify the severity of the disease according to Feldman [75].

effective whereas the other two compounds were inactive at doses up to 10 mg/kg. However, when injected subcutaneously, rifaximin displayed a good therapeutic efficacy (table 2). While confirming its antibacterial activity, these results clearly indicate that rifaximin, like gentamycin, is poorly absorbed after oral administration.

The lack of absorption and, consequently, the lack of 'systemic' therapeutic activity was also demonstrated in a model of experimental tuberculosis in the guinea pig [75]. Here again, oral rifampicin but not oral rifaximin did protect the animals from the development of the infection (table 3) [76].

A large number of human studies [71, 77–80] performed in patients with infectious diarrhea or other GI diseases (e.g. hepatic encephalopathy, small bowel

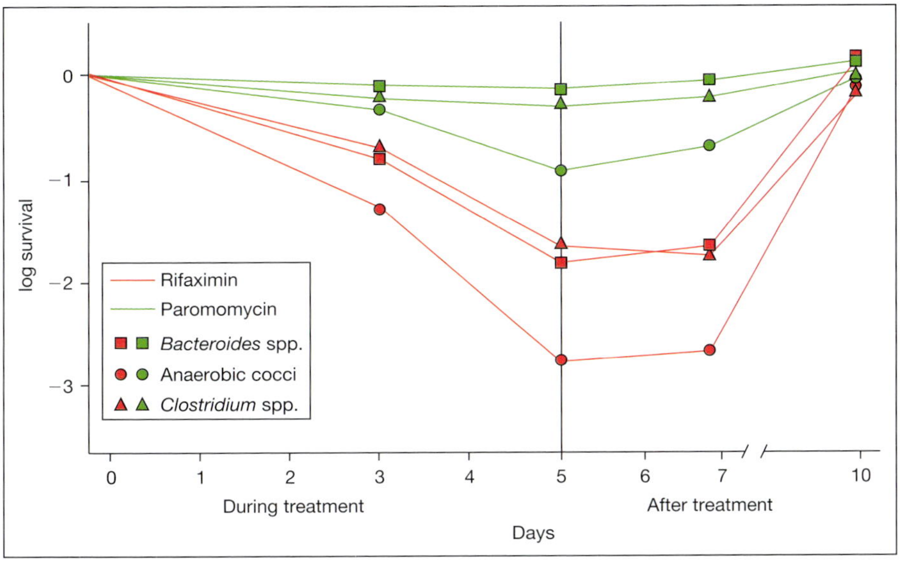

Fig. 4. Changes in anaerobic flora population following oral administration of rifaximin or paromomycin in patients with hepatic encephalopathy (from Testa et al. [81]).

bacterial overgrowth, IBD, colonic diverticular disease) have confirmed the antibacterial activity of rifaximin demonstrated in vitro and in laboratory animals.

In approximately 50% of patients with infectious diarrhea enrolled in clinical trials the most common organism isolated and presumed causative was *E. coli.* Treatment with the antibiotic led to clearance of the bacterium in 65–80% of the patients [33, 71]. Eradication of or decrease in microorganisms count in the feces was also reported for other Enterobacteriaceae after short-term rifaximin treatment [33, 71].

On the basis of log bacterial survival rates, the antibacterial activity of rifaximin was greater than that of paromomycin against *Enterococcus* spp., anaerobic cocci, *Bacterioides* spp. and *Clostridium* spp. isolated in fecal samples from 20 patients with subclinical hepatic encephalopathy (fig. 4) [81]. On the other hand, *E. coli* and *Klebsiella* spp. appeared more susceptible to paromomycin while both antibiotics showed equal potency against *Proteus* spp. [81]. Here again it should be pointed out that stool concentrations of rifaximin are 250–500 times higher than the MIC_{90} values [71], which makes the in vitro differences of activity between this and other antimicrobials meaningless from a clinical standpoint.

Repeated oral administration of an antibiotic that reaches very high concentrations within the GI lumen could have profound effects on intestinal flora

Table 4. Changes in fecal bacterial population after oral rifaximin administration in healthy volunteers (from Testa et al. [81])

Organisms		Weeks					
		0	1	2	4	8	12
E. coli	$\times 10^8$	2.9	0.46	2.5	2.7	3.0	3.0
Other enterobacters	$\times 10^7$	1.0	0.09	1.0	1.2	1.1	1.2
Enterococci	$\times 10^7$	5.6	0.08	3.1	5.7	5.6	4.9
Bacteroides spp.	$\times 10^9$	6.0	0.10	5.4	6.1	6.2	5.6
Clostridium spp.	$\times 10^8$	1.1	0.04	1.0	1.1	1.0	0.9
Anaerobic cocci	$\times 10^7$	6.1	0.02	5.6	6.0	6.2	5.8

Rifaximin (800 mg) was given in two daily doses for 5 days after the first stool collection.

[12, 13]. As expected, rifaximin markedly reduced fecal bacterial counts during oral intake but the effect was short-lasting since the bacterial population recovered within 1–2 weeks from the end of treatment (table 4) [82]. Most importantly, fungal colonization occurred very rarely. Indeed, *Candida albicans*, which has been implicated in the pathogenesis of antibiotic-associated diarrhea [82, 83], was isolated from the fecal samples of only 2 out of 10 patients given 1,200 mg of rifaximin daily [81] and in none of the volunteers taking 800 mg daily [82].

It is worthwhile mentioning that treatment with high-dose (600 mg, 3 times a day, for 14 days) rifaximin was also efficacious in resolving the clinical symptoms and clearing protozoan infections in HIV-1-infected patients with a CD4 count $\geq 200/mm^3$, who presented enteric and systemic symptoms due to *Cryptosporidium parvum* or *Blastocystis hominis* associated with enteropathogens [84].

In vivo Antimicrobial Resistance

Antimicrobial resistance to rifamycins develops rapidly both in vitro and in vivo [65, 85, 86]. As a consequence, all the three members of the family (i.e. rifampicin, rifabutin and rifapentine) are used clinically as components of combination therapies [65, 87]. Being structurally related, rifaximin could share this potential. And indeed resistance rates, recorded in fecal strains of Enterobacteriaceae, *Enterococcus, Bacteroides, Clostridium* and anaerobic cocci, ranged between 30 and 90% after short-term (5 days) antibiotic (800 mg daily) treatment [82]. A similar pattern was observed in 10 patients with hepatic encephalopathy after treatment with rifaximin 1,200 mg/day for 5 days [80].

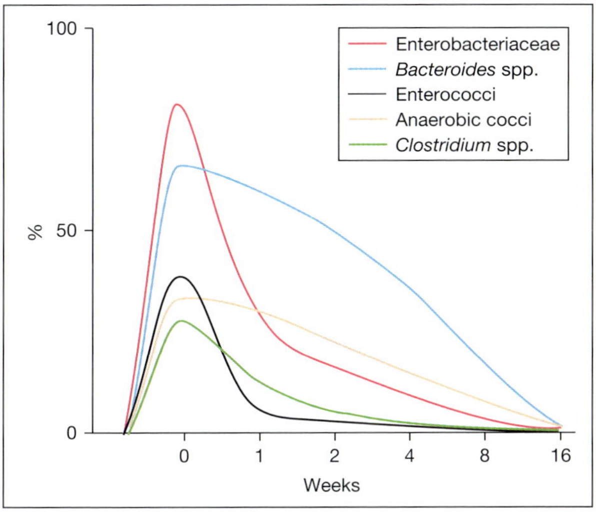

Fig. 5. Disappearance of rifaximin-resistant bacteria from the human intestine after stopping the antibiotic treatment (week 0) (from De Leo et al. [82]).

Nevertheless, a rapid disappearance of resistant bacteria was observed after stopping the antibiotic treatment (fig. 5). Different kinetics of disappearance were, however, observed. The aerobic species showed a more rapid return to the baseline 'sensitive' status whereas the anaerobic bacteria, especially the Gram-negative rods, regained sensitivity to rifaximin more slowly. In any case, 3 months after the end of treatment resistant strains were no longer detectable in the feces [82]. These results support the cyclic use of rifaximin that has been adopted by the investigators in the treatment of hepatic encephalopathy [77] and colonic diverticular disease [79].

However, DuPont and Jiang [88], by studying changes in the susceptibility of intestinal flora during a 3-day rifaximin course among US students with TD, failed to document the emergence of drug-resistant Gram-positive (e.g. enterococci) and Gram-negative (*E. coli*) organisms during treatment.

Since rifamycins are important drugs for the treatment of *M. tuberculosis* infection [36, 86, 87] the activity of rifaximin on and interference with this bacterium have been carefully studied. Indeed, a potential problem of the treatment with this antibiotic is represented by the possibility that even very low blood levels achieved by oral administration might be able to select mutants, cross-resistant to rifamycins [85], in patients treated for GI infections and harboring *M. tuberculosis.*

A study in the guinea pig with experimentally induced tuberculosis [44] did show that sensitivity to both rifampicin and rifaximin of the *Mycobacterium*

(H37RV strain) remained unchanged after 3 months of drug administration, the MIC values being virtually the same before and after treatment. The development of resistance to rifaximin of different strains of *M. tuberculosis*, isolated from patients with pulmonary and renal tuberculosis, was studied under extremely stringent conditions [45]. The drug was tested at very high concentrations (up to 270 ng/ml), largely exceeding those expected from intestinal absorption during an average course of therapy for enteric infections. These experiments showed a concentration-dependent subinhibitory effect of the antibiotic on *Mycobacterium* growth. One can, therefore, speculate that the circulating, albeit very low, levels of rifaximin could represent a stimulus for the selection of resistant mycobacterial strains [89]. However, measurement of both rifaximin and rifampicin MICs before and after successive exposure to rifaximin gave the same value in all the *Mycobacterium* strains examined [45].

All these data, taken together, do suggest that therapy with rifaximin in GI patients harboring *M. tuberculosis* should not represent a hazard to the treatment of pulmonary as well as extrapulmonary tuberculosis. A recent 10-year survey [90] in Italy showed that – in the period 1990–2000, during which rifaximin has been largely used – mycobacterial resistance to rifampicin has been quite stable. This finding is consistent with the idea that the likelihood of rifampicin resistance emerging in infected, but otherwise asymptomatic, individuals receiving this antibiotic is extremely low.

Rifampicin is currently employed prophylactically to eliminate pharyngeal carriage of *Neisseria meningitidis*, thereby lowering the potential risk of meningitis [91–93]. The selection of resistant *Neisseria* mutants could theoretically be the consequence of rifaximin use for GI infections. Here again, a recent study performed in Italy [94] found that all the meningococci isolated from asymptomatic carriers were susceptible to rifampicin, thus ruling out this possibility.

Pharmacokinetics and Drug Interactions

Animal Pharmacokinetics

The pharmacokinetic investigations on rifaximin were performed in the animal species (namely the rat and dog) in which the short- and long-term toxicological studies had been performed according to the OECD (Organization for Economic Co-operation and Development) guidelines. Experimental studies were performed by using unlabeled and labeled rifaximin that was purportedly synthesized [95] to allow the quantitation of minute amounts of the antibiotic within the body. Rifaximin was given to fed and fasted animals in order to ascertain whether the GI absorption, if any, of rifaximin could be modified by food intake. Rifampicin, another systemic rifamycin derivative, whose

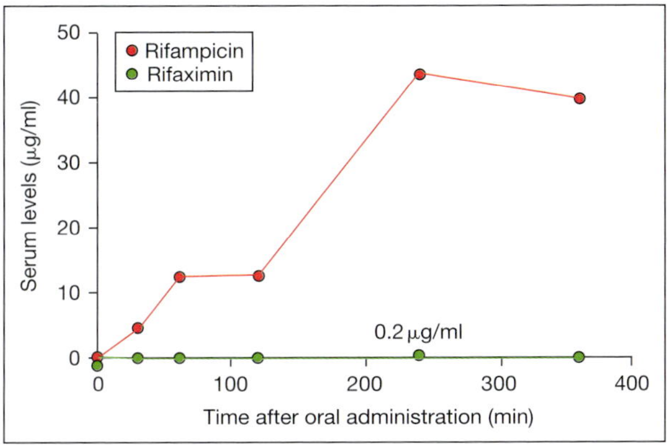

Fig. 6. Drug serum levels after oral administration of rifampicin (100 mg/kg) or rifaximin (100 mg/kg) to fed rats (from data in Venturini [97]).

pharmacokinetic properties are well known [36, 96], was used as a reference compound.

The first study was performed by Venturini [97, 98] in both rats and dogs by using a microbiological assay (i.e. agar diffusion test and *S. aureus* 209 P FDA as test organism). Conversely from rifampicin, whose serum levels were already detectable 30 min after the administration and still measurable after 48 h, only trace amounts (i.e. 0.2 μg/ml) of rifaximin were detected in serum of fed rats 4 h later (fig. 6). The amount of detectable antibiotic was reduced by 50% in fasted animals. Similar results have been obtained in dogs after oral administration of 25 mg/kg of both rifamycin derivatives [97, 98]. No detectable amount of rifaximin was found in serum at any time.

The negligible intestinal absorption of rifaximin was subsequently confirmed with the use of the labeled drug. After oral administration in rats the total radioactivity present in plasma was found to be no more than 0.1 and 2% of the administered dose after the intake of ^{3}H-labeled [99] and ^{14}C-labeled [59] compound, respectively.

Although theoretically safe, poorly absorbed antimicrobials could become 'absorbable' in the presence of mucosal inflammatory or ulcerative changes [100], like those occurring in IBD or when invasive bacteria colonize the intestine. To verify whether the presence of intestinal lesions would affect rifaximin absorption, the drug was given to rats with experimentally induced colitis [101]. The indomethacin-induced enteropathy did not affect intestinal absorption of rifaximin. However, under the same experimental conditions, systemic bioavailability of neomycin did increase [101].

The labeled rifaximin molecules were also employed to better evaluate the fecal and urinary excretion of the antibiotic, originally studied with the unlabeled drug [97]. The major route of excretion was in feces with all rats excreting more than 96 or 86% of the dose of the ^{3}H-labeled [99] and ^{14}C-labeled [59] rifaximin, respectively. In contrast, urinary recovery was found to be very low, i.e. less than 1%, thus confirming the insignificant systemic absorption of the drug. A small, sex-dependent recovery of radioactivity (1.72% in male and 0.5% in female) was recorded in bile [59], thereby proving evidence of an, albeit negligible, enterohepatic circulation of the drug. When the fecal and urinary counts were added to the radioactivity found after carcass digestion, the total radioactivity recovered over 7 days ranged between 95 and 100% [59, 99]. Similar findings have been reported in dogs [59].

The studies with radiolabeled rifaximin also showed that the greatest concentration of radioactivity is found in the GI tract [59, 99] that represents the therapeutic target organ. The radioactivity peak was reached at 0.5 h in the stomach, at 2 h in the small intestine and at 7 h in the cecum and large intestine. Other than in the GI tract, radioactivity counts were generally low and only the liver and kidneys contained more than 0.01% of the dose administered, a finding consistent with the results obtained with unlabeled rifaximin measured by a microbiological assay [97].

Specific studies directed to elucidate the metabolism of rifaximin have not been done since the compound does not reach the systemic circulation. Theoretically, it may be assumed that the small amount of circulating rifaximin is metabolized like the other rifamycin derivatives [36, 96], that is via the liver.

Human Pharmacokinetics

The pharmacokinetics of rifaximin after oral administration has been studied in healthy volunteers and patients with intestinal infections or IBD. The aim of these studies was to confirm the low, if any, systemic absorption of the drug; metabolism and excretion data are scant. In all these investigations a sensitive high-pressure liquid chromatographic (HPLC) method was used to measure rifaximin in body fluids.

After oral administration of 400 mg of rifaximin to fasted healthy volunteers blood drug concentration was found to be lower than the detection limit of the analytical method (i.e. 2.5 ng/ml) in half of them [102]. In the remaining subjects very low amounts were detected at some of the time intervals during the first 4 h after intake. Along the same lines, the urinary concentrations of the drug were very low and often undetectable. The effect of food on the absorption of the antibiotic was also evaluated [34] and a significant, albeit not clinically relevant, increase of bioavailabity was observed after a high-fat breakfast (table 5).

Table 5. Effect of food on the mean pharmacokinetic parameters following administration of a single rifaximin dose (400 mg) in 14 healthy volunteers (from FDA rifaximin label [34])

Parameter	Fasting	Fed
C_{max}, ng/ml	3.8 ± 1.32	9.63 ± 5.93
T_{max}, h	1.21 ± 0.47	1.90 ± 1.52
Half-life, h	5.85 ± 4.34	5.95 ± 1.88
AUC, ng·h/ml	18.35 ± 9.48	34.70 ± 9.23
Excreted in urine, %	0.023 ± 0.009	0.051 ± 0.017

*Each value represents the mean ± SD.

^{14}C-labeled rifaximin was administered as a single dose to 4 healthy male subjects [34]. The mean overall recovery of radioactivity in the urine and feces of 3 subjects during the 168 h after administration was 96.94 ± 5.64% of the dose. Radioactivity was excreted almost exclusively in the feces with only a small proportion of the dose (i.e. 0.32%) excreted in urine. Analysis of fecal extracts indicated that rifaximin was being excreted as unchanged drug [34]. The amount of radioactivity in urine (<0.4% of the dose) is consistent with animal data and shows that rifaximin is poorly absorbed from the GI tract and is almost exclusively and completely excreted in feces as unchanged drug.

Systemic absorption of rifaximin (200 mg 3 times daily) was also evaluated in 13 patients with shigellosis on days 1 and 3 of a 3-day course of treatment [34]. Rifaximin plasma concentrations were low and variable. There was no evidence of drug accumulation following repeated administration for 3 days (9 doses). Peak plasma rifaximin concentrations after 3 and 9 consecutive doses ranged from 0.81 to 3.4 ng/ml on day 1 and 0.68 to 2.26 ng/ml on day 3 [34]. Fecal excretion of the drug was also assessed in 39 patients with acute diarrhea after administration of 400 mg every 12 h for 3 consecutive days [42]. As shown in (figure 7), post-therapy stool rifaximin levels were high, decreasing gradually over a 5-day period. It is worthwhile mentioning that fecal drug concentrations largely exceeded the MIC values for the bacterial isolates obtained from patients with TD [42].

IBD being one of the therapeutic indications of rifaximin, its absorption was carefully studied in patients with mild-to-moderate ulcerative colitis (UC), after the administration of two tablets (i.e. 400 mg) orally [103]. As shown in table 6, in most plasma samples rifaximin concentrations were below the detection limits. Only in few patients was the drug detected during the first 8 h after administration. The total rifaximin amount recovered in the urine was only 0.009% of the dose. This figure fits well with the corresponding value (i.e. 0.007%) observed in healthy volunteers [102]. No correlation between disease activity and urinary

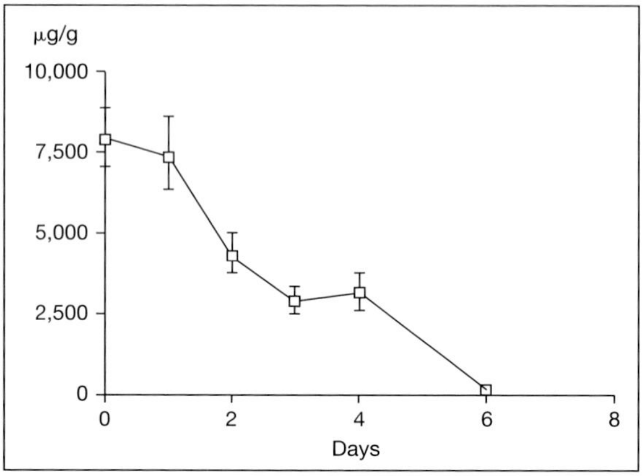

Fig. 7. Fecal concentration of rifaximin in patients with TD after treatment with 800 mg/day of the drug for 3 consecutive days. Each square refers to the mean of the values obtained from 39 subjects. Vertical bars are standard errors (from Jiang et al. [42]).

concentrations was found after repeated drug administration [104]. It is worthwhile mentioning that, even after 15 days of therapy of patients with resistant pouchitis with high dose (2 g daily) of rifaximin, together with ciprofloxacin (1 g daily), no plasma level of the antibiotic was detectable in any patient [105].

Since animal data indicated the presence of an enterohepatic circulation [59], the biliary concentration of rifaximin after oral preoperative administration of the drug (400 mg every 12 h) was evaluated in bile samples taken from patients undergoing cholecystectomy [106]. In 7 out of 13 subjects only trace amounts of the antibiotic were detected while the remaining ones had biliary concentrations ranging from 4.5 to 15.6 μg/ml. These figures are extremely low especially if compared to the biliary rifampicin concentrations (i.e. >150 μg/ml) observed after a single 450-mg oral dose [107]. Taking into account the bile volume, the highest biliary excretion was less than 0.2% [106].

Although the pharmacokinetics of rifaximin in patients with renal insufficiency has not been specifically studied, its very low renal excretion makes any dose adjustment unnecessary. The same holds true for patients with hepatic insufficiency. In fact, the mean peak drug plasma concentrations (i.e. 13.5 ng/ml) detected in subjects with hepatic encephalopathy patients given rifaximin 800 mg 3 times daily for 7 days [34, 108] were not dissimilar to those found in healthy subjects [102] and patients with IBD [98]. Indeed, in all the trials performed in this condition the drug has been well tolerated [33, 77].

Finally, drug absorption and excretion have not been evaluated in pediatric or geriatric populations. However, here again the tolerability of rifaximin in childhood and in the elderly has found to be extremely good [33].

Table 6. Plasma concentrations and urinary excretion of rifaximin in patients with UC given 400 mg of the drug (from Rizzello et al. [103])

Patient No.	Plasma concentrations, ng/ml					Urinary excretion							
	0 h	1 h	4 h	8 h	24 h	0–4 h		4–8 h		8–24 h		Total amount	
						Urine ml	Rifaximin ng · ml^{-1}	Urine ml	Rifaximin ng · ml^{-1}	Urine ml	Rifaximin ng · ml^{-1}	Ng	Total excretion, %
1	–	–	–	–	–	600	48.4	450	10.9	800	13.0	44,322	0.011
2	–	–	–	–	–	750	31.7	600	15.4	950	7.8	40,412	0.010
3	–	–	–	22.4	–	300	38.5	450	32.5	900	20.4	44,485	0.011
4				2.38		150	46.3	400	62.1	850	8.8	39,215	0.010
5	–	4.64	4.63	4.39	–	200	–	150	42.7	1,000	11.1	17,525	0.004
6			3.03			100	412.0	50	66.8	800	12.3	54,409	0.014
7	–	2.00	–	–	–	180	33.6	200	12.2	750	6.7	13,483	0.003
8	–	–	–	–	–	100	277.4	0	–	600	8.0	32,518	0.008
9				13.4		700	3.8	200	12.6	1,000	43.2	48,306	0.012
10	–	–	BLQ	–	–	200	6.5	200	8.5	450	4.6	5,053	0.001
11	–	4.38	BLQ	BLQ	–	600	59.9	100	44.0	1,700	26.6	85,534	0.021
12				BLQ		700	5.2	600	5.6	1,200	5.3	13,350	0.003
Mean												36,551	0.009
SD												22,244	0.006

BLQ = Below the limit of quantitation.
– = Not detected.

Drug-to-Drug Interactions

As new classes of antimicrobial drugs have become available, pharmacokinetic drug interactions with antimicrobials have become more common. Macrolides, fluoroquinolones, rifamycins, azoles and other agents can interact adversely with commonly used drugs, usually by altering their hepatic metabolism [109]. The mechanisms by which antimicrobial agents alter the biotransformation of other drugs are increasingly understood to reflect inhibition or induction of specific cytochrome P450 enzymes. Rifampicin and rifabutin induce several cytochromes P450, including CYP3A4, and can therefore enhance the metabolism of many other drugs [109].

By using in vitro preparations of human enzymes it is possible to predict those antibiotics that will adversely affect the metabolism of other drugs [110]. Such studies have shown that rifaximin, at concentrations ranging from 2 to 200 ng/ml, did not inhibit human hepatic cytochrome P450 isoenzymes: 1A2, 2A6, 2B6, 2C9, 2C19, 2D6, 2E1 and 3A4 [34]. In an in vitro hepatocyte induction model, rifaximin was shown to induce cytochrome P450 3A4 (CYP3A4) [34], an isoenzyme which rifampicin is known to induce [109].

Since rifampicin impairs the effectiveness of oral contraceptives (OCs) and pregnancies have been reported in women taking OCs and antibiotics [111], the interaction between an OC containing ethinyl estradiol and norgestimate and rifaximin was studied in 28 healthy female subjects given a short course of the drug [34]. Results of this study showed that the pharmacokinetics of single doses of ethinyl estradiol and norgestimate were not altered by concomitant antibiotic administration.

Midazolam and other benzodiazepines (e.g. alprazolam and triazolam) are selective substrates of CYP3A4 [110] and the concomitant administration of potent metabolic CYP3A4 inducers results in statistically significant pharmacokinetic changes and a consequent loss of therapeutic efficacy [112]. To evaluate the possible midazolam-rifaximin interaction an open-label, randomized, crossover trial was designed to assess the effect of oral rifaximin (200 mg thrice daily for 3 or 7 days) on the pharmacokinetics of a single dose of midazolam, administered either intravenously (2 mg) or orally (6 mg) [34]. No significant difference was observed in all the pharmacokinetic parameters of midazolam or its major metabolite, 1′-hydroxymidazolam, with or without simultaneous antibiotic therapy. These results, therefore, show that rifaximin does not significantly affect intestinal or hepatic CYP3A4 activity.

The lack of any significant in vivo interaction between rifaximin and human cytochrome P450 is also consistent with the absence of any significant induction of drug-metabolizing enzymes in the liver and the GI tract of rats given the antibiotic orally for 6 months [113]. When given for prevention or treatment of TD [70], rifaximin should, therefore, not affect the pharmacokinetics (and consequently pharmacodynamics) of other prophylactic drugs (e.g. antimalarials) [113].

General Pharmacology

The GI tract being the main therapeutic target of rifaximin, its potential effects on gastric secretion and GI motility have been investigated in rats and mice [59]. The antibiotic was given intraduodenally to pylorus-ligated rats (Shay rat) at doses ranging from 10 to 500 mg/kg, that is up to 50 times the therapeutic daily dose. No effect on pH and volume of gastric juice as well as on acid output and pepsin activity was observed.

Gastric emptying was studied in rats by means of a liquid meal labeled with phenol red [Scarpignato, unpubl. observations] while intestinal transit was evaluated in mice by means of the charcoal test meal [59]. Here again rifaximin was unable to influence either the emptying rate or intestinal motility. The drug could, however, be capable of correcting the GI motility derangement often observed in the presence of small intestinal bacterial overgrowth (SIBO) [114]. This is the case of patients with diabetes [115] or Crohn's disease [116], in whom the delayed intestinal transit, detected together with SIBO, was accelerated by a short-course treatment with rifaximin.

The effect of rifaximin on cardiovascular (CV) and respiratory systems was investigated in anesthetized rats and guinea pigs, respectively [59]. Rifaximin was given intraduodenally at doses up to 100 mg/kg and carotid pressure and flow as well as heart rate were continuously measured in rats while respiration amplitude and frequency were monitored in guinea pigs. The rifamycin derivative did not affect any of the measured parameters at any time after its administration.

Clinical pharmacological studies to specifically address the effect of rifaximin on GI or CV and respiratory functions have not been performed. However, while the most frequently reported, albeit few, adverse events associated with rifaximin administration were gastrointestinal in nature, no untoward reactions involving the CV or respiratory systems have been described [33, 117].

Clinical Use and Therapeutic Potential

Data from both experimental and clinical pharmacology clearly show that rifaximin is a nonsystemic antibiotic with a broad spectrum of antibacterial action covering Gram-positive and Gram-negative organisms, both aerobes and anaerobes. Being virtually nonabsorbed, its bioavailability within the GI tract is rather high with intraluminal and fecal drug concentrations that largely exceed

Table 7. Established and potential clinical indications for rifaximin

Established indications
Infectious diarrhea (including TD)
Hepatic encephalopathy
SIBO
IBD
Colonic diverticular disease
Potential indications
IBS and chronic constipation
C. difficile infection
Bowel preparation before colorectal surgery
H. pylori infection
Selective bowel decontamination in acute pancreatitis
Prevention of SBP in cirrhosis
Prevention of NSAID intestinal injury
Extra-GI indications
Skin infections
Bacterial vaginosis
Periodontal disease

the MIC values observed in vitro against a wide range of pathogenic organisms. The GI tract represents, therefore, the primary therapeutic target and GI infections the main indication [33, 71]. Since gut bacteria play a pathogenic role in several GI disorders (like for instance IBD or irritable bowel syndrome, IBS), the broad antimicrobial activity of rifaximin is also of value in these clinical conditions [33]. Thanks to the lack of transcutaneous absorption pointed out in both animal [118] and human [119] studies, its topical use in skin infections has also been investigated [120]. Finally, since the rifaximin spectrum of antibacterial action includes many organisms (e.g. *Bacteroides biviusdisiens*, *Gardnerella vaginalis*, *Haemophilus ducreyi*) causing genital infections [46], including *Trichomonas vaginalis* [46] and *Chlamydia trachomatis* [121], an attempt has been made to apply it locally in the treatment of bacterial vaginosis [120]. The growing list of therapeutic applications of rifaximin, for which there are published clinical studies, is shown in table 7. Amongst them, some are established indications for which the clinical trials so far performed have provided evidence for a substantial benefit of rifaximin. These include infectious diarrhea [71], hepatic encephalopathy [77], SIBO [78], colonic diverticular disease [79] and IBD [80]. For each of these indications a summary of scientific rationale and of available data, which the reader is referred to, has recently been published

[71, 77–80]. In this section, therefore, only the potential clinical GI use of rifaximin is discussed in detail.

IBS and Chronic Constipation

A thoughtful review of Lin [122] has put forward the hypothesis that SIBO could represent a framework to understand IBS. The possibility that SIBO may explain bloating, which is present in 92% of patients with IBS, is supported by a greater total hydrogen excretion after lactulose ingestion, by a correlation between the pattern of bowel movement and the type of excreted gas, a prevalence of abnormal lactulose breath tests in 84% of IBS patients, and a 75% improvement of IBS symptoms after eradication of SIBO. Altered GI motility and sensation, changed activity of the central nervous system, and increased sympathetic drive and immune activation may be understood as consequences of the host response to SIBO [115]. To further support the suggestion that abnormal enteric flora may be a contributing cause of IBS, two recent studies have shown that metronidazole [123] and neomycin [124] are both able to cause a significant symptomatic improvement in this condition.

Besides constipation-related IBS, several studies have also suggested abnormalities of colonic bacterial composition in chronic idiopathic constipation [125]. Here again antibiotic treatment with vancomycin [126, 127], rovamycin (in combination with diphetarsone, an amebicidal agent) [128, 129] or erythromycin [130], which, however, displays a prokinetic activity [131, 132], proved to be capable of reversing long-lasting constipation. Furthermore, the efficacy in both clinical conditions of probiotics [133–135] lends further support to the pathogenic role of bowel flora.

Since remarkable symptomatic improvement can be achieved in most patients, antibiotic therapy is obviously the cornerstone of the treatment of SIBO [136]. Ideally, the choice of an antimicrobial agent should be based on in vitro susceptibility testing of the bacteria in the small bowel of the individual patient. However, because it is impractical to obtain this information in most cases, the choice of the antibiotic is largely empiric and based on results of published series involving small intestinal cultures [137]. Whereas most patients with SIBO have aerobic and anaerobic overgrowth, in others malabsorption has been associated with overgrowth of purely aerobic flora. Therefore, the most effective antibiotic regimens generally include one or more drugs with activity against aerobic and anaerobic bacteria. The majority of drugs which proved to be effective, with the exception of neomycin and rifaximin, are systemic antimicrobials [78, 136] whose adverse events may limit their usefulness, especially in the long term. Benefits of therapy must indeed be weighed against the risks of long-term antibiotic use, such as diarrhea, *C. difficile* colitis, patient intolerance and bacterial resistance. Thanks to its efficacy (the highest amongst the tested antimicrobials, [78]) and safety, rifaximin currently represents the best pharmacological option for SIBO and associated GI disorders. A randomized, placebo-controlled, double-blind trial on the effect of rifaximin on SIBO and symptom relief in IBS is ongoing in the US.

C. difficile *Infection*

Progress in defining new treatments for *C. difficile* infection has been hindered by the heterogeneous nature of hospital-acquired diarrhea, and in particular by whether colitis and/or pseudomembranous colitis is present in individual cases. Study groups have usually been poorly defined in this context, and given the spontaneous resolution of symptoms in a proportion of cases the true efficacy of treatment approaches often remains uncertain. Enthusiasm to explore new treatment possibilities for *C. difficile* has been largely fuelled by the apparently high relapse rate of conventional (metronidazole or vancomycin) treatment [138].

There is a consensus amongst published recommendations for the management of *C. difficile* infection [19–21]. The most important first step in the treatment is cessation of the precipitating agent, most commonly antibiotics, if this is deemed to be medically appropriate. In mild disease, this is often sufficient for full recovery. In more severe disease, antimicrobial therapy directed against *C. difficile* is required. Oral metronidazole is recommended as the initial treatment of choice. Vancomycin, which has a comparable efficacy, represents the second-line therapy. Given the higher cost of oral vancomycin therapy and concern about the selection for vancomycin-resistant enterococci, metronidazole is preferred as the initial agent of choice. Vancomycin is appropriate for patients with contraindications or intolerance to metronidazole or for those who fail to respond to metronidazole. Other antibiotics such as glycopeptides [17, 22, 23] should be reserved for patients who cannot tolerate metronidazole or vancomycin or who are nonresponders [139, 140].

Rifaximin displays good antibacterial activity against *C. difficile* in vitro [47, 48], with MIC values lower than those of metronidazole and vancomycin (table 8). Furthermore, the microorganism showed a particularly low incidence of spontaneously resistant mutants ($<1 \cdot 10^{-9}$). The low incidence of resistant subpopulations selected by a concentration 8 times the MIC value suggests that the high levels of the drug that will be reached within the GI lumen may further prevent the selection of mutants [48]. Data from trials with antibiotics in TD and preoperative bowel decontamination suggest that poorly absorbed antimicrobials might have a decreased risk of causing antibiotic-associated diarrhea and *C. difficile*-associated disease [14]. In this connection rifaximin, which displays an intrinsic activity against this microorganism, should carry less of a risk.

Table 8. Activity of rifaximin, vancomycin and metronidazole against 93 clinical isolates of *C. difficile* (from Marchese et al. [48])

Antibiotic	Range mg/l	MIC_{50} mg/l	MIC_{90} mg/l	Susceptible[a] %
Rifaximin	0.004–128	0.004	128	74.1
Vancomycin	0.25–4	1	2	100
Metronidazole	0.06–0.25	0.125	0.25	100

[a]The breakpoint for susceptibility of rifaximin was assumed to be equal to that of rifampicin.

A randomized open trial, performed in patients with *C. difficile* pseudomembranous colitis, compared rifaximin (200 mg 3 times daily) to vancomycin (500 mg 2 times daily) and found the two drugs similarly effective [141]. The clearance of bacterial toxins was, however, more rapid with vancomycin. Further large double-blind clinical studies are needed to better define the role of rifaximin in the treatment of *C. difficile* infection.

Bowel Preparation for Colorectal Surgery

Effective management of intra-abdominal infections requires a combination of preoperative mechanical bowel preparation (MBP), antibiotic prophylaxis and appropriate surgical technique [142]. However, a recent meta-analysis of randomized clinical trials [143] concluded that there is limited evidence in the literature to support the use of mechanical bowel preparation in patients undergoing elective colorectal surgery. Although drugs are not a substitute for attention to detail and meticulous surgical technique, the judicious use of antibiotic prophylaxis can decrease the overall risk of infection, especially following clean-contaminated and contaminated operations [144]. The benefit of administering antimicrobial agents as a prophylaxis against postoperative infections has long been debated. Because of the high density of bacteria in the large intestine and rectum, there appears to be general agreement on the need for prophylactic antibacterial treatment for surgical procedures involving this area [145–147]. It has been estimated that, without prophylaxis or with inappropriate prophylaxis, the postoperative complication rate following colorectal surgery can range from 30 to 60% compared with less than 10% with suitable antibiotic prophylaxis [146]. However, the choice of an ideal agent(s) and route of administration remains controversial. It should provide coverage of all likely pathogens, including aerobic and anaerobic organisms [142, 146]. Both oral

Table 9. Effect of short-term preoperative treatment with rifaximin or placebo on fecal bacterial counts in 118 patients submitted to colonic open surgery (from Gruttadauria et al. [148])

Bacterial counts	Placebo		Rifaximin	
	Before	After	Before	After
Aerobic, CFU $\times 10^6$	3.9 ± 0.7	3.4 ± 0.4	4.2 ± 0.53	1.58 ± 2.5*
Anaerobic, CFU $\times 10^9$	89.1 ± 15.3	78.2 ± 21.3	70.2 ± 12.1	14.5 ± 0.1*

Rifaximin (200 mg thrice daily) or placebo were given in a double-blind, double-dummy fashion for 3 consecutive days in addition to mechanical bowel preparation, which can account for the decrease, albeit not significant, of anaerobic flora in the placebo group.

*$p < 0.001$ versus the pretreatment value.

and/or parenteral antibiotics have been used [for a review, *see* 147]. Two oral regimens are currently employed: (1) an aminoglycoside agent with erythromycin base and (2) an aminoglycoside agent with metronidazole. The regimen most often chosen in the United States is neomycin and erythromycin base. In Europe and Australia, however, physicians prefer kanamycin and metronidazole or neomycin and metronidazole [147].

Due to its pharmacokinetic and pharmacodynamic properties, rifaximin could be a suitable single oral agent for antibiotic prophylaxis in colorectal surgery. Indeed preoperative administration of 600 mg/daily [148] or 800mg/daily [149] for 3 days significantly reduces fecal counts of both aerobic and anaerobic bacteria (table 9). In two studies rifaximin was compared to parenteral gentamycin [148] or to oral paromomycin [149] and proved to be equally effective in the prevention of infectious complications of colonic surgery. An additional trial [150] evaluated the effect of adding rifaximin to intravenous cefotaxime (3 g daily for 5 days) in the prevention of bacterial infections after major colic surgery. Compared to the cephalosporin alone, the antibiotic combination was more effective. In all studies, rifaximin was tolerated extremely well. Nasogastric administration of rifaximin suspension (800 mg/day) for 5 postoperative days after colon surgery was attempted at our university hospital [151] and appeared to be as effective as preoperative oral administration in preventing infectious complications

In summary, 3-day preoperative treatment with rifaximin appears to be an effective antibiotic prophylaxis for patients submitted to colorectal surgery. However, this kind of prophylaxis should be compared with the convenience and efficacy of perioperative regimens [152, 153], such as those with an aminoglycoside or a cephalosporin, before gaining wider acceptance. Being perioperative antibiotics systemic drugs whose administration might be accompanied by adverse events, including life-threatening reactions [154], the use of a virtually unabsorbed antimicrobial would be the winner in terms of tolerability and safety [15]. A large, double-blind clinical trial comparing different prophylactic regimens in the same population of patients is eagerly waited to definitely assess the potential of rifaximin in colorectal surgery.

H. pylori *Infection*

H. pylori infection is a long-lasting, transmissible disease that has spread worldwide causing significant morbidity and mortality with a relevant economic impact. Since Warren and Marshall [155] first described the infectious etiology of peptic ulcer disease in 1984, a great deal of evidence has accumulated to suggest that *H. pylori* eradication therapy cures peptic ulcer disease [156] and can also be beneficial to other *H. pylori*-related diseases [157]. Having been classified as a definite 'type I carcinogen' [158], this Gram-negative, microaerophile bacterium needs to be eradicated from the host anyway [159, 160] since this can prevent the development of dyspeptic symptoms and peptic ulcer disease in healthy asymptomatic subjects [161] and that of gastric cancer in dyspeptic patients [162]. The survival capabilities of the *H. pylori* organism within the stomach make it, however, difficult to eradicate. The organism is able to survive over a wide pH spectrum. It is found within the gastric mucus layer, deep within the mucus-secreting glands of the antrum, attached to cells, and even within cells [56]. The organism must be eradicated from each of these potential niches and this is a daunting task for any single antibiotic. Initial attempts to cure the infection showed that the presence of antibiotic susceptibility in vitro did not necessarily correlate with successful treatment. It was rapidly recognized that therapy with a single antibiotic led to a poor cure rate and various antimicrobial mixtures were tried resulting in several effective combinations of antibiotics, bismuth, and antisecretory drugs [163].

Several European Guidelines [for a review, *see* 163] suggest the use of a 7-day triple therapy, comprising a proton pump inhibitor (or ranitidine bismuth citrate), clarithromycin and amoxycillin or metronidazole, as first-line therapy, whilst a 7-day quadruple therapy (proton pump inhibitor, bismuth salts, tetracycline, and metronidazole) is indicated for patients with eradication failure. However, increasing evidence suggests that the success rate following such regimens is decreasing in several countries. Indeed, some systematic reviews showed that standard triple therapies fail to eradicate *H. pylori* in up to 20% of patients [163]. Moreover, even lower cure rates have been observed in primary medical care settings, bacterial eradication being achieved in only

Table 10. Genes affected by point mutations or other genetic events leading to antibiotic resistance in *H. pylori* and the frequency of resistance (from Mégraud and Lamouliatte [166])

Antibiotic group	Genes affected	Frequency of resistance, %
Macrolides	23S rRNA	0–20
Metronidazole	*rdxA, frxA*	10–90
Quinolones	*gyrA*	0–10
Rifamycins	*rpoB*	0–5
Amoxicillin	PBP-1A	Few cases described
Tetracycline	16S rRNA	Few cases described

61–76% of patients [164]. As a consequence, new therapeutic combinations to cure *H. pylori* infection have been pioneered in the last few years. In addition, some effective rescue therapies have been developed in order to overcome treatment failures [165–167].

Although there are several reasons accounting for the lack of efficacy of eradication regimens, the main reason was found to be *H. pylori* resistance to antimicrobials (especially clarithromycin and metronidazole). The microorganism can become resistant to most antibiotics by chromosome mutation. This is the essential resistance mechanism found in this bacterial species, although genetic exchanges, especially transformation, have also been documented [166]. The genes affected by point mutations together with the frequency of resistance for the commonly used classes of antimicrobials are shown table 10.

Rifamycin derivatives (such as rifampicin, rifabutin and rifaximin) display antibacterial activity against *H. pylori* [51–54, 168, 169]. Rifabutin, whose oral bioavailability is rather low (i.e. 20%), is being increasingly used in some 'rescue' therapies after failed eradication attempts [170–172]. The prevalence *of H. pylori* resistance to this group of antibiotics is not exactly known but is probably extremely low as these drugs have – until recently – only been used in a limited number of patients to treat mycobacterial infections. On these grounds, some new rifamycin derivatives that display a potent bactericidal activity against *H. pylori* have been patented by different pharmaceutical companies. More interestingly, these compounds seem to be also active against those bacterial strains resistant to both metronidazole and clarithromycin [173].

Because of its antibacterial activity against microorganisms [51–54] and the lack of strains with primary resistance [52, 53], some preliminary studies

Table 11. Eradication rate and incidence of adverse events following administration of rifaximin and different rifaximin-based eradication regimens in *H. pylori*-positive patients (from Pretolani et al. [174])

Regimen	eradication rate %	adverse events %
Rifaximin 400 mg b.i.d.	40 (4/10)	0 (0/10)
Rifaximin + CBS 120 mg b.i.d.	50 (5/10)	20 (2/10)
Rifaximin + clarithromycin 500 mg b.i.d.	73 (8/11)	18 (2/11)
Rifaximin + metronidazole 250 mg t.i.d.	60 (6/10)	30 (3/10)

Drugs were given for 2 weeks and eradication checked 1 month after stopping treatment with rapid urease test and histology on biopsy samples taken from the antrum and the corpus.
CBS = Colloidal bismuth subcitrate.

[174–176] have explored the potential of rifaximin for *H. pylori* eradication. A first single-blind randomized study [174] evaluated the efficacy of rifaximin alone or in combination in *H. pylori*-positive patients with antral gastritis and found the dual therapy with clarithromycin particularly effective (table 11).

On the basis of these results, a triple therapy including rifaximin, amoxicillin and omeprazole was attempted [175]. However, results were disappointing since the eradication rate (i.e. 60%) did not differ from that observed with dual therapy. However, in this study high doses (600 mg 3 times daily) of rifaximin suspension (2%) were used, which proved in a subsequent study [176] to be less effective than the tablet formulation. In addition, large volumes of the suspension had to be taken, which might have lowered patients' compliance and, consequently, the eradication rate [175]. Moreover, in the above study, drugs were given on an empty stomach. Since a meal markedly prolongs gastric residence time of the drug and improves its intragastric distribution to the body and fundus [177], postprandial dosing seems a more suitable strategy for improving topical delivery and mixing (thanks to increased antral motility) of antimicrobials [177, 178], provided that binding to or inactivation by food does not occur. An additional finding that would suggest postprandial dosing is that eating is associated with desquamation of gastric surface cells and discharge of mucus [179], possibly exposing the organisms to higher concentrations of the antimicrobial agent, or exposing a higher percentage of the organisms to it.

In conclusion, rifaximin-based eradication regimens are promising but new antimicrobial combinations (with and without proton pump inhibitors) need to be explored in well-designed clinical trials including a large cohort of *H. pylori*-infected patients.

Selective Bowel Decontamination in Acute Pancreatitis

Acute necrotizing pancreatitis (ANP) still remains a life-threatening disease despite several improvements in diagnosis, prevention and treatment. Infectious complications are the most frequent and severe complications of acute pancreatitis with a mortality rate up to 80%. Bacterial infections, frequently caused by microorganisms of enteric origin, are often seen during the progression of severe ANP, concomitant with the potential development of multiple organ dysfunction [180]. The role of antibiotics in reducing infectious morbidity and mortality has been debated for decades because of a lack of supportive clinical data. Research completed over the past decade has helped to define the microbiology, establish the risk factors, and improve the understanding of the pathogenesis of infectious complications in patients with ANP [181]. These patients are at the greatest risk of developing an infection with enteric Gram-negative or Gram-positive bacteria 'translocated' from the bowel lumen into the necrotic pancreatic tissue [181, 182].

Bacterial translocation is defined as the passage of viable indigenous bacteria from the GI tract to extraintestinal sites, such as the mesenteric lymph node complex, liver, spleen and bloodstream [183]. Three major mechanisms promote bacterial translocation: intestinal bacterial overgrowth, deficiencies in host immune defenses and increased permeability or damage to the intestinal mucosal barrier [184]. These mechanisms can act in concert to promote synergistically the systemic spread of indigenous translocating bacteria to cause lethal sepsis.

Animal and human studies support the use of antibiotics for the prevention of infectious morbidity and mortality in severe ANP. The most effective antimicrobial agents are the fluoroquinolones, imipenem-cilastatin, and metronidazole, which achieve adequate penetration into pancreatic juice and necrotic tissue and inhibit the growth of enteric bacteria. Although a recent meta-analysis [185] suggested that prophylactic antibiotic administration reduces sepsis and mortality and this approach has been recommended by recent guidelines and consensus statements [186–191] on the treatment of ANP, the first double-blind, placebo-controlled trial [192] found no benefit of antibiotic prophylaxis with respect to the risk of developing infected pancreatic necrosis.

The route of antibiotic administration might be crucial. Animal studies [193, 194] have shown that enteral administration (either by oral or rectal route) of antimicrobials reduces the rate of bacterial translocation and early mortality in rats or mice with experimentally induced pancreatitis. Indeed, in patients with ANP, selective bowel decontamination with oral and rectal antibiotics decreased the infection rate [195].

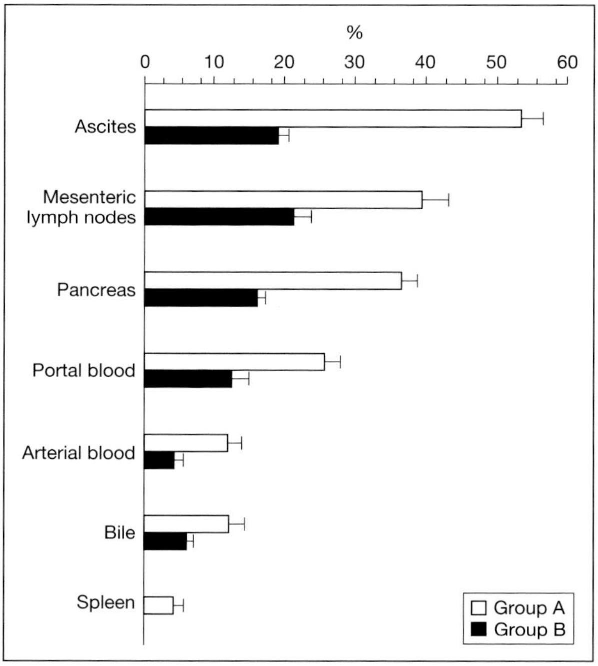

Fig. 8. Inhibition of bacterial translocation by rifaximin in the rat. Results of bacteriological culture (for aerobic and anaerobic bacteria) of tissues and biological fluids obtained from rats with taurocholate-induced ANP. Bars represent the percentage of positive biological samples. Horizontal lines are standard errors. Animals of group A received no treatment, while those of group B were given an enema of 30 ml warmed saline containing rifaximin (20 mg/kg) 1 h prior the induction of ANP (from Marotta et al. [196]).

Investigations performed in rats with experimental acute pancreatitis [196] or ulcerative colitis [197] have shown that both rectal and oral administration of rifaximin decreased colonic bacterial translocation towards mesenteric lymph nodes. In the model of ANP [196] not only was the intra-abdominal spread of enteric bacteria (fig. 8) significantly reduced but also the pancreatic damage was lessened by rifaximin treatment.

In addition to ANP where it is associated with GI dysmotility [198, 199], SIBO is present in a significant proportion of patients with chronic pancreatitis [200, 201]. Short-term rifaximin therapy was able to normalize the hydrogen breath test and improve symptoms (i.e. diarrhea and fecal fat excretion) in all patients studied (fig. 9) [201]. Bowel decontamination via administration of this 'topical' antibiotic could, therefore, be beneficial in both acute and chronic pancreatitis. Double-blind, placebo-controlled studies are to be performed to explore the rifaximin potential in this indication.

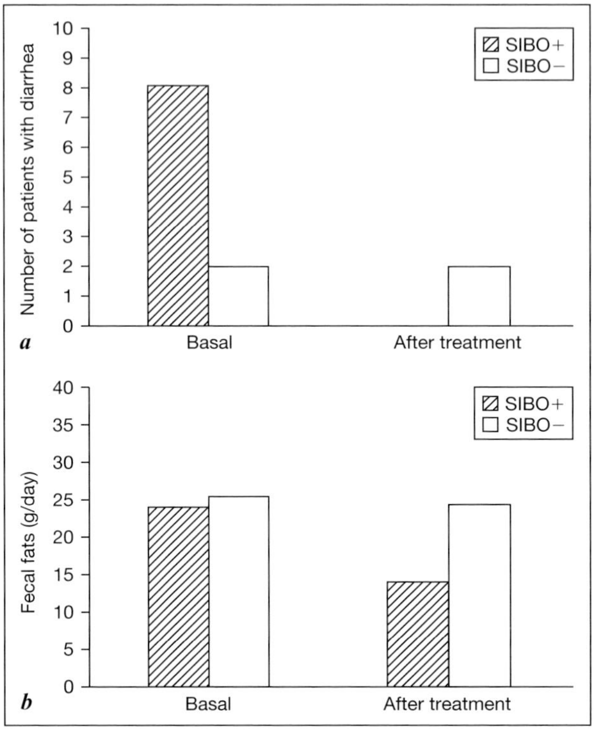

Fig. 9. Effect of short-term rifaximin administration (400 mg t.i.d. for 7 days) on diarrhea (***a***) and fecal fat excretion (***b***) in patients with chronic pancreatitis with and without SIBO (from Trespi and Ferrieri [201]).

Prevention of Spontaneous Bacterial Peritonitis in Cirrhosis

Spontaneous bacterial peritonitis (SBP) is a serious complication of cirrhotic ascites, arising most frequently in those with advanced liver disease. Its development leads to a further reduction in the effective arterial blood volume, and it has a mortality rate equivalent to that of a variceal bleed [202]. Since hepatic blood flow and function are age-dependent [203], SBP could be particularly severe in the elderly.

SBP is considered a bacterial infection of a previously sterile ascitic fluid in the absence of any intra-abdominal, surgically treatable source of infection [204]. Independent predictors of the development of bacterial infections in hospitalized cirrhotic patients are poor liver synthetic function and admission for GI hemorrhage [205]. Diagnosis of SBP is established by a polymorphonuclear cell count in ascitic fluid $\geq$250 cells/mm^3. The organism responsible for the infection is isolated in 60–70% of the cases. The remaining cases are considered to be a variant of SBP (culture-negative SBP) and are treated in the same way as those with a positive culture. The SBP resolution rate ranges between 70 and 90%, and hospital survival between 50 and 70% [206]. An early diagnosis and the use of a more adequate antibiotic therapy are the most probable reasons for the improvement in the prognosis for SBP in recent decades [205, 206]. Despite the resolution of the infection, SBP may trigger severe complications such as renal impairment, GI bleeding and accentuation of hepatic insufficiency, which are responsible for the associated mortality. Patients recovering from an episode of SBP should actually be considered as potential candidates for liver transplantation [206].

An in vitro [207] study on 124 aerobic bacterial pathogens obtained from patients with SBP showed that most isolates were Gram-negative organisms, and that *E. coli* and *Klebsiella pneumoniae* were responsible for 63% of the episodes evaluated. The fluoroquinolones (ciprofloxacin and ofloxacin) and the 'fourth-generation' cephalosporin cefpirome were the most active agents against the Gram-negative bacteria. Although the International Ascites Club (IAC) [208] suggested the use of intravenous cefotaxim or oral ofloxacin as the antimicrobial treatment of choice, a recent systematic review [209, 210] found no convincing evidence concerning efficacy of antibiotics in the treatment of SBP, and identified several gaps that warrant future research. Since bacterial translocation, depressed activity of the reticuloendothelial phagocytic system and decreased antibacterial capacity of ascitic fluid seem to be the main steps in the pathogenesis of ascitic fluid infection [211], antimicrobial prophylaxis seems, however, indicated.

It is now well established that the gut is the source of most of the bacteria that eventually cause SBP [212]. As cirrhosis develops in animals, Gram-negative bacteria increase in numbers in the gut [213]. Furthermore, the gut of animals and patients with advanced cirrhosis is more permeable to bacteria than the normal gut and more permeable than the gut in less advanced cirrhosis [214, 215]. Once bacteria reach a critical concentration in the gut lumen, they 'spill over', and escape from the gut, 'translocating' to mesenteric lymph nodes. Then, they can enter lymph, blood, and eventually ascitic fluid [216]. If the ability of the ascitic fluid to assist macrophages and neutrophils in killing the errant bacteria is deficient, uncontrolled growth occurs [214]. Bacterial translocation is facilitated by SIBO that in turn is facilitated by disorders in intestinal motility. Bacterial overgrowth and alterations in intestinal motility have both been shown to be more frequent in cirrhosis, particularly in patients with the most severe liver disease [217, 218]. In summary, SBP is the result of a failure of the gut to contain bacteria and a failure of the immune system to kill the virulent bacteria once they have escaped from the gut. Treating SIBO should, therefore, prevent bacterial translocation and, consequently, SBP in

Table 12. Prophylaxis of SBP with rifaximin in patients with alcoholic cirrhosis (from Trespi et al. [224])

	Cumulative incidence		
	Rifaximin (n = 27)	Controls (n = 25)	p value
Cirrhotic patients developing SPB	3/27 (11.1)	10/25 (40.0)	0.0246
Cirrhotic patients with SIBO developing SPB	1/11 (9.0)	8/9 (88.9)	0.0009

Figures in parentheses represent percentage.

cirrhosis. Indeed, selective intestinal decontamination with antibiotics reduces gut bacterial counts, reduces translocation rates, can prevent SBP in high-risk subgroups, and can improve the hyperdynamic circulatory state of these patients [208, 219, 220]. Selective intestinal decontamination can even improve the survival of rats with cirrhosis and ascites [221]. Although several guidelines [222] including those of the IAC [208] suggest long-term prophylaxis with oral norfloxacin, the growing microbial resistance to quinolones [223] and the well-known adverse effects of systemic antimicrobials [154], often amplified in patients with an impairment of the liver function, call for alternative effective and safe treatment. Thanks to its activity against the microorganisms often responsible for SBP and its safety profile, rifaximin could represent a suitable antibiotic for long-term prophylaxis in cirrhotics. In this connection, the efficacy of this rifamycin derivative, given for a week, monthly over a period of 12 months, in the prevention of SBP was prospectively evaluated in patients with alcoholic cirrhosis [224]. The incidence of peritonitis was significantly reduced by the antibiotic treatment. Rifaximin did correct SIBO in 91% of patients and in all of them the occurrence of SBP was prevented (table 12). Since these are the promising results of an open trial, a larger, double-blind, controlled study is needed to confirm these data and select the best dose regimen and duration.

Prevention of Nonsteroidal Anti-Inflammatory Drug-Induced Enteropathy

Nonsteroidal anti-inflammatory drugs (NSAIDs) are widely prescribed medicines. Although these compounds represent a very effective class of drugs, their use is associated with a broad spectrum of untoward reactions in the liver, kidney, skin and gut. GI problems constitute a wide range of different clinical pictures, ranging from symptoms such as dyspepsia, heartburn and abdominal discomfort to more serious events, like peptic ulcer and its life-threatening complications, bleeding and perforation [225]. Although the upper GI toxicity of NSAIDs is well documented, the fact that NSAID damage extends beyond the duodenum is less well recognized. Upper GI effects are indeed the most known and most feared adverse events, but it is evident that NSAID therapy is also associated with lower GI complications: 10–15% of NSAID users experience diarrhea [226]. Furthermore, in patients taking long-term NSAIDs [227–230] there is an increased risk of intestinal erosion, ulceration and perforation. The hitherto small number of reports of toxic effects of NSAIDs to the small bowel may reflect primarily a lack of diagnostic tools. Indeed, push enteroscopy [231] and endoscopic capsule [232] have only recently been available to clinicians. Nevertheless, a host of small bowel manifestations have now been documented, ranging from strictures causing dramatic small-bowel obstruction and severe bleeding to low-grade NSAID 'enteropathy', a syndrome comprising increased intestinal permeability and low-grade inflammation with blood and protein loss. The enteropathy, although not dramatic, may add to existing GI problems, especially in rheumatic patients, and contribute to iron deficiency anemia or hypoalbuminemia. NSAID use has also been associated with onset or relapse of IBD [227–230].

Animal studies indicate that the pathogenesis of NSAID small intestinal toxicity involves multiple interactions dependent on enterohepatic circulation, epithelial permeability, neutrophil infiltration and bacterial infection [233]. Several investigations [234–238] have suggested that bacterial flora may play a role in the pathogenesis of NSAID bowel injury and Robert and Asano [239] did show more than 25 years ago that germ-free rats are resistant to indomethacin-induced intestinal lesions. A recent paper [238] found an unbalanced growth of Gram-negative bacteria in the ileum of NSAID-treated animals and showed that heat-killed *E. coli* cells and their purified lipopolysaccharide caused a deterioration of NSAID-induced ulcers. Additional studies demonstrated that antimicrobials, such as tetracycline [234], kanamycin [236, 237], metronidazole [235, 237] and neomycin plus bacitracin [237], attenuate NSAID enteropathy, thus giving further support to the pathogenic role of enteric bacteria. The evidence from animal experiments has been confirmed in human studies, showing that metronidazole, an antimicrobial mainly targeted against anaerobic organisms [240], significantly prevented indomethacin-induced increase of intestinal permeability in healthy volunteers [241] and reduced inflammation and blood loss in rheumatic patients taking NSAIDs (table 13) [242]. Although metronidazole is able to protect against mitochon-drial uncoupling induced by indomethacin [243], it does not possess any 'intrinsic' anti-inflammatory activity [244]. Its beneficial effect on NSAID enteropathy is, therefore, likely to be due to the antibacterial action. In this

Table 13. Reduction of intestinal inflammation and blood loss by metronidazole in patients on NSAIDs (from Bjarnason et al. [242])

Parameter	Metronidazole 800 mg/day		Significance p
	Before	After	
Fecal excretion of ^{111}In-labeled neutrophils, %	4.7 ± 1.30	1.5 ± 0.36	<0.0001
Fecal excretion of ^{51}Cr-labeled red cells, ml	2.6 ± 0.44	0.9 ± 0.13	<0.01
5-hour urinary excretion ratio ^{51}Cr-EDTA/*L*-rhamnose	0.133 ± 0.012	0.1154 ± 0.017	NS

Intestinal inflammation was assessed by fecal excretion of ^{111}In-labeled neutrophils while blood loss was quanti-tated via fecal excretion of ^{51}Cr-labeled red cells. The urinary excretion ratio or ^{51}Cr-EDTA/*L*-rhamnose was used as an index of intestinal permeability.

connection, an elegant study [245] with microbiological cultures of luminal aspirates was able to show that small intestinal permeability is increased in subjects with SIBO. This finding can easily explain how antibacterial agents, by correcting SIBO, could counterbalance intestinal permeability changes which set in motion a series of pathophysiological events leading to gross lesion formation.

An indirect proof of the role exerted by gut bacteria in the pathogenesis of NSAID enteropathy is represented by the similarities between indomethacin-induced intestinal damage and Crohn's disease [234, 246]. Not only are these lesions anatomically (both macro- and microscopically) similar [246], but also sensitive to the same drugs, e.g. sulfasalazine [234, 247], steroids [234, 247], immuno-suppressive compounds [248], and antibiotics [234–237].

There is now a huge amount of data suggesting a pathogenetic role of bacteria in Crohn's disease [249, 250]. As a consequence, antibiotics, including rifaximin [80], proved to be effective in both inducing and maintaining remission from the disease [251, 252]. All these data, taken together, are consistent with the hypothesis that rifaximin, by correcting SIBO, would prevent or lessen NSAID enteropathy. Conversely to metronidazole [253], this rifamycin derivative is virtually unabsorbed by the GI tract and is devoid of any carcinogenic potential, being therefore more suitable for long-term use. One could actually speculate that cyclic antibiotic administration, getting rid of enteric pathogenic bacteria, would protect in this way the intestine from the damaging effect of anti-inflammatory compounds. This could be particularly useful in elderly patients, in whom a coexistence of osteoarthritis and colonic diverticular disease [254] would make rifaximin administration very cost-effective. Studies to explore this appealing clinical use are on the way in our laboratory.

Safety and Tolerability

Some toxicological investigations of rifaximin were performed at the beginning of the 1980s and some additional studies have recently been completed. The old tests did not comply with good laboratory practice principles since they were carried out before 1986. However, overall, the experiments were sufficiently accurate to permit adequate assessment of the drug toxicity [59], particularly in view of its very limited oral absorption.

The studies were performed by the route proposed for human therapy, that is oral, and also by the intravenous route as required by the guidelines; the animal species and the protocols used are considered as the best fitted for the different kinds of tests [59].

Acute and Chronic Toxicity in Animals

The single-dose toxicity studies were performed in two mammalian species, rat and mouse, by the route used in clinical practice, that is oral, as well as that ensuring adequate systemic exposure to the drug, that is intravenous. The subacute (3 months) toxicity studies were correctly carried out in the two animal species (rat, dog) in which also the pharmacokinetics was studied. Since in accordance with the International Conference on Harmonization (CPMP/ICH/286/95), 3-month toxicity studies support clinical trials for up to 1 month's duration (the longest duration of drug administration in clinical use), chronic toxicity studies have not been performed.

The acute oral treatment of rats and mice did not induce any important behavioral change. Only at the highest dose (2,000 mg/kg) was some excitement observed in rats, but no animal died. The LD_{50} was, therefore, considered $>$2,000 mg/kg. Since only one mouse given that dose died, the lethal oral dose in that species was established to be 2,000 mg/kg [59, 255].

In subacute toxicity studies only the highest rifaximin dose (i.e. 100 mg/kg, corresponding to 25 times the therapeutic dose in humans) induced mild toxic effects (like, for instance, acute gastroenteritis) connected to the topical GI action of the drug [59, 255]. A dose-dependent increase of the total cholesterol value was recorded in female animals [255], most likely due to an alteration of biliary acid metabolism consequent to the antibiotic effect on gut flora [256].

Table 14. Adverse events with an incidence ≥2% among patients receiving rifaximin (600 mg daily) or placebo in placebo-controlled studies (from rifaximin FDA label [34])

MedDRA preferred term	Patients, n	
	Rifaximin tablets (600 mg/day; n = 320)	Placebo (n = 228)
Flatulence	36 (11.3)	45 (19.7)
Headache	31 (9.7)	21 (9.2)
Abdominal pain NOS	23 (7.2)	23 (10.1)
Rectal tenesmus	23 (7.2)	20 (8.8)
Defecation urgency	19 (5.9)	21 (9.2)
Nausea	17 (5.3)	19 (8.3)
Constipation	12 (3.8)	8 (3.5)
Pyrexia	10 (3.1)	10 (4.4)
Vomiting NOS	7 (2.2)	4 (1.8)

Adverse events include those that may be attributable to the underlying disease. Figures in parentheses represent percentage. MedDRA = Medical Dictionary for Regulatory Activities (http:// www.meddramsso.com/NewWeb2003/medra_overview/index. htm); NOS = not otherwise specified.

All these data, taken together, do suggest that rifaximin is devoid of any toxic effect in experimental animals.

Genotoxicity

It is clear today that no single test is capable of detecting all genotoxic agents. Therefore, the usual approach is to perform a standard battery of in vitro and in vivo tests for genotoxicity [257]. The Ames *Salmonella*/microsome mutagenicity assay (Ames test) is a short-term bacterial reverse mutation assay specifically designed to detect a wide range of chemical substances that can produce genetic damage that leads to gene mutations [258]. The test employs several histidine-dependent *Salmonella* strains each carrying different mutations in various genes in the histidine operon. Indeed, rifaximin was assessed with the Ames test in five different strains *of Salmonella typhimurium* with and without metabolic activation [59, 255]. Being an antibiotic, the drug was considerably toxic to all the five bacterial strains but was not mutagenic since there was no increase in the number of revertants. Furthermore, no mutagenic activity was detected by using the gene conversion test on *Saccharomyces cerevisiae* or the gene mutation test on *Schizosaccharomyces pombe* [59, 255, 259].

Additional studies were performed with eukaryotic cell systems (i.e. Chinese hamster ovary cells, rat bone marrow cells and human lymphocytes) and none of them revealed a genotoxic potential [59]. No carcinogenicity tests have been done, but the short duration of patient treatment and the nature of the drug itself, which is virtually unabsorbed, do not raise any concern for carcinogenic potential.

Reproductive Toxicity

In the early investigations oral administration of rifaximin did not induce any toxic effect on the reproductive ability of rats, on the embryo-fetal development of rats and rabbits and on the peri- and postnatal development of rats [59, 260, 261]. However, more recent embryo-fetal toxicity studies, performed in rabbits [262], revealed that fetuses from treated animals display an increased incidence of linked skeletal anomalies and variants associated with vertebral and rib configuration. Because of these findings the US FDA put rifaximin – like many other antimicrobial agents [263] – in the pregnancy category C[1] [34]. In the above experiments, however, the food intake of the female rabbits was significantly decreased during the first half of the treatment period and remained lower, but not significantly so, throughout the experiment. As a consequence, body weight loss for the majority of treated females was evident in the first few days of the treatment period. Subsequent body weight gains were, however, similar to control values but, overall, body weight gain of the rifaximin-treated group for the gestation period remained below that seen in the control group rabbits [262]. A similar reduction in body weight gain through prepairing and gestation was observed in rats given rifaximin [264]. These apparent effects on body weight were considered a reflection of the antimicrobial action of the drug on the intestinal flora (with consequent impairment of nutrient absorption) and, therefore, connected to its primary pharmacological action [264]. On the other hand, it is well known that maternal nutrition does affect fetal development [265] and that malnutrition can actually potentiate the teratogenic effects of some drugs, like for instance aspirin [266]. As a matter of fact, a careful examination of fetuses made it possible to conclude that the types and incidences of the observed skeletal anomalies are unrelated to maternal treatment with rifaximin [267]. It is worthwhile mentioning that the rabbit is generally not considered a suitable species for the study of teratological effects of antibiotics because its susceptibility to them can make clinical signs difficult to interpret [268]. It is however reassuring that a population-based

[1] Animal reproduction studies have shown an adverse effect on the fetus; however, there are no adequate and well-controlled studies in humans, but potential benefits may warrant the use of the drug in pregnant women despite potential risks.

case-control study [269] showed that maternal exposure to antituberculosis drugs during pregnancy does not reveal a detectable teratogenic risk to the fetus. It is, therefore, very unlikely that the minute amounts of absorbed rifaximin, which will never be taken throughout the full gestation period, affect fetal development in humans.

No studies evaluating the excretion of rifaximin into breast milk and its bioavailability to the infant have been performed. However, due to its very limited, if any, absorption from the GI tract and its physicochemical characteristics any milk excretion of the drug is unlikely [270].

Tolerability Profile in Humans

An evaluation of the rifaximin tolerability profile observed in almost 1,000 patients from 30 clinical trials was unable to identify a definite pattern of intolerance [33]. Very few adverse events have been reported during short-tem treatment with the drug, the most frequently reported being gastrointestinal in nature (e.g. flatulence, nausea, abdominal pain and vomiting). It is worthwhile to emphasize that the detection of GI adverse reactions could have been difficult in rifaximin trials since the symptoms of the underlying diseases were often similar to the GI complaints observed after drug treatment.

The safety of rifaximin, 200 mg 3 times daily, was evaluated more recently in 320 patients from two placebo-controlled clinical trials [34]. All the adverse events for either rifaximin or placebo that occurred at a frequency $\geq 2\%$ are shown in table 14. With the exception of flatulence, which occurred significantly ($p = 0.0071$) less frequently after drug treatment, the adverse event profile of rifaximin overlapped that of placebo.

Prolonged therapy with high doses of the antibiotic has been associated with infrequent urticarial skin reactions [33]. A significant increase in serum potassium and sodium concentrations, although within the physiological range, has been observed after the drug. Since rifaximin was employed mainly for the treatment of diarrheal diseases, this finding could likely be connected to the electrolyte disturbances of underlying conditions.

Postmarketing Surveillance

The excellent safety profile observed in clinical trials has been confirmed by the postmarketing surveillance program [117]. More than 8.5 million patients have been treated in Italy and abroad with rifaximin since its introduction to the market. During the overall postmarketing period, 26 adverse reactions (17 cases of patients) were reported to the manufacturer, of which only 4 were judged to be serious. They consisted in 1 case of angioneurotic edema, 1 of cutaneous rash and 2 of urticaria.

In summary, rifaximin appears to be extremely safe with a very favorable risk-to-benefit ratio.

Conclusions and Perspectives for the Future

Rifaximin was first described in 1982 and was introduced into the Italian market 5 years later. Taking into account its excellent activity against a broad range of enteropathogens, the first 'logical' indication for this GI-targeted antibiotic was the treatment of infectious diarrhea in both adults and children. However, the appreciation of the pathogenic role of gut bacteria in several organic and functional GI diseases [12, 13] has increasingly broadened its clinical use.

Being virtually unabsorbed, this antimicrobial has little value outside the area of enteric infections, thus minimizing both antimicrobial resistance and systemic adverse events. It proved to be safe in all patient populations, including young children. Although pregnant women were purportedly excluded from controlled trials, clinical experience does suggest that the use of a nonabsorbable antibiotic, when strictly needed, represents the safest choice in this physiological condition. In this connection, it was shown that treatment with oral neomycin, a poorly absorbed aminoglucoside, during pregnancy presents no detectable teratogenic risk to the human fetus [271]. Rifaximin, therefore, possesses almost all the characteristics of the 'ideal' antibiotic targeted at the GI tract [272].

As shown in table 7, there are established and potential clinical indications for this peculiar drug. In all these conditions, many of which share SIBO as a common feature, gut bacteria represent the specific target of rifaximin. The drug can be used alone (like, for instance, in the treatment of infectious diarrhea) or as add-on medication (as in the management of IBD) and given short-term (single course of treatment) or long-term (repeated courses of therapy, i.e. cyclically).

Although rifaximin has stood the test of time, it still attracts the attention of both basic scientists and clinicians as attested by the regular number of publications which appear every year in the medical literature (fig. 10). As a matter of fact, with the advancement of the knowledge on microbial-gut interactions in health and disease novel indications and new drug regimens are being explored.

Besides widening the clinical use, the research on rifaximin is also focused on the synthesis of new derivatives [173, 273] and on the development of original formulations, like soft capsules [274] and a gum-like device [275], designed for the controlled and continuous release of rifaximin. The former preparation, being bioadhesive, could be particularly useful in the *Helicobacter* eradication from the stomach whereas the latter should make the treatment of infections of the oral cavity possible, thus expanding the spectrum of clinical use.

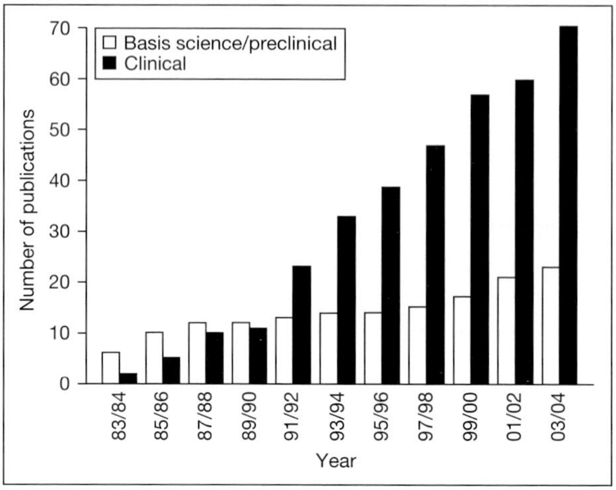

Fig. 10. Cumulative number of preclinical and clinical publications on rifaximin (courtesy of Lorin Johnson, PhD). Only papers quoted in Medline are presented.

All this ongoing research clearly indicates that the final chapter on this stimulating antibiotic has not yet been written.

Acknowledgments

We are indebted to Professor Claudio Rossi (Department of Chemical and Biosystem Sciences, University of Siena) and Professor Paolo Colombo (Department of Pharmaceutical Sciences, University of Parma) for their critical reading of the manuscript.

References

1 Vedantam G, Hecht DW: Antibiotics and anaerobes of gut origin. Curr Opin Microbiol 2003;6:457–561.
2 Fantry L: Gastrointestinal infections in the immunocompromised host. Curr Opin Gastroenterol 2001;17:40–45.
3 Stagg AJ, Hart AL, Knight SC, Kamm MA: Microbial-gut interactions in health and disease. Interactions between dendritic cells and bacteria in the regulation of intestinal immunity. Best Pract Res Clin Gastroenterol 2004;18:255–270.
4 Lu L, Walker WA: Pathologic and physiologic interactions of bacteria with the gastrointestinal epithelium. Am J Clin Nutr 2001;73(suppl):1124S–1130S.
5 Brito GAC, Alcantara C, Carneiro-Filho BA, Guerrant RL: Pathophysiology and impact of bacterial and protozoal infections: New approaches to therapy. Chemotherapy 2005;51(suppl1):23–25.
6 Procop GW: Gastrointestinal infections. Infect Dis Clin North Am 2001;15:1073–1108.
7 Pithie AD, Ellis CJ: Antibiotics and the gut. Aliment Pharmacol Ther 1989;3:321–332.
8 Li E, Stanley SL Jr: The role of newer antibiotics in gastroenterology. Gastroenterol Clin North Am 1992;21:613–629.

9 Renner F, Mittermayer H, Hafner M, Schofl R: Prophylaxis with antibiotics in gastrointestinal endoscopy. Z Gastroenterol 2002;40:1–7.
10 Norrby SR: Principles for targeted antibiotic use in urinary tract and enteric infections: A review with special emphasis on norfloxacin. Scand J Infect Dis 1986;18(suppl 48):7–19.
11 Van den Hazel SJ, Speelman P, Tytgat GNJ, Dankert J, Van Leeuwen DJ: Role of antibiotics in the treatment and prevention of acute and recurrent cholangitis. Clin Infect Dis 1994;19: 279–286.
12 Hart AL, Stagg AJ, Frame M, Graffner H, Glise H, Falk P, Kamm MA: Review article: The role of the gut flora in health and disease, and its modification as therapy. Aliment Pharmacol Ther 2002; 16:1383–1393.
13 Guarner F, Malagelada JR: Gut flora in health and disease. Lancet 2003;361:512–519.
14 Surawicz CM: Antibiotic-associated diarrhea and pseudomembranous colitis: Are they less common with poorly absorbed antimicrobials? Chemotherapy 2005;51(suppl 1):81–89.
15 DuPont HL: Community-acquired diarrheal disease in western countries: Applications of nonabsorbable oral antibiotic therapy. Adv Stud Med 2003;3(suppl A):S945–S950.
16 Cheung RP, DiPiro JT: Vancomycin: An update. Pharmacotherapy 1986;6:153–169.
17 Brogden RN, Peters DH: Teicoplanin: A reappraisal of its antimicrobial activity, pharmacokinetic properties and therapeutic efficacy. Drugs 1994;47:823–854.
18 Toscano WA Jr, Storm DR: Bacitracin. Pharmacol Ther 1982;16:199–210.
19 Zimmerman MJ, Bak A, Sutherland LR: Review article: Treatment of *Clostridium difficile* infection. Aliment Pharmacol Ther 1997;11:1003–1012.
20 Surawicz CM, McFarland LV: Pseudomem branous colitis: Causes and cures. Digestion 1999;60:91–100.
21 Poutanen SM, Simor AE: *Clostridium difficile*- associated diarrhea in adults. CMAJ 2004;171:51–58.
22 McCafferty DG, Cudic P, Frankel BA, Barkallah S, Kruger RG, Li W: Chemistry and biology of the ramoplanin family of peptide antibiotics. Biopolymers 2002;66:261–284.
23 Ramoplanin: A 16686, a 16686a, MDL 62198. Drugs R D 2002;3:61–64.
24 Montecalvo MA: Ramoplanin: A novel antimicrobial agent with the potential to prevent vancomycin-resistant enterococcal infection in high-risk patients. J Antimicrob Chemother 2003;51 (suppl 3):31–35.
25 Simon HJ: Streptomycin, kanamycin, neomycin and paromomycin. Pediatr Clin North Am 1968;15:73–83.
26 Wright GD, Berghuis AM, Mobashery S: Aminoglycoside antibiotics. Structures, functions, and resistance. Adv Exp Med Biol 1998;456:27–69.
27 Berk DP, Chalmers T: Deafness complicating antibiotic therapy of hepatic encephalopathy. Ann Intern Med 1970;73:393–396.
28 Lerner SA, Matz GJ: Aminoglycoside ototoxicity. Am J Otolaryngol 1980;1:169–179.
29 Kavanagh KT, McCabe BF: Ototoxicity of oral neomycin and vancomycin. Laryngoscope 1983;93:649–653.
30 Appel GB, Neu HC: The nephrotoxicity of antimicrobial agents (second of three parts). N Engl J Med 1977;296:722–728.
31 Kunin CM, Chalmers TC, Leevy CM, Sebastyen SC, Lieber CS, Finland M: Absorption of orally administered neomycin and kanamycin with special reference to patients with severe hepatic and renal disease. N Engl J Med 1960;262:380–385.
32 Stockwell M: Gentamicin ear drops and ototoxicity: Update. CMAJ 2001;164:93–94.
33 Gillis JC, Brogden RN: Rifaximin. A review of its antibacterial activity, pharmacokinetic properties and therapeutic potential in conditions mediated by gastrointestinal bacteria. Drugs 1995;49: 467–484.
34 Rifaximin label approved on 05/25/2004 (http://www.fda.gov/cder/foi/label/2004/21361_xifaxan_lbl.pdf).
35 Lal R, Lal S: Recent trends in rifamycin research. Bioessays 1994;16:211–216.
36 Burman WJ, GallicanoK, Peloquin C: Comparative pharmacokinetics and pharmacodynamics of the rifamycin antibiotics. Clin Pharmacokinet 2001;40:327–341.
37 Brufani M, Cellai L, Marchi E, Segre A: The synthesis of 4-deoxypyrido[1′,2′-1,2]imidazo [5,4-c]rifamycin SV derivatives. J Antibiot (Tokyo) 1984;37:1611–1622.

38 Marchi E, Montecchi L, Venturini AP, Mascellani G, Brufani M, Cellai L: 4-Deoxypyrido [1′,2′:1,2]imidazo[5,4-c]rifamycin SV derivatives. A new series of semisynthetic rifamycins with high antibacterial activity and low gastroenteric absorption. J Med Chem 1985;28:960–963.
39 De Angelis L: L-105. Drugs Future 1982;7:260–261.
40 Brufani M, Cellai L, Cerrini S, Fedeli W, Marchi E, Segre A, Vaciago A: X-ray crystal structure of 4-deoxy-3′-bromopyrido[1′,2′-1,2]imidazo[5,4-c]rifamycin SV. J Antibiot (Tokyo) 1984;37: 1623–1627.
41 Cellai L, Cerrini S, Segre A, Battistoni C, Cossu G, Mattogno G, Brufani M, Marchi E: A study of structure-activity relationships in 4-deoxypyrido[1′,2′-1,2]imidazo[5,4-c]rifamycin SV derivatives by electron spectroscopy for chemical analysis and ^{1}H NMR. MolPharmacol 1985;27:103–108.
42 Jiang ZD, Ke S, Palazzini E, Riopel L, Dupont H: In vitro activity and fecal concentration of rifaximin after oral administration. Antimicrob Agents Chemother 2000;44:2205–2206.
43 Jiang ZD, DuPont HL: Rifaximin: In vitro and in vivo antibacterial activity. A review. Chemotherapy 2005;51(suppl 1):67–72.
44 Malvisi Stracciari J, Venturini AP, Anfossi P, Marchi E, Stracciari GL: Sensitivity to rifaximin and rifampicin of *Mycobacterium tuberculosis* isolated from guinea pigs treated orally with rifaximin. Chemioterapia (Florence) 1987;6:82–84.
45 Soro O, Pesce A, Raggi M, Debbia EA, Schito GC: Selection of rifampicin-resistant *Mycobacterium tuberculosis* does not occur in the presence of low concentrations of rifaximin. Clin Microbiol Infect 1997;3:147–151.
46 Hoover WW, Gerlach EH, Hoban DJ, Eliopoulos GM, Pfaller MA, Jones RN: Antimicrobial activity and spectrum of rifaximin, a new topical rifamycin derivative. Diagn Microbiol Infect Dis 1993;16:111–118.
47 Ripa S, Mignini F, Prenna M, Falcioni E: Invitro antibacterial activity of rifaximin against *Clostridium difficile, Campylobacter jejunii* and *Yersinia* spp. Drugs Exp Clin Res 1987;13:483–488.
48 Marchese A, Salerno A, Pesce A, Debbia EA, Schito GC: In vitro activity of rifaximin, metronidazole and vancomycin against *Clostridium difficile* and the rate of selection of spontaneously resistant mutants against representative anaerobic and aerobic bacteria, including ammonia-producing species. Chemotherapy 2000;46:253–266.
49 Gomi H, Jiang ZD, Adachi JA, Ashley D, Lowe B, Verenkar MP, Steffen R, DuPont HL: Invitro antimicrobial susceptibility testing of bacterial enteropathogens causing traveler's diarrhea in four geographic regions. Antimicrob Agents Chemother 2001;45:212–216.
50 Sierra JM, Navia MM, Vargas M, Urassa H, Schellemberg D, Gascon J, Vila J, Ruiz J: In vitro activity of rifaximin against bacterial enteropathogens causing diarrhoea in children under 5 years of age in Ifakara, Tanzania. J Antimicrob Chemother 2001;47:904–905.
51 Mignini F, Falcioni E, Prenna M, Santacroce F, Ripa S: In vitro antibacterial activity of rifaximin against *Campylobacter pylori (Campylo bacter pyloridis).* Chemioterapia (Florence) 1989;1 (suppl4):222–223.
52 Mégraud F, Bouffant F, Camou Juncas C: Invitro activity of rifaximin against *Helicobacter pylori.* Eur J Clin Microbiol Infect Dis 1994;13:184–186.
53 Holton J, Vaira D, Menegatti M, Barbara L: The susceptibility of *Helicobacter pylori* to the rifamycin, rifaximin. J Antimicrob Chemother 1995;35:545–549.
54 Quesada M, Sanfeliu I, Junquera F, Segura F, Calvet X: Evaluation *of Helicobacter pylori* susceptibility to rifaximin (in Spanish). Gastroenterol Hepatol 2004;27:393–396.
55 Scarpignato C, Pelosini I: Bismuth compounds for eradication *of Helicobacter pylori:* Pharmacology and safety. Progr Basic Clin Pharmacol 1999;11:87–126.
56 Scarpignato C, Pelosini I: Antisecretory drugs for eradication *of Helicobacter pylori:* Antibacterial activity and synergism with antimicrobial agents. Progr Basic Clin Pharmacol 1999;11:136–180.
57 Scrascia M, Forcillo M, Maimone F, Pazzani C: Susceptibility to rifaximin of *Vibrio cholerae* strains from different geographical areas. J Antimicrob Chemother 2003;52:303–305.
58 Lancini GC, Sartori G: Rifamycins LXI: In vivo inhibition of RNA synthesis of rifamycins. Experientia 1968;24:1105–1106.
59 Dayan AD: Rifaximin (Normix®) Preclinical Expert Report. London, submitted to Medicines and Healthcare Products Regulatory Agency, 1997.

60 Umezawa H, Mizuno S, Yamazaki H, Nitta K: Inhibition of DNA-dependent RNA synthesis by rifamycins. J Antibiot (Tokyo) 1968;21:234–236.
61 Struelens MJ: How Europe is facing up to antibiotic resistance. Euro Surveill 2004;9:1 (http://www.eurosurveillance.org/em/v09n01/0901–221.asp).
62 Hamilton-Miller JM: Antibiotic resistance from two perspectives: Man and microbe. Int J Antimicrob Agents 2004;23:209–212.
63 Collignon PJ: 11: Antibiotic resistance. Med J Aust 2002;177:325–329.
64 Gould IM: A review of the role of antibiotic policies in the control of antibiotic resistance. J Antimicrob Ther 1999;43:459–465.
65 al-Orainey IO: Drug resistance in tuberculosis. J Chemother 1990;2:147–151.
66 Spratt BG: Resistance to antibiotics mediated by target alterations. Science 1994;264:388–393.
67 Smith CA, Baker EN: Aminoglycoside antibiotic resistance by enzymatic deactivation. Curr Drug Targets Infect Disord 2002;2:143–160.
68 Joyce M, Woods CW: Antibacterial susceptibility testing in the clinical laboratory. Infect Dis Clin North Am 2004;18:401–434.
69 Smaill F: Antibiotic susceptibility and resistance testing: An overview. Can J Gastroenterol 2000;14:871–875.
70 Gemmel GC, Lorian V: Effects of low concentrations of antibiotics on bacterial ultrastructure, virulence, and susceptibility to immunodefenses: Clinical significance; in Lorian V (ed): Antibiotics in Laboratory Medicine, ed 4. Baltimore, Williams & Wilkins, 1996, pp 397–452.
71 Ericsson CD, DuPont HL: Rifaximin in the treatment of infectious diarrhea. Chemotherapy 2005;51(suppl 1):73–80.
72 Berti T, Benoni G, Miglioli PA, Velo GP: Intestinal antibacterial activity of a new rifamycin derivative: Compound L-105. Chemioterapia (Florence) 1982;1(suppl 4):106A.
73 Miglioli PA, Allerberger F, Calabrò GB, Gaion RM: Effects of daily oral administration of rifaximin and neomycin on faecal aerobic florain rats. Pharmacol Res 2001;44:373–375.
74 Venturini AP, Marchi E: In vitro and in vivo evaluation of L/105, a new topical intestinal rifamycin. Chemioterapia (Florence) 1986;5:257–262.
75 Feldman WH: A scheme for numerical recording of tuberculous changes in experimentally infected guinea-pig. Annu Rev Turbec 1943;48:248.
76 Lucchesi M, Marchi E, Venturini AP: Antimy-cobacterial activity of rifaximin (L/105) in experimental tuberculosis in the guinea pig. Chemioterapia (Florence) 1984;3:371–372.
77 Zeneroli ML, Avallone R, Corsi L, Venturini I, Baraldi C, Baraldi M: Management of hepatic encephalopathy: Role of rifaximin. Chemotherapy 2005;51(suppl 1):90–95.
78 Di Stefano M, Corazza GR: Treatment of small intestinal bacterial overgrowth and related symptoms by rifaximin. Chemotherapy 2005;51(suppl 1):103–109.
79 Papi C, Koch M, Capurso L: Management of diverticular disaease: Is there room for rifaximin? Chemotherapy 2005;51(suppl 1):110–114.
80 Gionchetti P, Rizzello F, Morselli C, Romagnoli R, Campieri M: Inflammatory bowel disease: Does rifaximin offer any promise? Chemotherapy 2005;51(suppl 1):96–102.
81 Testa R, Eftimiadi C, Sukkar GS, De Leo C, Rovida S, Schito GC, Celle G: A non-absorbable rifamycin for treatment of hepatic encephalopathy. Drugs Exp Clin Res 1985;11:387–392.
82 De Leo C, Eftimiadi C, Schito GC: Rapid disappearance from the intestinal tract of bacteria resistant to rifaximin. Drugs Exp Clin Res 1986;12:979–981.
83 Lacour M, Zunder T, Huber R, Sander A, Daschner F, Frank U: The pathogenetic significance of intestinal *Candida* colonization – A systematic review from an interdisciplinary and environmental medical point of view. Int J Hyg Environ Health 2002;205:257–268.
84 Amenta M, Dalle Nogare ER, Colomba C, Prestileo TS, Di Lorenzo F, Fundaro S, Colomba A, Ferrieri A: Intestinal protozoa in HIV-infected patients: Effect of rifaximin in *Cryptosporidium parvum* and *Blastocystis hominis* infections. J Chemother 1999;11:391–395.
85 Gillespie SH: Evolution of drug resistance in *Mycobacterium tuberculosis:* Clinical and molecular perspective. Antimicrob Agents Chemother 2002;46:267–274.
86 Kapusnik JE, Parenti F, Sande MA: The use of rifampicin in staphylococcal infections – A review. J Antimicrob Chemother 1984;13(suppl C):61–66.

87 Frieden TR, Sterling TR, Munsiff SS, Watt CJ, Dye C: Tuberculosis. Lancet 2003;362: 887–899.
88 DuPont HL, Jiang Z-D: Influence of rifaximin treatment on susceptibility of intestinal gram-negative flora and enterococci; Clin Microbiol Infect 2004;10:1009–1011.
89 Murray BE, Hodel-Christian SL: Bacterial resistance: Theoretical and practical considerations, mutations to antibiotic resistance, characterization of R plasmid, and detection of plasmid-specific genes; in Lorian V (ed): Antibiotics in Laboratory Medicine, ed 4. Baltimore, Williams & Wilkins, 1996.
90 Fietta A, Cascina A, Meloni F, Morosini M, Casali L, Bono L, Minoli L, Marone P: A 10-year survey *of Mycobacterium tuberculosis* isolates in Pavia and their drug resistance: A comparison with other Italian reports. J Chemother 2002;14:33–40.
91 Girgis N, Sultan Y, Frenck RW Jr, El-Gendy A, Farid Z, Mateczun A: Azithromycin compared with rifampin for eradication of nasopharyngeal colonization by *Neisseria meningitidis*. Pediatr Infect Dis J 1998;17:816–819.
92 Cuevas LE, Kazembe P, Mughogho GK, Tillotson GS, Hart CA: Eradication of nasopharyngeal carriage of *Neisseria meningitidis* in children and adults in rural Africa: A comparison of ciprofloxacin and rifampicin. J Infect Dis 1995;171:728–731.
93 Schwartz B, Al-Tobaiqi A, Al-Ruwais A, Fontaine RE, A'ashi J, Hightower AW, Broome CV, Music SI: Comparative efficacy of ceftriaxone and rifampicin in eradicating pharyngeal carriage of group A *Neisseria meningitidis*. Lancet 1988;i:1239–1242.
94 Cresti S, Giordano I, Donati E, Giaccherini R, Barberi A, Cellesi C: Prevalence and chemosusceptibility of *Neisseria meningitidis* and *Haemophilus influenzae* in a population of central Italy. New Microbiol 2003;26:281–288.
95 Cellai L, Colosimo M, Marchi E: Synthesis of ^3H labeled rifamycin L 105. J Label Comp Radiopharm 1983;20:1287–1296.
96 Kenny MT, Strates B: Metabolism and pharmacokinetics of the antibiotic rifampin. Drug MetabRev1981;12:159–218.
97 Venturini AP: Pharmacokinetics of *L*/105, a new rifamycin, in rats and dogs, after oral administration. Chemotherapy (Basel) 1983;29:1–3.
98 Venturini AP: L/105: Report on pharmacokinetics in rats, dogs after oral administration and adverse reactions. Chemioterapia (Florence) 1983;2(suppl5):162–163.
99 Cellai L, Colosimo M, Marchi E, Venturini AP, Zanolo G: Rifaximin (L/105), a new topical intestinal antibiotic: Pharmacokinetic study after single oral administration of ^3H-rifaximin to rats. Chemioterapia (Florence) 1984;3:373–377.
100 Breen KJ, Bryant RE, Levinson JD, Schemker S: Neomycin absorption in man: Studies of oral and enema administration and effect of intestinal ulceration. Ann Intern Med 1972;76:211–218.
101 Venturini AP: Gastrointestinal absorption of rifaximin (L/105) in experimentally-induced colitis in the rat (in Italian). Riv Tossicol Sper Clin (Rome) 1986;16:119A.
102 Descombe JJ, Dubourg D, Picard M, Palaz-zini E: Pharmacokinetic study of rifaximin after oral administration in healthy volunteers. Int J Clin Pharmacol Res 1994;14:51–56.
103 Rizzello F, Gionchetti P, Venturi A, Ferretti M, Peruzzo S, Raspanti X, Picard M, Canova N, Palazzini E, Campieri M: Rifaximin systemic absorption in patients with ulcerative colitis. Eur J Clin Pharmacol 1998;54:91–93.
104 Gionchetti P, Rizzello F, Ferrieri A, Venturi A, Brignola C, Ferretti M, Peruzzo S, Miglioli M, Campieri M: Rifaximin in patients with moderate or severe ulcerative colitis refractory to steroid-treatment: A double-blind, placebo-controlled trial. Dig Dis Sci 1999;44:1220–1221.
105 Gionchetti P, Rizzello F, Venturi A, Ugolini F, Rossi M, Brigidi P, Johansson R, Ferrieri A, Poggioli G, Campieri M: Antibiotic combination therapy in patients with chronic, treatment-resistant pouchitis. Aliment Pharmacol Ther 1999;13:713–718.
106 Verardi S, Verardi V: Bile rifaximin concentration after oral administration in patients undergoing cholecystectomy. Farmaco 1990;45:131–135.
107 Acocella G: Clinical pharmacokinetics of rifampicin. Clin Pharmacokinet 1978;3:108–127.
108 Williams R, James OF, Warnes TW, Morgan MY: Evaluation of the efficacy and safety of rifaximin in the treatment of hepatic encephalopathy: A double-blind, randomized, dose-finding multicentre study. Eur J Gastroenterol Hepatol 2000;12:203–208.

109 Gillum JG, Israel DS, Polk RE: Pharmacokinetic drug interactions with antimicrobial agents. Clin Pharmacokinet 1993;25:450–482.
110 Fry RF: Probing the world of cytochrome P450 enzymes. Mol Interv 2004;4:157–162.
111 Dickinson BD, Altman RD, Nielsen NH, Sterling ML: Council on Scientific Affairs, American Medical Association: Drug interactions between oral contraceptives and antibiotics. Obstet Gynecol 2001;98:853–860.
112 Yuan R, Flockhart DA, Balian JD: Pharmacokinetic and pharmacodynamic consequences of metabolism-based drug interactions with alprazolam, midazolam, and triazolam. J Clin Pharmacol 1999;39:1109–1125.
113 Steffen R, Sack DA, Riopel L, Jiang ZD, Sturchler M, Ericsson CD, Lowe B, Waiyaki P, White M, DuPont HL: Therapy of travelers' diarrhea with rifaximin on various continents. Am J Gastroenterol 2003;98:1073–1078.
114 Husebye E: The pathogenesis of gastrointestinal bacterial overgrowth. Chemotherapy 2005; 51(suppl1):1–22.
115 Cuoco L, Montalto M, Jorizzo RA, Santarelli L, Arancio F, Cammarota G, Gasbarrini G: Eradication of small intestinal bacterial over growth and oro-cecal transit in diabetics. Hepatogastroenterology 2002;49:1582–1586.
116 Tursi A, Brandimarte G, Giorgetti G, Nasi G: Assessment of orocaecal transit time in different localization of Crohn's disease and its possible influence on clinical response to therapy. Eur J Gastroenterol Hepatol 2003;15:69–74.
117 Palazzini E: Periodic Safety Update Report for Rixamin (January 1987–December 2003). Bologna, Alfa Wassermann, 2004.
118 Venturini AP, Bertoli D, Marchi E: Transcutaneous absorption of a topical rifamycin preparation: Rifaximin (L/105). Drugs Exp Clin Res 1987;13:231–232.
119 Berlo JA, Debruyne HJ, Gortz JP: A prospective study in healthy volunteers of the topical absorption of a 5% rifaximin cream. Drugs Exp Clin Res 1994;20:205–208.
120 Pelosini I, Scarpignato C: Rifaximin, a peculiar rifamycin derivative: Established and potential clinical use outside the gastrointestinal tract. Chemotherapy 2005;51(suppl1):122–130.
121 Prasad ES, Wenman WM: In vitro activity of rifaximin, a topical rifamycin derivative, against *Chlamydia trachomatis*. Diagn Microbiol Infect Dis 1993;16:135–136.
122 Lin HC: Small intestinal bacterial over growth: A framework for understanding irritable bowel syndrome. JAMA 2004;292:852–858.
123 Nayak AK, Karnad DR, Abraham P, Mistry FP: Metronidazole relieves symptoms in irritable bowel syndrome: The confusion with so-called 'chronic amebiasis'. Indian J Gastroenterol 1997; 16:137–139.
124 Pimentel M, Chow EJ, Lin HC: Normalization of lactulose breath testing correlates with symptom improvement in irritable bowel syndrome. A double-blind, randomized, placebo-controlled study. Am J Gastroenterol 2003;98:412–419.
125 Madden JA, Hunter JO: A review of the role of the gut microflora in irritable bowel syndrome and the effects of probiotics. Br J Nutr 2002;88(suppl 1):S67–S72.
126 Andrews PJ, Barnes P, Borody TJ: Chronic constipation reversed by restoration of bowel flora. A case and a hypothesis. Eur J Gastroenterol Hepatol 1992;4:245–247.
127 Celik AF, Tomlin J, Read NW: The effect of oral vancomycin on chronic idiopathic constipation. Aliment Pharmacol Ther 1995;9:63–68.
128 Bernay P, Houver A, Carraz M, Castel G: Study of fecal flora in constipated patients. Their modification by treatment with rovamycin-diphetarsone (in French). J Med Lyon 1967;48: 847–854.
129 Chabanon MR: Contribution to the clinical study of 6,753 in the treatment of chronic constipation (rovamycin-diphetarsone) (in French). J Med Lyon 1967;48:263–268.
130 Bellomo-Brandao MA, Collares EF, da-Costa-Pinto EA: Use of erythromycin for the treatment of severe chronic constipation in children. Braz J Med Biol Res 2003;36:1391–1396.
131 Sharma SS, Bhargava N, Mathur SC: Effect of oral erythromycin on colonic transit in patients with idiopathic constipation. A pilot study. Dig Dis Sci 1995;40:2446–2449.
132 Scarpignato C, Pelosini I: Management of irritable bowel syndrome: Novel approaches to the pharmacology of gut motility. Can J Gastroenterol 1999;13(suppl A):50A–65 A.

133 Hamilton-Miller JMT: Probiotics in the management of irritable bowel syndrome: A review of clinical trials. Microb Ecol Health Dis 2001;13:211–215.
134 Ouwehand AC, Lagstrom H, Suomalainen T, Salminen S: Effect of probiotics on constipation, fecal azoreductase activity and fecal mucin content in the elderly. Ann Nutr Metab 2002;46:159–162.
135 Koebnick C, Wagner I, Leitzmann P, Stern U, Zunft HJ: Probiotic beverage containing *Lactobacillus casei* Shirota improves gastrointestinal symptoms in patients with chronic constipation. Can J Gastroenterol 2003;17:655–659.
136 Singh VV, Toskes PP: Small bowel bacterial overgrowth: Presentation, diagnosis, and treatment. Curr Gastroenterol Rep 2003;5:365–372.
137 Bouhnik Y, Alain S, Attar A, Flourie B, Raskine L, Sanson-Le Pors MJ, Rambaud JC: Bacterial populations contaminating the upper gut in patients with small intestinal bacterial overgrowth syndrome. Am J Gastroenterol 1999;94:1327–1331.
138 Wilcox MH, Spencer RC: *Clostridium difficile* infection: Responses, relapses and reinfections. J Hosp Infect 1992;22:85–92.
139 de Lalla F, Nicolin R, Rinaldi E, Scarpellini P, Rigoli R, Manfrin V, Tramarin A: Prospective study of oral teicoplanin versus oral van comycin for therapy of pseudomembranous colitis and *Clostridium difficile-associated* diarrhea. Antimicrob Agents Chemother 1992;36:2192–2196.
140 Wenisch C, Parschalk B, Hasenhundl M, Hirschl AM, Graninger W: Comparison of vancomycin, teicoplanin, metronidazole, and fusidic acid for the treatment of *Clostridium difficile-associated* diarrhea. Clin Infect Dis 1996;22:813–818.
141 Boero M, Berti E, Morgando A, Verme G: Treatment of *Clostridium difficile-associated* colitis: Results of an open randomized study with rifaximin versus vancomycin. Microbiol Med (Milan) 1990;5:74–77.
142 Sganga G: New perspectives in antibiotic prophylaxis for intra-abdominal surgery. J Hosp Infect 2002;50(suppl A): S17–S21.
143 Bucher P, Mermillod B, Morel P, Soravia C: Does mechanical bowel preparation have a role in preventing postoperative complications in elective colorectal surgery? Swiss Med Wkly 2004;134: 69–74.
144 Barie PS: Surgical site infections: Epidemiology and prevention. Surg Infect (Larchmt) 2002;3(suppl1):S9–S21.
145 Gorbach SL: Antimicrobial prophylaxis for appendectomy and colorectal surgery. Rev Infect Dis 1991;13(suppl 10):S815–S820.
146 DiPiro JT: Short-term prophylaxis in clean-contaminated surgery. J Chemother 1999;11:551–555.
147 Nichols RL, Choe EU, Weldon CB: Mechanical and antibacterial bowel preparation in colon and rectal surgery. Chemotherapy 2005;51(suppl1):115–121.
148 Gruttadauria G, La Barbera F, Cutaia G, Salanitri G: Prevention of infection in colonic surgery by rifaximin. A controlled, prospective, randomized trial. Eur Rev Med Pharmacol Sci 1987;9:101–105.
149 Verardi S, Verardi V, Fusillo M: Rifaximin effectiveness evaluation in the preparation of large intestine to surgery. Eur Rev Med Pharmacol Sci 1986;8:267–270.
150 Bresadola F, Intini S, Anania G, Noce L, Cedolini C, De Anna D, Ferrieri A: Chemotherapeutic prophylaxis in the preparation of the large intestine for surgical interventions: Rifaximin P.O. vs cephalosporin I.V. (in Italian). Ann Ital Chir 1992;63:201–207.
151 Salcuni PE, Palazzini E: An evaluation of the therapeutic activity and tolerance of rifaximin, administered by stomach probe, in patients after colorectal surgery. Aggiornamenti Med Chir 1988;6:1–7.
152 Esposito S: Is single-dose antibiotic prophylaxis sufficient for any surgical procedure? J Chemother 1999;11:556–564.
153 Platt R: Antibiotic prophylaxis in clean surgery: Does it work? Should it be used if it does? New Horiz 1998;6(2 suppl):S53–S57.
154 Cunha BA: Antibiotic side effects. Med Clin North Am 2001;85:149–185.
155 Marshall BJ, Warren JR: Unidentified curved bacilli in the stomach of patients with gastritis and peptic ulceration. Lancet 1984;i:1311—1315.
156 Leodolter A, Kulig M, Brasch H, Meyer-Sabellek W, Willich SN, Malfertheiner P: A meta-analysis comparing eradication, healing and relapse rates in patients with *Helicobacterpylori*-associated gastric or duodenal ulcer. Aliment Pharmacol Ther 2001;15:1949–1958.

157 Bazzoli F, BianchiPorro G, Bianchi MG, Molteni M, Pazzato P, Zagari RM: Treatment of *Helicobacter pylori* infection. Indications and regimens: An update. Dig Liver Dis 2002;34:70–83.
158 International Agency for Research on Cancer: Infection with *Helicobacter pylori;* in Schistosomes, Liver Flukes and *Helicobacter pylori.* Lyon, IARC, 1994, pp 177–202.
159 Misiewicz JJ: Is the only good *Helicobacter* a dead *Helicobacter*? Helicobacter 1997;2(suppl1): S89–S91.
160 Graham DY: The only good *Helicobacter pylori* is a dead *Helicobacter pylori.* Lancet 1997; 350:70–71.
161 Vaira D, Vakil N, Rugge M, Gatta L, Ricci C, Menegatti M, Leandro G, Holton J, Russo VM, Miglioli M: Effect of *Helicobacter pylori* eradication on development of dyspeptic and reflux disease in healthy asymptomatic subjects. Gut 2003;52:1543–1547.
162 Uemura N, Okamoto S, Yamamoto S, Matsumura N, Yamaguchi S, Yamakido M, Taniyama K, Sasaki N, Schlemper RJ: *Helicobacter pylori* infection and the development of gastric cancer. N Engl J Med 2001;345:784–789.
163 Scarpignato C: Towards the ideal regimen for *Helicobacter pylori* eradication: The search continues. Dig Liver Dis 2004;36:243–247.
164 Della Monica P, Lavagna A, Masoero G, Lombardo L, Crocella L, Pera A: Effectiveness of *Helicobacter pylori* eradication treatments in a primary care setting in Italy. Aliment Pharmacol Ther 2002;16:1269–1275.
165 Gisbert JP, Pajares JM: *Helicobacter pylori* 'rescue' regimen when proton pump inhibitor-based triple therapies fail. Aliment Pharmacol Ther 2002;16:1047–1057.
166 Mégraud F, Lamouliatte H: The treatment of refractory *Helicobacter pylori* infection. Aliment Pharmacol Ther 2003;17:1333–1343.
167 Parente F, Cucino C, Bianchi Porro G: Treatment options for patients with *Helicobacter pylori* infection resistant to one or more eradication attempts. Dig Liver Dis 2003;35:523–528.
168 Pilotto A, Franceschi M, Rassu M, Furlan F, Scagnelli M: In vitro activity of rifabutin against strains *of Helicobacter pylori* resistant to metronidazole and clarithromycin. Am J Gastroenterol 2000;95:833–834.
169 Heep M, Beck D, Bayerdorffer E, Lehn N: Rifampin and rifabutin resistance mechanism in *Helicobacter pylori.* Antimicrob Agents Chemother 1999;43:1497–1499.
170 Gisbert JP, Calvet X, Bujanda L, Marcos S, Gisbert JL, Pajares JM: 'Rescue' therapy with rifabutin after multiple *Helicobacter pylori* treatment failures. Helicobacter 2003;8:90–94.
171 Wong WM, Gu Q, Lam SK, Fung FM, Lai KC, Hu WH, Yee YK, Chan CK, Xia HH, Yuen MF, Wong BC: Randomized controlled study of rabeprazole, levofloxacin and rifabutin triple therapy vs. quadruple therapy as second-line treatment for *Helicobacter pylori* infection. Aliment Pharmacol Ther 2003;17:553–560.
172 Perri F, Festa V, Clemente R, Quitadamo M, Andriulli A: Rifabutin-based 'rescue therapy' for *Helicobacter pylori* infected patients after failure of standard regimens. Aliment Pharmacol Ther 2000;14:311–316.
173 Zullo A, Hassan C, Campo S, Morini S: Evolving therapy for *Helicobacter pylori* infection. Exp Opin Ther Patents 2004;14:1453–1464.
174 Pretolani S, Bonvicini F, Brocci E, Cilla D, Pasini P, Baldini L, Epifanio G, Miglio F, Gasbarrini G: Effect of rifaximin, a new non-absorbed antibiotic, in the treatment *of Helicobacter pylori* infection. Acta Gastroenterol Belg 1993;56:144A.
175 De Giorgio R, Stanghellini V, Barbara G, Guerrini S, Ferrieri A, Corinaldesi R: Rifaximin and *Helicobacter pylori* eradication. Eur Rev Med Pharmacol Sci 1997;1:105–110.
176 Dell'Anna A, Azzarone P, Ferrieri A: A randomized openly comparative study between rifaximin suspension versus rifaximin pills for the eradication of *Helicobacter pylori.* Eur Rev Med Pharmacol Sci 1999;3:105–110.
177 Atherton JC, Washington N, Bracewell MA, Sutton LJ, Greaves JL, Perkins AC, Hawkey CJ, Spiller RC: Scintigraphic assessment of the intragastric distribution and gastric emptying of an encapsulated drug: The effect of feeding and of a proton pump inhibitor. Aliment Pharmacol Ther 1994;8:489–494.
178 Gottfries J, Svenheden A, Alpstein M, Bake B, Larsson A, Idstrom JP: Gastrointestinal transit of amoxicillin-modified release tablets and a placebo tablet including pharmacokinetic assessments of amoxicillin. Scand J Gastroenterol 1996;31:49–53.

179 Grant R, Grossman MI, Ivy AC: Histological changes in the gastric mucosa during digestion and their relationship to mucosal growth. Gastroenterology 1953;25:218–231.
180 Butturini G, Salvia R, Bettini R, Falconi M, Pederzoli P, Bassi C: Infection prevention in necrotizing pancreatitis: An old challenge with new perspectives. J Hosp Infect 2001;49:4–8.
181 Isenmann R, Beger HG: Bacterial infection of pancreatic necrosis: Role of bacterial translocation, impact of antibiotic treatment. Pancreatology 2001;1:79–89.
182 Dervenis C, Smailis D, Hatzitheoklitos E: Bacterial translocation and its prevention in acute pancreatitis. J Hepatobiliary Pancreat Surg 2003;10:415–418.
183 Berg RD: Bacterial translocation from the gastrointestinal tract. Adv Exp Med Biol 1999;473:11–30.
184 Juvonen PO, Alhava EM, Takala JA: Gut permeability in patients with acute pancreatitis. Scand J Gastroenterol 2000;35:1314–1318.
185 Sharma VK, Howden CW: Prophylactic antibiotic administration reduces sepsis and mortality in acute necrotizing pancreatitis: A meta-analysis. Pancreas 2001;22:28–31.
186 Banks PA: Practice guidelines in acute pancreatitis. Am J Gastroenterol 1997;92:377–386.
187 Glazer G, Mann D: United Kingdom guidelines for the management of acute pancreatitis. Gut 1998;42:S1–S13.
188 Dervenis C, Johnson CD, Bassi C, Bradley EL 3rd, Imrie CW, McMahon MJ, Modlin I: Diagnosis, objective assessment of severity, and the management of acute pancreatitis. Int J Pancreatol 1999;25:195–210.
189 Rünzi M, Layer P, Büchler MW, Beger HG, Ell C, Fölsch UR, Goebell H, Hopt UT, Lankisch PG, Schmidt WE, Schmiegel W, Schölmerich J: The therapy of acute pancreatitis. General guidelines. Working group of the Society for Scientific-Medical Specialties (in German). Z Gastroenterol 2000;38:571–580.
190 Société Nationale Francaise de Gastro-Entérologie: French Consensus Conference on Acute Pancreatitis: Conclusions and recommendations. Eur J Gastroenterol Hepatol 2001;13:S1–S13.
191 Uhl W, Warshaw A, Imrie CW, Bassi C, McKay CJ, Lankisch PG, Carter RC, DiMagno EP, Banks PA, Whitcomb DC, Dervenis C, Ulrich CD, Satake K, Ghaneh P, Hartwig W, Werner J, McEntee G, Neoptolemos JP, Büchler MW: IAP-guidelines for the surgical management of acute pancreatitis. Pancreatology 2002;2:565–573.
192 R, Runzi M, Kron M, Kahl S, Kraus D, Jung N, Maier L, Malfertheiner P, Goebell H, Beger HG: German Antibiotics in Severe Acute Pancreatitis Study Group: Prophylactic antibiotic treatment in patients with predicted severe acute pancreatitis: A placebo-controlled, double-blind trial. Gastroenterology 2004;126:997–1004.
193 Gianotti L, Munda R, Gennari R, Pyles R, Alexander JW: Effect of different regimens of gut decontamination on bacterial translocation and mortality in experimental acute pancreatitis. Eur J Surg 1995;161:85–92.
194 de las Heras G, Forcelledo JL, Gutierrez JM, Calvo J, Obaya S, Fernandez Fernandez F, Mayorga M, Aguero J, Pons Romero F: Selective intestinal bacterial decontamination in experimental acute pancreatitis (in Spanish). Gastroenterol Hepatol 2000;23:461–465.
195 Luiten EJ, Hop WC, Lange JF, Bruining HA: Controlled clinical trial of selective decontamination for the treatment of severe acute pancreatitis. Ann Surg 1995;222:57–65.
196 Marotta F, Geng TC, Wu CC, Barbi G: Bacterial translocation in the course of acute pancreatitis: Beneficial role of nonabsorbable antibiotics and lactitol enemas. Digestion 1996;57:446–452.
197 Fiorucci S, Distrutti E, Mencarelli A, Barbanti M, Palazzini E, Morelli A: Inhibition of intestinal bacterial translocation with rifaximin modulates lamina propria monocytic cells reactivity and protects against inflammation in a rodent model of colitis. Digestion 2002;66:246–256.
198 Wang X, Gong Z, Wu K, Wang B, Yuang Y: Gastrointestinal dysmotility in patients with acute pancreatitis. J Gastroenterol Hepatol 2003;18:57–62.
199 Van Felius ID, Akkermans LM, Bosscha K, Verheem A, Harmsen W, Visser MR, Gooszen HG: Interdigestive small bowel motility and duodenal bacterial overgrowth in experimental acute pancreatitis. Neurogastroenterol Motil 2003;15:267–276.
200 Casellas F, Guarner L, Vaquero E, Antolin M, de Gracia X, Malagelada JR: Hydrogen breath test with glucose in exocrine pancreatic insufficiency. Pancreas 1998;16:481–486.
201 Trespi E, Ferrieri A: Intestinal bacterial over growth during chronic pancreatitis. Curr Med Res Opin 1999;15:47–52.

202 Mowat C, Stanley AJ: Spontaneous bacterial peritonitis – Diagnosis, treatment and prevention. Aliment Pharmacol Ther 2001;15:1851–1859.
203 Anand BS: Drug treatment of the complications of cirrhosis in the older adult. Drugs Aging 2001;18:575–585.
204 Garcia-Tsao G: Current management of the complications of cirrhosis and portal hypertension: Variceal hemorrhage, ascites, and spontaneous bacterial peritonitis. Gastroenterology 2001;120: 726–748.
205 Navasa M, Rodes J: Bacterial infections in cirrhosis. Liver Int 2004;24:277–280.
206 Fernandez J, Bauer TM, Navasa M, Rodes J: Diagnosis, treatment and prevention of spontaneous bacterial peritonitis. Baillières Best Pract Res Clin Gastroenterol 2000;14:975–990.
207 Sader HS, Runyon BA, Erwin ME, Jones RN: Antimicrobial activity of 11 newer and investigational drugs tested against aerobic isolates from spontaneous bacterial peritonitis. Diagn Microbiol Infect Dis 1995;21:105–110.
208 Rimola A, Garcia-Tsao G, Navasa M, Piddock LJ, Planas R, Bernard B, Inadomi JM: Diagnosis, treatment and prophylaxis of spontaneous bacterial peritonitis: A consensus document. J Hepatol 2000;32:142–153.
209 Soares-Weiser K, Brezis M, Leibovici L: Antibiotics for spontaneous bacterial peritonitis in cirrhotics. Cochrane Database Syst Rev 2001;3:CD002232.
210 Soares-Weiser K, Paul M, Brezis M, Leibovici M: Antibiotic treatment for spontaneous bacterial peritonitis. BMJ 2002;324:100–102.
211 Guarner C, Soriano G: Spontaneous bacterial peritonitis. Semin Liver Dis 1997;17:203–217.
212 Garcia-Tsao G, Wiest R: Gut microflora in the pathogenesis of the complications of cirrhosis. Best Pract Res Clin Gastroenterol 2004;18:353–372.
213 Guarner C, Runyon BA, Young S, Heck M, Sheikh MY: Intestinal bacterial overgrowth and bacterial translocation in an experimental model of cirrhosis in rats. J Hepatol 1997;26:1372–1378.
214 Runyon BA, Squier SU, Borzio M: Translocation of gut bacteria in rats with cirrhosis to mesenteric lymph nodes partially explains the pathogenesis of spontaneous bacterial peritonitis. J Hepatol 1994;21:792–796.
215 Cirera I, Bauer TM, Navasa M, Vila J, Grande L, Taura P, Fuster J, Garcia-Valdecasas JC, Lacy A, Suarez MJ, Rimola A, Rodes J: Bacterial translocation of enteric organisms in patients with cirrhosis. J Hepatol 2001;34:32–37.
216 Runyon BA: Patients with deficient ascitic fluid opsonic activity are predisposed to spontaneous bacterial peritonitis. Hepatology 1988;8:632–635.
217 Morencos FC, de las Heras G, Ramos M, Lopez-Arias MJ, Ledesma F, Pons F: Small bowel bacterial overgrowth in patients with alcoholic cirrhosis. Dig Dis Sci 1995;40:1252–1256.
218 Chang CS, Chen GH, Lien HC, Yeh HZ: Small intestine dysmotility and bacterial overgrowth in cirrhotic patients with spontaneous bacterial peritonitis. Hepatology 1998;28:1187–1190.
219 Runyon BA, Borzio M, Young S, Squier SU, Guarner C, Runyon MA: Effect of selective intestinal decontamination with norfloxacin on spontaneous bacterial peritonitis, translocation, and survival in an animal model of cirrhosis. Hepatology 1995;21:1719–1724.
220 Rasaratnam B, Kaye D, Jennings G, Dudley F, Chin-Dusting J: The effect of selective intestinal decontamination on the hyperdynamic circulatory state in cirrhosis. Ann Intern Med 2003;139:186–193.
221 Guarner C, Runyon BA, Heck M, Young S, Sheikh MY: Effect of long-term trimethoprim/sulfamethoxazole prophylaxis on ascites formation, bacterial translocation, spontaneous bacterial peritonitis and survival incirrhotic rats. Dig Dis Sci 1999;44:1957–1962.
222 Gines P, Navasa M: Antibiotic prophylaxis for spontaneous bacterial peritonitis: How and whom? J Hepatol 1998;29:490–494.
223 Thomson KS: Minimizing quinolone resistance: Are the new agents more or less likely to cause resistance? J Antimicrob Chemother 2000;45:719–723.
224 Trespi E, Colla C, Belloni G, Pollino MG, Magnani L, Panizza P, Venturini A: Efficacy of rifaximin as a prophylactic agent for the prevention of spontaneous bacterial peritonitis in alcoholic patients. Ital J Gastroenterol Hepatol 1999;31:534A.
225 Scarpignato C, Bjarnason I, Bretagne J-F, De Pouvourville G, García Rodríquez LA, Goldstein JL, Müller PA, Simon B: Working Team Report: Towards a GI safer antiinflammatory therapy. Gastroenterol Int 1999;12:186–215.

226 Henry DA: Side-effects of non-steroidal antiinflammatory drugs. Baillières Clin Rheumatol 1988;2: 425–454.
227 Bjarnason I, Hayllar J, Macherson AJ, Russell AS: Side effects of nonsteroidal anti-inflammatory drugs on the small and large intestine in humans. Gastroenterology 1993;104:1832–1847.
228 Aabakken L: Small-bowel side-effects of non steroidal anti-inflammatory drugs. Eur J Gastroenterol Hepatol 1999;11:383–388.
229 Davies NM, Saleh JY: Detection and prevention of NSAID enteropathy. J Pharm Pharm Sci 2000;3:137–155.
230 Lanas A, Panes J, Pique JM: Clinical implications of COX-1 and/or COX-2 inhibition for the distal gastrointestinal tract. Curr Pharm Des 2003;9:2253–2266.
231 Rossini FP, Pennazio M: Small-bowel endoscopy. Endoscopy 2002;34:13–20.
232 Chutkan R, Toubia N: Effect of nonsteroidal anti-inflammatory drugs on the gastrointestinal tract: Diagnosis by wireless capsule endoscopy. Gastrointest Endosc Clin N Am 2004;14:67–85.
233 Reuter BK, Davies NM, Wallace JL: Nonsteroidal anti-inflammatory drug enteropathy in rats: Role of permeability, bacteria, and enterohepatic circulation. Gastroenterology 1997;112: 109–117.
234 Banerjee AK, Peters TJ: Experimental nonsteroidal anti-inflammatory drug-induced enteropathy in the rat: Similarities to inflammatory bowel disease and effect of thromboxane synthetase inhibitors. Gut 1990;31:1358–1364.
235 Davies NM, Jamali F: Pharmacological protection of NSAID-induced intestinal permeability in the rat: Effect of tempo and metronidazole as potential free radical scavengers. Hum Exp Toxicol 1997;16:345–349.
236 Koga H, Aoyagi K, Matsumoto T, Iida M, Fujishima M: Experimental enteropathy in athymic and euthymic rats: Synergistic role of lipopolysaccharide and indomethacin. Am J Physiol 1999;276:G576–G582.
237 Kinouchi T, Kataoka K, Bing SR, Nakayama H, Uejima M, Shimono K, Kuwahara T, Akimoto S, Hiraoka I, Ohnishi Y: Culture supernatants of *Lactobacillus acidophilus* and *Bifidobacterium adolescentis* repress ileal ulcer formation in rats treated with a nonsteroidal antiinflammatory drug by suppressing unbalanced growth of aerobic bacteria and lipid peroxidation. Microbiol Immunol 1998;42:347–355.
238 Hagiwara M, Kataoka K, Arimochi H, Kuwahara T, Ohnishi Y: Role of unbalanced growth of gram-negative bacteria in ileal ulcer formation in rats treated with a nonsteroidal anti-inflammatory drug. J Med Invest 2004;51:43–51.
239 Robert A, Asano T: Resistance of germfree rats to indomethacin-induced intestinal lesions. Prostaglandins 1977;14:333–341.
240 Freeman CD, Klutman NE, Lamp KC: Metronidazole. A therapeutic review and update. Drugs 1997;54:679–708.
241 Davies GR, Wilkie ME, Rampton DS: Effects of metronidazole and misoprostol on indomethacin-induced changes in intestinal permeability. Dig Dis Sci 1993;38:417–425.
242 Bjarnason I, Hayllar J, Smethurst P, Price A, Gumpel MJ: Metronidazole reduces intestinal inflammation and blood loss in non-steroidal anti-inflammatory drug induced enteropathy. Gut 1992;33:1204–1208.
243 Leite AZ, Sipahi AM, Damiao AO, Coelho AM, Garcez AT, Machado MC, Buchpiguel CA, Lopasso FP, Lordello ML, Agostinho CL, Laudanna AA: Protective effect of metronidazole on uncoupling mitochondrial oxidative phosphorylation induced by NSAID: A new mechanism. Gut 2001;48:163–167.
244 Ganrot-Norlin K, Stalhandske T, Karlstrom R: Lack of antiinflammatory activity of metronidazole. Acta Pharmacol Toxicol (Copenh) 1981;49:130–133.
245 Riordan SM, McIver CJ, Thomas DH, Duncombe VM, Bolin TD, Thomas MC: Luminal bacteria and small-intestinal permeability. Scand J Gastroenterol 1997;32:556–563.
246 Anthony A, Pounder RE, Dhillon AP, Wake-field AJ: Similarities between ileal Crohn's disease and indomethacin experimental jejunal ulcers in the rat. Aliment Pharmacol Ther 2000;14: 241–245.
247 Del Soldato P, Foschi D, Varin L, Daniotti S: Indomethacin-induced intestinal ulcers inrats: Effects of salicylazosulfapyridine and dexamethasone. Agents Actions 1985;16:393–396.

248 Matsumoto T, Iida M, Nakamura S, Hizawa K, Kuroki F, Fujishima M: Preventive effect of immunosuppressive agents against indomethacin-induced small intestinal ulcers inrats. Dig Dis Sci 1994;39:787–795.
249 Linskens RK, Huijsdens XW, Savelkoul PH, Vandenbroucke-Grauls CM, Meuwissen SG: The bacterial flora in inflammatory bowel disease: Current insights in pathogenesis and the influence of antibiotics and probiotics. Scand J Gastroenterol 2001;36(suppl 234):29–40.
250 Tamboli CP, Neut C, Desreumaux P, Colombel JF: Dysbiosis in inflammatory bowel disease. Gut 2004;53:1–4.
251 Sartor RB: Therapeutic manipulation of the enteric microflora in inflammatory bowel diseases: Antibiotics, probiotics, and prebiotics. Gastroenterology 2004;126:1620–1633.
252 Wild GE: The role of antibiotics in the management of Crohn's disease. Inflamm Bowel Dis 2004;10:321–323.
253 Bendesky A, Menendez D, Ostrosky-Wegman P: Is metronidazole carcinogenic? Mutat Res 2002;511:133–144.
254 Kadam UT, Jordan K, Croft PR: Clinical comorbidity in patients with osteoarthritis: A case-control study of general practice consulters in England and Wales. Ann Rheum Dis 2004;63: 408–414.
255 Borelli G, Bertoli D: Acute, subacute, chronictoxicity and mutagenicity studies of rifaximin (L/105) in rats. Chemioterapia (Florence) 1986;5:263–267.
256 Mackie RI, White BA, Bryant MP: Lipid metabolism in anaerobic ecosystems. Crit Rev Microbiol 1991;17:449–479.
257 Kramer PJ: Genetic toxicology. J Pharm Pharmacol 1998;50:395–405.
258 Mortelmans K, Zeiger E: The Ames Salmonella/microsome mutagenicity assay. Mutat Res 2000;455:29–60.
259 Murthy MS: Induction of gene conversion in diploid yeast by chemicals: Correlation with mutagenic action and its relevance in genotoxicity screening. Mutat Res 1979;64:1–17.
260 Bertoli D, Borelli G: Teratogenic action of Rifaximin in the rat and rabbit and its effect on perinatal development in the rat. Boll Soc Ital Biol Sper 1984;60:1079–1085.
261 Bertoli D, Borelli G: Fertility study of rifaximin (L/105) in rats. Chemioterapia (Florence) 1986;5:204–207.
262 Burns LM: Rifaximin: Study of Effects on Embryo-Fetal Toxicity in the Rabbit by Oral Gavage Administration. Final Report. Eye, Huntington Life Sciences, 1998.
263 Physicians' Desk Reference: Use-in-Pregnancy Ratings, ed 58. Montvale, Medical Economics Company, 2004.
264 Fulcher SM: Rifaximin Combined Study of Effects on Fertility and Embryo-Fetal Toxicity in CD Rats by Oral Gavage Administration. Eye, Huntington Life Sciences, 2000.
265 Wu G, Bazer FW, Cudd TA, Meininger CJ, Spencer TE: Maternal nutrition and fetal development. J Nutr 2004;134:2169–2172.
266 Hamed MR, al-Assy YS, Ezzeldin E: Influence of protein malnutrition on teratogenicity of acetylsalicylic acid in rats. Hum Exp Toxicol 1994;13:83–88.
267 Meyers D: Rifaximin: Study of Effect on Embryo-Fetal Toxicity in the Rabbit by Oral Gavage Administration. Report Amendment 1. Eye, Huntington Life Sciences, 2001.
268 European Commission – Enterprise and Industry DG – Pharmaceutical Unit: Detection of Toxicity to Reproduction for Medicinal Products Including Toxicity to Male Fertility (Directive 75/318/ EEG – June 1996). Available at: http://pharmacos.eudra.org/F2/eudralex/vol-3/pdfs-en/ 3bs4aen.pdf.
269 Czeizel AE, Rockenbauer M, Olsen J, Sorensen HT: A population-based case-control study of the safety of oral anti-tuberculosis drug treatment during pregnancy. Int J Tuberc Lung Dis 2001;5: 564–568.
270 Ito S, Lee A: Drug excretion into breast milk – Overview. Adv Drug Deliv Rev 2003;55:617–627.
271 Czeizel AE, Rockenbauer M, Olsen J, Sorensen HT: A teratological study of aminoglycoside antibiotic treatment during pregnancy. Scand J Infect Dis 2000;32:309–313.
272 DuPont HL, Ericsson CD: Prevention and treatment of traveler's diarrhea. New Engl J Med 1993;328:1821–1827.
273 Martini S, Bonechi C, Corbini G, Donati A, Rossi C: Solution structure of rifaximin and its synthetic derivative rifaximin OR determined by experimental NMR and theoretical simulation methods. Bioorg Med Chem 2004;12:2163–2172.

274 Wanlian Pharmaceutical Co.: Rifaximin Soft Capsule Composition. Patent No. CN1451386, 2002.
275 Dalseno R, Chiarelli P: Controlled and Continued Delivery of Rifaximin and/or Other Substances. Patent No. WO200441240, 2003.

Note Added in Proof

The antibacterial activity of rifaximin has recently been confirmed in a clinical pharmacological study [1]. Two groups of healthy volunteers pretreated with either rifaximin (200 mg t.i.d. for 3 days) or placebo were challenged after the 4th dose of the antibiotic with *Shigella flexneri* 2a (1,000–1,500 CFU). The incidence of diarrhea was 0% in the rifaximin group compared with 60% in the placebo group ($p = 0.001$ at Fisher's exact test). The results of this study support the use of rifaximin in the *prevention* of infectious diarrhea in the traveler (TD). And indeed, DuPont et al. [2] have just reported that even once daily administration of rifaximin is able to prevent TD. The same team of investigators [3] has shown that up to 28% of the patients who developed TD still complain of chronic symptoms (namely loose stools, abdominal pain and fecal urgency) 6 months after the travel and that 11% of them met the Rome II criteria for irritable bowel syndrome. These findings underline the high incidence of postinfectious complications of TD and call for the use of antibiotic prophylaxis to prevent long-lasting complaints in the returning traveler.

References

1 Taylor DN, MacKenzie R, Durbin A, Carpenter C, Atzinger CB, Haake R, Bourgeois AL: Double-blind, placebo-controlled trial to evaluate the use of rifaximin (200 mg TID) to prevent diarrhea in volunteers challenged with *Shigella flexneri* 2a (2457T). Am J Trop Med Hyg 2004;71(suppl 4): 1–303 [Abstract #2079].
2 DuPont HL, Jiang ZD, Ericsson CD, de la Cabada F, Shi K, DuPont MW, Martinez-Sandoval F: Rifaximin, a nonabsorbed (0.5%) antibiotic, prevents travelers diarrhea (TD). Gastroenterology 2004;126(suppl 2):A12.
3 Okhuysen PC, Jiang ZD, Carlin L, Forbes C, DuPont HL: Post-diarrhea chronic intestinal symptoms and irritable bowel syndrome in North American travelers to Mexico. Am J Gastroenterol 2004;99:1774–1778.

Prof. Carmelo Scarpignato, MD, DSc, PharmD, FCP, FACG
Laboratory of Clinical Pharmacology, School of Medicine and Dentistry
University of Parma, Via Volturno, 39, IT-43100 Parma (Italy)
Tel. +39 0521 903863, eFax +1 603 8435621, E-Mail scarpi@tin.it

This chapter should be cited as follows:

Scarpignato C, Pelosini I: Rifaximin, a Poorly Absorbed Antibiotic: Pharmacology and Clinical Potential. Chemotherapy 2005;51(suppl 1):36–66.

Scarpignato C (ed): Rifaximin: A Poorly Absorbed Antibiotic.
Pharmacology and Clinical Use.

Rifaximin: In vitro and in vivo Antibacterial Activity

A Review

Zhi-Dong Jiang[a], *H.L. DuPont*[a,b]

[a]Center for Infectious Diseases, University of Texas-Houston School of Public Health,
[b]St. Luke's Episcopal Hospital and Baylor College of Medicine, Houston, Tex., USA

Abstract

In vitro inhibitory activity of rifaximin is directed against Gram-positive and Gram-negative, aerobic and anaerobic bacteria. It is effective in the treatment of gastrointestinal infections when given orally because of the high concentration of the drug remaining in the gut lumen. Laboratory investigations have been carried out to assess the in vitro activity of rifaximin on different bacterial strains isolated from both human and domestic animals. The objective of this project is to review the in vitro and in vivo activity of rifaximin against bacterial infection with Gram-negative rods, Gram-positive rods and Gram-positive cocci and their resistance to rifaximin. The available data suggest that rifaximin is active in vitro and in vivo in the treatment of bacterial infection of adults and children.

Introduction

Rifaximin (4-deoxy-4′-methylpyrido-[1′,2′-1′2′] imidazo[5,4-C] rifamycin SV) is a semisynthetic antibiotic molecule belonging to the rifamycin group [1] and synthesized by Alfa Wassermann (Bologna, Italy). Contrary to its structural analogue, rifaximin's chemical and physical properties do not allow its absorption following oral administration [2]. This feature prompted researchers to investigate the drug as a topical antimicrobial agent capable of acting against intestinal bacteria without causing systemic side effects.

Rifaximin is available in Europe for the treatment of acute intestinal bacterial infections, hepatic encephalopathy, bacterial overgrowth syndrome, diverticular disease of the colon, and for the prevention of infections after colorectal surgery [3, 4]. Rifaximin is also licensed in Mexico, Asia and Northern Africa and has recently been approved in USA for the treatment of traveler's diarrhea.

Rifaximin shows in vitro activity against a broad range of enteric pathogens. The minimal inhibitory concentration (MIC) at which 90% of isolates are inhibited (MIC_{90}) is 16–50 μg/ml for the various bacterial enteropathogens [5]. Ordinarily, isolates at this level of susceptibility would be considered 'resistant'. However, the drug is active against bacterial enteropathogens in vivo, which is explained by the extremely high luminal levels of the drug when it is administered orally. The fecal levels were in the range of 4,000–8,000 μg/g stool in a previous study [5]. The objective of this project is to review the in vitro and in vivo activity of rifaximin against bacterial infection.

Mechanism of Action

The mechanism of action of rifaximin depends on the inhibition of DNA-dependent RNA polymerase of the target microorganisms, leading to the suppression of initiation of chain formation in RNA synthesis.

Pharmacology

Animal and human studies have demonstrated that rifaximin has very poor intestinal absorption after oral administration, so that blood and urine concentrations of rifaximin are practically undetectable [6]. Rifaximin excretion is almost completely by the fecal route [5]. Therefore, when rifaximin is administered by the oral route, it acts locally at the intestinal level and eliminates the bacterial organisms that are causing the infection. The important antibacterial activity of rifaximin appears to be directly related to the high intestinal concentration of the drug and inhibition of bacterial growth. The drug has been used successfully in the treatment of infectious diarrhea in adults and children [7, 8], with low potential for inducing resistance by infecting bacterial strains [9].

Gram-Negative Rods Identified from Patients with Gastrointestinal Diseases

Diarrhea affects approximately 40% of travelers to tropical and semitropical areas of the developing world [10]. In up to 50–80% of patients with travelers' diarrhea, enteric bacterial pathogens are identified as the cause [11]. The important causes of travelers' diarrhea include enterotoxigenic *Escherichia coli*

Table 1. In vitro susceptibility to rifaximin (MIC) of enteric pathogens isolated from patients with bacterial diarrhea from multiple areas of the world [Mathewson et al., unpubl. data] [17, 18]

Species	Number of isolates	MIC_{50} μg/ml	MIC_{90} μg/ml	MIC range μg/ml
Aeromonas spp.	27	16	128	16 to > 256
Campylobacter jejuni	54	12.5	>100	0.78 to > 100
Campylobacter spp.	35	32	128	0.25 to > 256
Enteroaggregative *E. coli*	50	64	128	16 to > 256
Enterohemorrhagic *E. coli*	17	64	>256	32 to > 256
Enteroinvasive *E. coli*	20	64	128	8 to > 256
ETEC	153	64	128	8 to 256
ETEC with LT	50	64	256	8 to > 256
ETEC with ST	76	64	128	8 to > 256
ETEC with ST and LT	27	64	128	32 to > 256
Plesiomonas shigelloides	25	64	256	16 to > 256
Salmonella spp.	53	64	128	8 to > 256
Shigella spp.	88	64	128	32 to > 256
Vibrio spp.[1]	25	128	128	8 to 128
Yersinia spp.	91	12.5	25	0.2 to 25

LT = Heat-labile toxin; ST = heat-stable toxin.
[1] *Vibrio* spp. include non-cholera-causing vibrios.

(ETEC) [11], enteroaggregative *E. coli* [12], *Salmonella* spp., *Shigella* spp., *Campylobacter* spp., *Plesiomonas shigelloides*, *Aeromonas* spp. and non-cholera-causing vibrios [11]. Since bacterial agents appear to be responsible for most causes of travelers' diarrhea and an important part of more severe diarrhea in children and adults in developing countries and industrialized regions, antimicrobial agents have become important for the treatment of this disease. Previous studies have shown that nonabsorbable antibacterial drugs were highly effective in treating travelers' diarrhea [13–15].

When bacterial isolates from patients with travelers' diarrhea from four geographic areas were tested [16], rifaximin was shown to have an MIC at which 50% of the isolates tested were inhibited (MIC_{50}) of 12.5–128 μg/ml. The MIC_{90} was 25 to >256 μg/ml. The results of in vitro susceptibility testing of specific enteric bacterial pathogens to rifaximin from three published studies [Mathewson et al., unpubl. data] [17, 18] are given in table 1. Differences were seen for individual enteric bacterial pathogens but no overall pattern of increased or decreased susceptibility was seen with the tested pathogens.

Table 2. Activity of rifaximin (μg/ml) against isolates of *H. pylori* according to the pH of the culture medium [20, 21]

Number of strains	pH 6.0			pH 7.2		
	MIC_{50}	MIC_{90}	MIC range	MIC_{50}	MIC_{90}	MIC range
30	4	4	0.5–8	1	2	0.25–4
43	2	8	0.5–8	NA	NA	NA

NA = Not available.

Helicobacter pylori has received much attention as a cause of gastritis, peptic ulcer and gastric cancer. In developing countries, the organism is acquired early in childhood, and up to 90% of children are infected by the age of 5 [19]. As the evidence linking *H. pylori* and gastric disease is impressive, eradication of *H. pylori* could reduce the rate of duodenal ulcer relapse and possibly gastric cancer. Megraud et al. [20] studied 43 *H. pylori* strains isolated from patients with gastritis for in vitro rifaximin activity (table 2). Rifaximin, amoxicillin and colloidal bismuth subcitrate all appeared to be active against *H. pylori* [20]. The MIC of rifaximin was influenced by the pH of the culture medium, with the agent being more active at basic pH. In another study, a total of 20 patients with *H. pylori* chronic gastritis were enrolled in a clinical trial of rifaximin. The trial demonstrated efficacy of rifaximin as treatment for *H. pylori* infection without important clinical side effects [21].

Gram-Positive Rods – *Mycobacterium* Identified from Patients with Tuberculosis

Tuberculosis remains a major global public health problem. The World Health Organization estimates that there are 8 million new cases of tuberculosis and 3 million deaths directly attributable to tuberculosis each year [22]. Drug resistance is a serious problem worldwide. In a study in New York City, 33% of patients with tuberculosis were infected by organisms resistant to at least one antituberculosis drug, and 19% were infected by organisms resistant to both INH and rifampin [23], the first-line drugs in the treatment of tuberculosis.

Mycobacteria are also killed in vitro, as expected from an antibiotic sharing the properties of the rifamycin family [24]. In a study by Soro et al. [25],

Table 3. In vitro antibacterial activity of rifaximin against anaerobic bacteria [24, 27, 28]

	Number of isolates	Source of isolates	MICs, μg/ml		
			MIC range	MIC_{50}	MIC_{90}
Bifidobacterium spp.	6	Cirrhotic patients, Italy	0.4–50	0.8	6.2
Clostridium difficile	4	Cirrhotic patients, Italy	0.2–0.8	0.2	0.8
Clostridium difficile	93	Human, Italy	0.004–128	0.004	128
Clostridium perfringens	15	Various clinical material, unknown location	Unknown	Unknown	4
Clostridium spp.	26	Cirrhotic patients, Italy	0.0125 to >100	0.4	50
Propionibacterium spp.	10	Cirrhotic patients, Italy	0.025–12.5	0.2	12.5

the MIC of rifaximin was determined for five *Mycobacterium tuberculosis* isolates from patients with tuberculosis. MIC concentrations were studied at 6, 20, 90 and 270 μg/ml, respectively. No resistant organisms were found. Growing *M. tuberculosis* in the presence of varying doses of rifaximin did not induce the occurrence of rifampicin-resistant strains [25]. In addition to this, experimental tubercular infection in the guinea pig was found not to be affected by an oral treatment course with rifaximin, therefore confirming the lack of absorption of the molecule after oral administration [26].

Anaerobic Bacteria – *Clostridium*

Rifaximin has been shown to possess good antibacterial activity against a variety of anaerobic bacteria (table 3) [24, 27, 28]. Anaerobes have been shown to be capable of producing ammonia (especially *Clostridia*), which has been incriminated in the pathogenesis of hepatic encephalopathy [29]. The authors suggested that since rifaximin is a nonabsorbable and effective antibiotic against anaerobic flora, it would be an ideal treatment for patients with compromised hepatic function. *Eubacterium* is inhibited by rifaximin with an MIC_{90} $\leq$2 μg/ml [27].

Gram-Positive Cocci

Streptococcus, Enterococcus and *Straphylococcus* are clinically the most important of the Gram-positive cocci. Table 4 shows the range of MIC of

Table 4. In vitro activity of rifaximin against Gram-positive cocci [27, 30, 31]

	Number tested	MIC_{50}, μg/ml	MIC_{90}, μg/ml	MIC range, μg/ml
Staphylococcus aureus	51	0.015	>8	≤0.01 to >8
Staphylococcus epidermidis	20	≤0.015	≤0.015	≤0.015
Staphylococcus haemolyticus	10	≤0.015	≤0.015	≤0.015 to >8
Enterococcus faecalis	21	2	8	0.5 to >8
Enterococcus faecium	11	2	>8	≤0.015 to >8
Enterococcus spp.	10	0.25	2	≤0.015 to >4
Streptococcus group A	19	0.12	0.25	≤0.03 to 0.25
Streptococcus group B	20	0.12	0.25	0.06 to 0.25
Streptococcus groups C, F and G	14	≤0.03	0.06	≤0.03 to 0.5
Streptococcus pneumoniae	30	≤0.03	0.06	≤0.03 to >4

rifaximin for 206 Gram-positive cocci where the MIC_{50} was ≤0.015–2 μg/ml for the tested strains [27, 30, 31]. The MIC_{90} was ≤0.015 to >8 μg/ml. Since Gram-positive cocci cause severe systemic infection, an orally administered drug without absorption would play no role in the therapy of these infections.

In vivo Rifaximin Activity in Intestinal Infections

Antimicrobial agents play an important role in the treatment of enteric infections caused by certain pathogens [32]. Several studies have been carried out to assess the effectiveness of rifaximin for eradication of causative bacterial enteropathogens [15, 33]. ETEC was the principal pathogen identified in these studies, since the target populations were travelers from industrialized countries to developing countries. The microbiologic eradication rates for rifaximin versus ciprofloxacin were not statistically significant. Furthermore, rifaximin has been shown to shorten the duration of bacterial diarrhea in children and diarrhea due to ETEC, *Shigella* and *Salmonella* in nontravelers and to shorten the duration of excretion of the infecting organism [8].

Interestingly, in a small study on patients with AIDS, rifaximin was found to be effective against infectious diarrhea with stool cultures positive for protozoal pathogens, such as *Cryptosporidium parvum* and *Blastocystis hominis* [34]. The favorable effects of rifaximin on protozoal diarrhea have been also reported in a recent multi-center study on patients with travelers' diarrhea [33]. In fact, patients with pretreatment stools positive for *Cryptosporidium* infections obtained a clinical improvement with rifaximin significantly superior to the placebo-treated subjects.

Rifaximin Resistance

Two concerns with all antimicrobial agents intended for oral administration are the risk of depleting normal gut flora and the potential to induce antibacterial resistance. These aspects have been studied in several trials.

Minimal effects on intestinal flora were seen with rifaximin administration [9, 35]. In an early study, performed on healthy volunteers who received a short-term (5 days) rifaximin treatment, the observed changes in bowel flora returned to baseline levels within 1–2 weeks [9]. In a recent investigation fecal samples of patients with ulcerative colitis given three 10 day courses of the antibiotic were cultured and the different microbial species quantitated. Despite the high dose (i.e. 1800 mg daily) of rifaximin used there was only a minor change in bacterial counts which reverted back to pre-treatment values during the washout period [35]. It appears therefore that administration of this antibiotic does not disrupt intestinal microbial ecology.

Development of resistance to rifaximin is primarily due to a chromosomal one-step alteration in the drug target, DNA-dependent RNA polymerase. This differs from the plasmid-mediated resistance commonly acquired by bacteria to aminoglycoside antibiotics such as neomycin [36]. In a recent study, we found no acquisition of rifaximin resistance in 27 rifaximin-treated subjects colonized by *Enterococcus* [37]. The MIC_{50} and MIC_{90} for the treatment group (rifaximin at a dose of either 400 or 200 mg twice daily for 3 days) were similar (16–64 μg/ml). In two published studies, rifaximin resistance was shown to occur in the bacterial flora of individuals who received treatment with rifaximin at a dose of 800 mg/day for 5 days [9, 27]. Within 1–2 weeks after the end of rifaximin treatment, resistance rates appeared to have decreased to less than 20% of the intestinal flora. The resistant strains detected during treatment appeared to be unstable and unable to persistently colonize the intestinal tract.

The available data suggest that bacterial resistance does not seem to be a major concern of the therapy with rifaximin. However, further monitoring of the occurrence of bacterial resistance to rifaximin would help to clearly define its clinical importance.

Conclusion

The available in vitro and in vivo studies suggest that rifaximin is active in the treatment of intestinal infections of adults and children.

References

1 Marchi E, Mascellani G, Montecchi L, Brufani M, Cellai L: L/105, a new semisynthetic derivative of rifamycin SV, synthesis and structure-activity relationship. Chemioterapia 1983;2:38.

2 Venturini AP: L/105: Report on pharmacokinetics in rats, dogs, after oral administration and adverse reactions. Proceedings of III Mediterranean Congress of Chemotherapy, 21–24 September 1982 – Dubrovnik, Yugoslavia. Chemioterapia 1983;2(suppl 5):162–163.

3 Gillis J, Brogden R: Rifaximin. A review of its antibacterial activity, pharmacokinetic properties and therapeutic potential in conditions mediated by gastrointestinal bacteria. Drugs 1995;49:467–484.

4 Corazza GR, Ventrucci M, Strocchi A, Sorge M, Pranzo L, Pezzilli R, Gasbarrini G: Treatment of small intestine bacterial overgrowth with rifaximin, a non-absorbable rifamycin. J Int Med Res 1988;16:312–316.

5 Jiang ZD, Ke S, Palazzini E, Riopel L, DuPont HL: In vitro activity and fecal concentration of rifaximin after oral administration. Antimicrob Agents Chemother 2000;44:2205–2206.

6 Venturini AP: Pharmacokinetics of L/105, a new rifamycin, in rats and dogs, after oral administration. Chemotherapy 1983;29:1–3.

7 DuPont HL, Jiang ZD, Ericsson CD, Mathewson JJ, Adachi J, Palazzini E, Riopel LM, Ashley D, Martinez-Sandoval F: Rifaximin for the treatment of travelers' diarrhea: A randomized, double-blind clinical trial versus ciprofloxacin. Clin Infect Dis, submitted.

8 Sanfilippo A, Raciti Longo G, Raciti Longo A: Clinical experience with rifaximin in pediatric diarrhea syndromes. Med Praxis 1984;5:375–379.

9 De-Leo C, Eftimiadi C, Schito GC: Rapid disappearance from the intestinal tract of bacteria resistant to rifaximin. Drugs Exp Clin Res 1986;12:979–981.

10 von Sonnenburg F, Tornieporth N, Waiyaki P, Lowe B, Peruski LF Jr, DuPont HL, Mathewson JJ, Steffen R: Risk and aetiology of diarrhoea at various tourist destinations. Lancet 2000;356:133–134.

11 Jiang ZD, Lowe B, Vernekar MP, Ashley D, Steffen R, Tornieporth N, von Sonnenburg F, Svennerholm AM, Waiyaki P, DuPont HL: Prevalence of enteric pathogens among international travelers with diarrhea acquired in Kenya (Mombasa), India (Goa), or Jamaica (Montego Bay). J Infect Dis 2002;185:497–502.

12 Adachi J, Jiang ZD, Mathewson JJ, Verenkar MP, Thompson S, Martinez-Sandoval F, Steffen R, Ericsson CD, DuPont HL: Enteroaggregative *Escherichia coli* as a major etiologic agent in traveler's diarrhea in 3 regions of the world. Clin Infect Dis 2001;32:1706–1709.

13 DuPont HL, Ericsson CD, Mathewson JJ, de la Cabada FJ, Conrad D: Oral aztreonam, a poorly absorbed yet effective therapy for bacterial diarrhea in US travelers to Mexico. JAMA 1992;267: 1932–1935.

14 Ericsson CD, DuPont HL, Sullivan P, Galindo E, Evans DG, Evans DJ Jr: Bicozamycin, a poorly absorbable antibiotic, effectively treats travelers' diarrhea. Ann Intern Med 1983;98:20–25.

15 DuPont HL, Ericsson CD, Mathewson JJ, Palazzini E, DuPont MW, Jiang ZD, Mosavi A, de la Cabada FJ: Rifaximin: A nonabsorbed antimicrobial in the therapy of travelers' diarrhea. Digestion 1998;59:708–714.

16 Gomi H, Jiang ZD, Adachi JA, Ashley D, Lowe B, Verenkar MP, Steffen R, DuPont HL: In vitro antimicrobial susceptibility testing of bacterial enteropathogens causing travelers' diarrhea in four geographic regions. Antimicrob Agents Chemother 2001;45:212–216.

17 Sierra JM, Ruiz J, Navia MM, Vargas M, Gascon J, Vila J: In vitro activity of rifaximin against enteropathogens producing traveler's diarrhea. Antimicrob Agents Chemother 2001;45:643–644.

18 Mignini F, Falcioni E, Prenna M, Santacroce F, Ripa S: Antibacterial activity of rifaximin against *Clostridium difficile, Campylobacter jejuni* and *Yersinia* spp. J Chemother 1989;1:220–222.

19 Ng BL, Ng HC, Goh KT, Ho B: *Helicobacter pylori* in familial clusters based on antibody profile. FEMS Immunol Med Microbiol 2001;30:139–142.

20 Megraud F, Bouffant F, Camou-Juncas C: In vitro activity of rifaximin against *Helicobacter pylori.* Eur J Clin Microbiol Infect Dis 1994;13:184–186.

21 Dell'Anna A, Azzarone P, Ferrieri A: A randomized openly comparative study between rifaximin suspension versus rifaximin pills for the eradication of *Helicobacter pylori.* Eur Rev Med Pharmacol Sci 1999;3:105–110.

22 Raviglione MC, Snider DE, Kochi A: Global epidemiology of tuberculosis. Morbidity and mortality of a worldwide epidemic. JAMA 1995;273:241–242.
23 Frieden TR, Sterling T, Pablos-Mendez A, Kilburn JO, Cauthen GM, Dooley SW: The emergence of drug-resistant tuberculosis in New York City. N Engl J Med 1993;328:521–526.
24 Lamanna A, Orsi A: In vitro activity of rifaximin and rifampicin against some anaerobic bacteria. Chemioterapia 1984;3:365–367.
25 Soro O, Pesce A, Raggi M, Debbia E, Shito C: Selection of rifampicin-resistant *Mycobacterium tuberculosis* does not occur in the presence of low concentrations of rifaximin. Clin Microbiol Infect 1997;3:147–151.
26 Lucchesi M, Marchi E, Venturini AP: Antimycobacterial activity of rifaximin (L/105) in experimental tuberculosis in the Guinea pig. Chemioterapia 1984;3:371–372.
27 Eftimiadi C, Deleo C, Schito GC: Treatment of hepatic encephalopathy with L/105, a new non-absorbable rifamycin. Drugs Exp Clin Res 1984;10:691–696.
28 Marchese A, Salerno A, Pesce A, Debbia EA, Schito GC: In vitro activity of rifaximin, metronidazole and vancomycin against *Clostridium difficile* and the rate of selection of spontaneously resistant mutants against representative anaerobic and aerobic bacteria, including ammonia-producing species. Chemotherapy 2000;46:253–266.
29 Crossley IR, Wardle EN, Williams R: Biochemical mechanisms of hepatic encephalopathy. Clin Sci (Lond) 1983;64:247–252.
30 Hoover W, Gerlach E, Hoban D, Eliopoulos G, Pfaller M, Jones R: Antimicrobial activity and spectrum of rifaximin. A new topical rifamycin derivative. Diagn Microbiol Infect Dis 1993;16:111–118.
31 Venturini AP, Marchi E: In vitro and in vivo evaluation of L/105, a new topical intestinal rifamycin. Chemioterapia 1986;5:257–262.
32 DuPont HL, Reves R, Galindo R, Sullivan P, Wood L, Mendiola J: Treatment of travelers' diarrhea with trimethoprim/sulfamethoxazole and with trimethoprim alone. N Engl J Med 1982;307: 841–844.
33 Steffen R, Sack DA, Riopel L, Jiang Z-D, Sturchler M, Ericsson CD, Lowe B, Waiyaki P, White M, DuPont HL: Therapy of travelers' diarrhea with rifaximin on various continents. Am J Gastroenterol 2003;98:1073–1078
34 Amenta M, Dalle Nogare ER, Colomba D, Prestileo TS, Di Lorenzo F, Fundaro S, Colomba A, Ferrieri A: Intestinal protozoa in HIV-infected patients: Effect of rifaximin in Cryptosporidium parvum and Blastocystis hominis infections. J Chemother 1999;11:391–395.
35 Brigidi P, Swennen E, Rizzello F, Bozzolasco M, Matteuzzi D: Effect of rifaximin administration on the intestinal microbiota in patients with ulcerative colitis. J Chemother (Florence) 2002;14(3): 290–295.
36 Neu HC: The crisis in antibiotic resistance. Science 1992;257:1064–1073.
37 DuPont HL, Jiang ZD: Influence of rifaximin treatment on the susceptibility of intestinal Gram-negative flora and enterococci. Clin Microbiol Infect 2004;10:1009–1011.

Dr. Zhi-Dong Jiang
University of Texas School of Public Health
1200 Herman Pressler Room 706, Houston, TX 77030 (USA)
Tel. +1 713 500 9375, Fax +1 713 500 9364, E-Mail zjiang@sph.uth.tmc.edu

This chapter should be cited as follows:

Jianga Z-D, DuPont HL: Rifaximin: In vitro and in vivo Antibacterial Activity – A Review. Chemotherapy 2005;51(suppl 1):67–72.

Scarpignato C (ed): Rifaximin: A Poorly Absorbed Antibiotic.
Pharmacology and Clinical Use.

Rifaximin in the Treatment of Infectious Diarrhea

Charles D. Ericsson[a], *Herbert L. DuPont*[a,b]

[a]Department of Internal Medicine and Division of Infectious Diseases, University of Texas Houston Medical School, [b]St. Luke's Episcopal Hospital and Baylor College of Medicine, Houston, Tex., USA

Abstract

Rifaximin matches the criteria for an ideal agent for the treatment of infectious diarrhea. It has excellent activity against a broad range of enteropathogens. It is nonabsorbable, which may help explain its excellent side effect profile and lack of emergence of resistance because of high stool levels that are not likely to reach subinhibitory levels before the target Gram-negative bacilli are killed. It has shown excellent efficacy in numerous clinical trials of bacterial diarrhea. Because of the lack of systemic absorption and minimal adverse reactions, rifaximin should be useful in treating hosts such as pregnant women in whom the currently favored fluoroquinolones are contraindicated. Uses limited to enteric indications and its inherently low propensity to induce sustainable resistance among Gram-negative flora favor the sustained usefulness of rifaximin in the treatment of enteric infectious syndromes.

Introduction

Antibiotics have a recognized role in the treatment of culture-proven bacterial causes of symptomatic enteric infection such as *Shigella* spp., *Campylobacter jejuni* and *Salmonella typhi*. The use of antibiotics in the treatment of nontyphoidal salmonellosis is controversial, but the consensus is generally not to treat with antibiotics unless the patient is elderly or has another condition that predisposes to bacteremia. Also, when infection with enterohemorrhagic *Escherichia coli* is suspected in children, the consensus is not to use antibiotics because of the concern of increasing the risk of hemolytic uremic syndrome.

While fluid replacement remains the classic cornerstone of the treatment of diarrhea, especially in children, empiric antibiotic treatment is logical in certain situations. Children and adults with diarrhea and signs and symptoms suggestive of dysentery (fever, tenesmus, bloody, mucoid stools) can be given empiric antibiotics awaiting culture results. Severe diarrhea is more likely to be associated with bacterial causes. Some hosts and groups commonly have bacterial causes of their diarrhea even without clinical evidence of invasive pathogens, and the empiric use of antibiotics can be supported in such cases. Examples include diarrhea in patients with AIDS, in those with the so-called 'gay bowel syndrome' and in those traveling from developed to developing regions of the world.

As proposed in earlier publications, an ideal antimicrobial agent for the treatment of bacterial causes of infectious diarrhea would have the following features [1, 2]: (1) excellent activity against a broad range of bacterial enteropathogens; (2) nonabsorbable; (3) favorable side effect profile; (4) efficacious in the treatment of infectious diarrhea; (5) major indication is enteric disease, and (6) does not easily develop resistance or promote cross-resistance.

Is rifaximin, a rifampin-like antimicrobial agent that inhibits bacterial synthesis of RNA, an ideal agent for the treatment of bacterial diarrhea? A critical examination of all the theoretic points suggests that it is the case.

Activity against Enteropathogens

First, rifaximin does have excellent activity against a broad range of enteropathogens. A problem is the definition of activity. Typically, a clinically acceptably low minimal inhibitory concentration (MIC) of an antibiotic is defined in terms of the pharmacokinetics of the antibiotic measured in serum. For some antibiotics (e.g. aminoglycosides), success is predicted by how much the concentration achieved in serum exceeds the MIC. For others (e.g. betalactam antibiotics), success is predicted by the percentage of the dosing interval that the serum level remains above the MIC. If an antibiotic like rifaximin is not absorbed, achieves concentrations in stool that far exceed the MIC of an organism and persists in stool at levels that exceed the MIC for days, clinical efficacy against the enteropathogen can be predicted.

When rifaximin is taken at clinical doses of 400 mg twice a day for 3 days, stool concentrations are high over the ensuing 5 days [3]. In that study, peak stool concentrations averaged nearly 8,000 μg/g, and remained in the range of 2–3,000 μg/g on days 4 and 5 after cessation of antibiotics [3]. In this same study, the authors measured the MIC at which 50% of the isolates were inhibited (MIC_{50}) and the MIC at which 90% of the isolates were inhibited (MIC_{90}) for 145 bacterial enteropathogens. The exact number of enterotoxigenic *E. coli* (ETEC), *Salmonella*, *Shigella* and other enteropathogens was not specified, but 50% of all bacterial isolates were inhibited at 12.5 μg/g and 90%

Table 1. Rifaximin MIC_{90} values for common enteropathogens causing travelers' diarrhea

Enteropathogen	Gomi et al. [4]		Sierra et al. [5]		DuPont et al. [6]		Peak stool concentration[3]/ MIC_{90}
	n	MIC_{90}, μg/g	n	MIC_{90}, μg/g	n	MIC_{90}, μg/g	
ETEC (Enterotoxic *E. coli*)	97	32	38	16	72	32	250–500
EAEC	75	32	28	16	–	–	250–500
Salmonella spp.	46	64	14	4	9	16–32	125–2,000
Shigella spp.	36	64	64	16	11	32–64	125–500
Campylobacter jejuni	9	32	12	512	–	–	15–250
Others	21[1]	4	11[2]	8	–	–	1,000–2,000

Gomi et al. [4] studied patients with diarrhea acquired in India, Mexico, Jamaica and Kenya, Sierra et al. [5] studied diarrhea in travelers returning to Spain from multiple locations, and DuPont et al. [6] studied patients with diarrhea acquired in Mexico. EAEC = Enteroaggregative *E. coli.*

[1]Includes noncholera vibrios, *Plesiomonas shigelloides* and *Aeromonas* spp.

[2]*Aeromonas* spp.

[3]7,961 μg/g [3].

were inhibited at 50 μg/g. The MIC ranges for ETEC and *Salmonella* were 0.098–200 μg/g. The MIC range for *Shigella* was 1.25–200 μg/g. Peak stool concentrations of rifaximin exceeded the MICs of these enteropathogens by 40- to over 80,000-fold. Defining susceptible as a ratio of stool concentration to MIC exceeding 1 during the anticipated dosing interval of 3–5 days, diarrheal illness caused by all of the 145 enteropathogens would be predicted to respond to treatment by rifaximin. As shown in table 1, Gomi et al. [4] determined the rifaximin MICs of 284 bacterial enteropathogens from four different locations around the world: India, Mexico, Jamaica and Kenya. Sierra et al. [5] determined the MICs of organisms causing diarrhea in travelers returning to Spain from various regions of the world. Table 1 also includes selected organisms from a comparative study of rifaximin versus ciprofloxacin in the treatment of travelers' diarrhea conducted by DuPont et al. [6] in Mexico. Taken in aggregate, these data show a consistent theme. Rifaximin MICs for common enteropathogens are similar from disparate regions of the world. Most MICs hover in the 32–64 μg/g range. Even relatively high MICs for *Campylobacter* noted by Sierra et al. [5] (but not by Gomi et al. [4]) are exceeded 15- to 250-fold by the concentrations of rifaximin achieved in stool.

Finally, one report of diarrhea in HIV-positive patients indicated that rifaximin might well prove useful in the treatment of protozoal causes of infectious diarrhea [4]. Thirteen patients had infections with *Cryptosporidium parvum.*

Lack of Absorption

The second feature of an ideal antibiotic for infectious diarrhea is that it should not be absorbed. Among 18 adult volunteers who received a 400-mg dose, no rifaximin was detected in serum 4 h later in 9 subjects, and the highest detected levels in the remaining 9 subjects was 5.3 ng/ml. The mean recovery in urine from a 400-mg dose was 0.007% in the first 24 h with a negligible amount detected in the second 24 h after the dose [7]. Furthermore, absorption of rifaximin is only minimally affected by colonic inflammation. Twelve subjects with mild to moderate ulcerative colitis took 400-mg doses. In only 4 subjects were levels ranging from 2 to 4.6 ng/ml noted irregularly, and 2 further subjects had single values of 13.4 and 22.4 ng/ml measured. The mean recovery in urine in the first 24 h was 0.009% [8]. That rifaximin is virtually non-absorbed is clear from these and other studies [9]. The reason that this is potentially important is that adverse reactions can be predicted to be higher for drugs with systemic absorption. A nonabsorbed drug should prove to be safe for special hosts like children and pregnant women.

Lack of absorption, however, was once considered to weigh against the predicted efficacy of an antibiotic in the treatment of bacterial diarrhea. Haltalin et al. [10] many years ago compared the efficacy of ampicillin with a non-absorbable aminoglycoside in the treatment of shigellosis. When the patients in the aminoglycoside arm failed to respond as those treated with ampicillin, the authors concluded that only an absorbable drug should be used in the treatment of bacterial diarrhea. It was later realized that poorly absorbed antimicrobials could be of value in the treatment of enteric infections. Indeed, oral bicozamycin and aztreonam proved to be efficacious in treating bacterial diarrhea, including cases caused by *Shigella* [11, 12].

Favorable Side Effect Profile

As might be expected from a nonabsorbed drug, the side effect profile of rifaximin has been shown to be excellent. Gillis and Brogden [9] summarized multiple studies in their excellent review of rifaximin. Although 963 patient experiences from 30 clinical studies were summarized, not all studies discussed drug tolerance specifically. Overall, only a handful of adverse events were recorded: 5 cases of flatulence, 2 of abdominal pain, 1 of nausea and 2 cases of vomiting in children. Overall, gastrointestinal side effects are estimated to occur in less than 1% of persons taking rifaximin. Other rare adverse events, like urticarial rash, headache, leg edema and weight loss, have been reported but often not considered drug-related by the investigators.

Efficacy in the Treatment of Infectious Diarrhea

Tables 2A and B summarize the results of clinical studies that assessed the efficacy of rifaximin in the treatment of bacterial diarrhea. Many of the studies suffer from small numbers and not uniform definitions of diarrhea. In the studies of DuPont et al. [6, 13], acute diarrhea was defined as three or more unformed stools passed in a 24-hour period accompanied by at least one symptom of enteric disease such as abdominal cramps, nausea or vomiting. While most of the studies allude to the treatment of bacterial diarrhea, some are not accompanied by convincing stool bacteriology, with notable exceptions indicated by asterisks in the table. The studies, many of which were not rigorously assessed, included many different doses of rifaximin, ranging from as low as 400 mg to as high as 1,600 mg/day in divided doses. We determined the time to 50% reduction of the mean frequency of passage of unformed stools in an effort to compare the studies meaningfully. This median duration of diarrhea is the figure that best reflects the nonparametric statistics that would be performed when comparing therapeutic arms in a study and was chosen as a figure that could be derived from the published data and would permit a degree of comparison. Regarding adverse event data, most of the studies simply noted no adverse events, implying most likely that they passively recorded adverse events complained of by the subject rather than actively inquiring about possible adverse events and indicating when the incidence exceeded those reported in the placebo or control drug arm of the study.

Despite such limitations, the data are uniformly favorable and generally indicate that treatment with rifaximin successfully limits the course of bacterial and travelers' diarrhea to 1–2 days (fig. 1). In the case of travelers' diarrhea, for which bacterial causes are well known, when treatment with rifaximin was compared to treatment with either trimethoprim-sulfamethoxazole or ciprofloxacin (fig. 2), equivalent efficacy was noted. The average post-treatment duration of travelers' diarrhea was 35 h in one study [6] and 27 in another [13]. While data on the time required to clear bacteria from stool are lacking in most trials, the studies of DuPont et al. [6, 13] indicate that pathogens are removed from stool as effectively with rifaximin as with trimethoprim-sulfamethoxazole or ciprofloxacin and that the vast majority of pathogens were eradicated from stool when stool cultures were repeated at the conclusion of the therapeutic course.

While in patients with travelers' diarrhea due to *E. coli* the efficacy of the antibiotic was uniformly high, the cure rate was significantly lower when invasive pathogens (e.g. *Campylobacter jejuni*) causing fever and/or dysentery were present (DuPont, unpublished observations).

Rifaximin appeared to be effective and safe in both adults and children. Not only do these data support the efficacy of a nonabsorbable antibiotic in the

Table 2A. Summary of clinical studies of the efficacy of rifaximin in the treatment of acute infectious diarrhea: study design

Study	Design	Population	Definition of diarrhea	Enteropathogens	Medications				
					Rifaximin		Control		
					n	Daily dose (duration)	Drug	n	Dose (duration)
Luttichau et al. [20]*	Open label	Adults	Acute diarrhea	11 EPEC 4 *Shigella* 4 *Salmonella* 1 *Yersinia*	20	800–1,200 mg (5 days)	NA	NA	NA
Alvisi et al. [21]	Open label	Adults	Acute diarrhea or bacterial super-infection of intestinal inflammatory diseases	1 *Yersinia* 2 patients with no pathogen Various nonclassic enteric flora[1]	20	800 mg (5–10 days)	NA	NA	NA
Fiorentino et al. [22]*	Open label	Older children and adults	Acute diarrhea	11 EPEC 7 *Salmonella* 1 *Shigella* 3 patients with no pathogen	22	600–1,200 mg (3–5 days)	NA	NA	NA

Table 2A. (continued)

Study	Design	Population	Definition of diarrhea	Enteropathogens	Medications				
					Rifaximin		Control		
					n	Daily dose (duration)	Drug	n	Dose (duration)
Lombardo and Santangelo [23]	Open label	Children	Acute and chronic bacterial diarrhea	*E. coli* in almost all cases	31	>20 months: 200 mg load then 400 mg/day <20 months: 100 mg load then 200 mg/day (5 days)	NA	NA	NA
Sanfilippo et al. [24]	Randomized, placebo-controlled, double-blind	Children	Acute diarrhea	Rifaximin/control 10/8 *E.coli* 2/2 *Shigella* Various nonclassic enteric flora	20	20–40 mg/kg/day (4 days)	Placebo	17	Matched placebo (4 days)
Vinci et al. [25]*	Randomized, placebo-controlled, double-blind	Adults	Acute diarrhea	Rifaximin/control 10/7 *E.coli* 8/5 ETEC 6/6 *Shigella* 1/2 *Salmonella* Various nonclassic enteric flora	20	600 mg/day (5 days)	Placebo	20	Matched placebo (5 days)

Della Marchina et al. [26]*	Randomized, placebo-controlled, double-blind	Elderly adults (>73 years)	Acute diarrhea	Rifaximin/control 28/30 *E.coli* 6/4 *Shigella* 8/9 *Salmonella* 4/3 *Yersinia* Various nonclassic enteric flora	63	600 mg/day (7 days)	Placebo	58	Matched placebo (7 days)
De Castro et al. [27]*	Randomized 2:1 to rifaximin vs. oral rehydration, not blinded	Children	Acute episode of recurrent diarrhea occurring between cycles of antibiotic prophylaxis for UTIs	Rifaximin/control 10/6 *Salmonella* 8/6 *Shigella* 6/1 *Yersinia* 4/2 *Campylobacter* 2/1 EPEC	30	400 mg/day (3–5 days)	Oral rehydration	16	NA
Alvisi et al. [28]	Randomized, active drug-controlled, double-blind	Adults	Acute 'secretory' diarrhea	Various nonclassic enteric flora	22	800 mg/day (5 days)	Neomycin	21	1 g/day (5 days)
Stornello and Salanitri [29]*	Randomized, active drug-controlled, not double-blind	Children	Acute diarrhea	Rifaximin/control 8/7 EPEC 2/3 *Salmonella* Various nonclassic enteric flora	20	200 mg load then 400 mg/day (3–6 days)	Neomycin	20	<6 years: 125,000 IU/day 6–12 years: 375,000 IU/day (3–6 days)

Table 2A. (continued)

Study	Design	Population	Definition of diarrhea	Enteropathogens	Medications				
					Rifaximin		Control		
					n	Daily dose (duration)	Drug	n	Dose (duration)
Palermo et al. [30]	Randomized, active drug-controlled, not double-blind	Older children and adults	Acute diarrhea	Various nonclassic enteric flora	29	800 mg/day (4–7 days)	Neomycin plus nalidixic acid capsules	20	1–2 capsules, 3–4 times/day (4–7 days)
Mazzitelli et al. [31]	Randomized, active drug-controlled, not double-blind	Adults	Acute diarrhea	Various nonclassic enteric flora	20	400–800 mg/day (7 days)	Neomycin	20	1.5 g/day (7 days)
Beseghi and De Angelis [32]*	Consecutive patient randomized, active drug-controlled, not double-blind	Children	Acute diarrhea	Rifaximin/control 9/7 *Salmonella* 5/10 EPEC	14	400 mg/day (3–5 days)	Neomycin plus bacitracin	17	5 ml, 4 times/day (3–5 days)

Frisari et al. [33]*	Consecutive patient randomized, active drug-controlled, not double-blind	Children	Acute diarrhea	Rifaximin/control 11/9 *Salmonella* 6/6 *Campylobacter* 3/3 *Shigella* 0/4 EPEC 1/0 *Salmonella* + *Campylobacter*	24	400 mg/day (3–5 days)	Paromomycin	25	500 mg/day (4–5 days)
DuPont et al. [13]*	Randomized, active drug-controlled, double-blind	Adults	Acute travelers' diarrhea	Rifaximin/control 12/6 ETEC 7/1 *Shigella*, *Salmonella*, *Campylobacter*	55	18: 600 mg/day 18: 1,200 mg/day 19: 1,800 mg/day	Trimethoprim-sulfamethoxazole	17	320 mg trimethoprim + 1,600 mg sulfamethozazole/day
DuPont et al. [6]*	Randomized, active drug-controlled, double-blind	Adults	Acute travelers' diarrhea	NA	93	800 mg/day	Ciprofloxacin	94	1 g/day

Table 2B. Summary of clinical studies of the efficacy of rifaximin in the treatment of acute infectious diarrhea: study outcome

Study	Outcome of rifaximin treatment		
	Clinical efficacy	Adverse drugs event	Bacteriologic cure
Luttichau et al. [20]	50% reduction in stool frequency by end of day 1**	None	90%
Alvisi et al. [21]	50% reduction in stool frequency by day 4	None	89 % (16/18) of original isolates eradicated
Fiorentino et al. [22]	50% reduction in stool frequency between day 1 and 2**	None	63% (7 *Salmonella* not eradicated despite clinical improvement)
Lombardo and Santangelo [23]	50% reduction in stool frequency between day 3 and 4	None	69% eradicated or markedly diminished
Sanfilippo et al. [24]	50% reduction in stool frequency between day 3 and 4; $p < 0.05$	None	90% of *Shigella* eradicated
Vinci et al. [25]	50% reduction in stool frequency by end of day 1; $p < 0.05$**	None	86%
Della Marchina et al. [26]	50% reduction in stool frequency by end of day 2; $p < 0.05$**	None	89%
De Castro et al. [27]	>50% reduction in stool frequency by the end of day 1; 50% reduction in the control group at day 5; $p < 0.05$**	None	93%
Alvisi et al. [28]	50% reduction in stool frequency by end of day 2 in both treatment groups	None	85%
Stornello and Slanitri [29]	50% reduction in stool frequency between day 3 and 4 in both treatment groups**	Oral rifaximin therapy discontinued in 1 child due to vomiting	90%

Palermo et al. [30]	50% reduction in stool frequency by end of day 1 in both treatment groups	Self-limiting urticarial rash	100%
Mazzitelli et al. [31]	Baseline frequency lacking; patients passing 1–2 loose stools/day by day 2–3 of treatment	None	70%
Beseghi and De'Angelis [32]	>50% reduction in stool frequency by end of day 1 in rifaximin group vs. 25% reduction in control group**	None	93%
Frisari et al. [33]	Significant improvement in both groups by day 2*	None	90%
DuPont et al. [13]	50% well at 35 h**	Minimal eosinophilia (5, 7 and 9%) in 3 subjects; 1 patient with posttreatment AST of 74; otherwise well tolerated	80%
DuPont et al. [6]	50% well at 27 h compared to 25 h for ciprofloxacin; $p = 0.3$**	Well tolerated in both groups	Not available

EPEC = Enteropathogenic *E. coli*; NA = not applicable; UTI = urinary tract infections; AST = aspartate amino transferase.

*Indicates studies that documented a substantial number of cases of bacterial diarrhea; ** denotes studies with substantial isolation of bacterial enteropathogens.

[1]Nonclassic enteric flora includes *E. coli* with the designation of enteropathogenic *E. coli* or other recognized diarrheogenic *E. coli*, *Klebsiella, Proteus*, *Enterobacter*, *Pseudomonas* and *Enterococcus.*

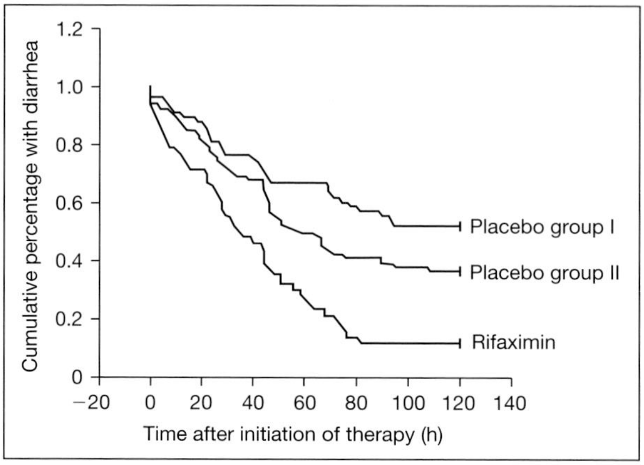

Fig. 1. Comparative effectiveness of treatment of patients with travelers' diarrhea. Percentage of subjects who continued to have diarrhea by hour after treatment in subjects receiving one of three doses of rifaximin compared with two similar placebo-treated groups studied earlier using identical study methods (from DuPont et al. [13]).

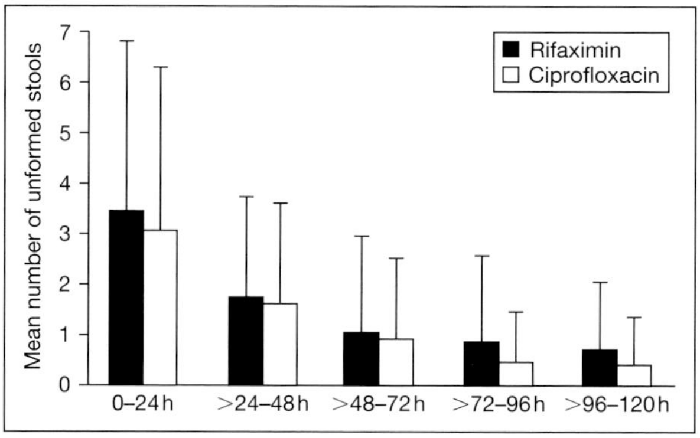

Fig. 2. Mean number of unformed stools passed per day of study by subjects with travelers' diarrhea taking rifaximin (400 mg twice a day) or ciprofloxain (500 mg twice a day). The mean values for the two treatment groups were comparable for each day of the study (from DuPont et al. [6]).

treatment of diarrhea, the lack of absorption and degree of safety reported to date support the likelihood that rifaximin will be safe to use in pregnant women. Currently, the drugs of choice for the treatment of bacterial diarrhea, especially travelers' diarrhea, are the fluoroquinolones, which are contraindicated in pregnancy. While rifaximin will likely never be adequately studied in pregnancy, it should be safe.

One published study supports the use of rifaximin in the treatment of diarrhea with protozoal causes [14]. In this small study, Amenta et al. [14] showed that diarrhea in patients with AIDS and from protozoal causes, including *Giardia lamblia* and *C. parvum*, responded favorably to treatment with rifaximin. In the Kenya arm of a recently reported multicenter trial of the treatment of diarrhea in travelers, rifaximin shortened the illness of European travelers with *Cryptosporidium* infection [15]. Further work should be done in these populations.

Finally, while a nonabsorbable antimicrobial agent has theoretic advantages as a choice for the treatment of infectious diarrhea, such an agent should not be used to treat hosts thought to have or be at risk for bacteremic disease (e.g. seriously immunocompromized patients).

Major Indication for Rifaximin Is Enteric Disease

As outlined in the excellent review by Gilles and Brogden [9], the current indications for rifaximin include surgical prophylaxis and the treatment of hepatic encephalopathy, infectious diarrhea and intestinal bacterial overgrowth syndromes. As such, rifaximin is aimed only at enteric flora. Owing to its lack of absorption, rifaximin will likely not be used for other conditions or indications. Such limited indications should help preserve the activity of the agent, since overuse for common conditions like urinary or respiratory tract infections will naturally not occur. Limited use should help retard the development of resistance among enteric flora.

Rifaximin Does Not Develop Resistance or Promote Cross-Resistance

While the emergence of rifaximin-resistant strains has been observed during the course of treatment, these strains disappear from the intestinal flora within 1–2 weeks of cessation of rifaximin [16]. It has been shown that in vitro, the emergence of resistant Gram-positive flora could be induced, but the emergence of aerobic Gram-negative flora was rare [Schito, personal communication]. Furthermore, emergence of resistance was much less common under anaerobic conditions that mimic the environment of the gut. Also, subinhibitory concentrations of an antibiotic encourage the emergence of resistance, a situation much less likely to occur in the gut because of the huge concentrations of rifaximin in stool.

Three studies have addressed the possibility of inducing cross-resistance to *Mycobacterium tuberculosis* during the use of rifaximin. In an experimental guinea pig model of *M. tuberculosis*, rifaximin was administered in an effort to induce resistance among *M. tuberculosis* strains of human origin. Not only did no resistance develop, cross-resistance to rifampin also did not occur [17, 18]. In another approach, *M. tuberculosis* strains were subjected to subinhibitory concentrations of rifaximin. No induction of resistance or cross-resistance to rifampin occurred [19].

Conclusion

Rifaximin appears to be an ideal agent for the treatment of infectious watery diarrhea. It has shown excellent efficacy in numerous clinical trials of bacterial diarrhea. Its excellent side effect profile and lack of systemic absorption predict that it should be useful in treating hosts for whom the currently favored fluoroquinolones are contraindicated. Uses limited to enteric indications and its inherently low propensity to induce sustainable resistance among Gram-negative flora favor the sustained usefulness of rifaximin in the treatment of enteric syndromes.

References

1 DuPont HL, Copperstock M, Corrado ML, Fekety R, Murray DM: Evaluation of new anti-infective drugs for the treatment of acute infectious diarrhea. Clin Infect Dis 1992;15(suppl 1): S228–S235.

2 DuPont HL, Ericsson CD: Prevention and treatment of travelers' diarrhea. N Engl J Med 1993; 328:1821–1827.

3 Jiang Z-D, Ke S, Palazzini E, Riopel L, DuPon HL: In vitro activity and fecal concentration of rifaximin after oral administration. Antimicrob Agents Chemother 2000;44:2205–2206.

4 Gomi H, Jiang Z-D, Adachi JA, Ashley D, Lowe B, Verenkar MP, Steffen R, DuPont HL: In vitro antimicrobial susceptibility testing of bacterial enteropathogens causing traveler's diarrhea in four geographic regions. Antimicrob Agents Chemother 2001;45:212–216.

5 Sierra JM, Ruiz J, Navia MM, Vargas M, Gascon J, Vila J: In vitro activity of rifaximin against enteropathogens producing traveler's diarrhea. Antimicrob Agents Chemother 2001;45:643–644.

6 DuPont HL, Jiang Z-D, Ericsson CD, Adachi JA, Mathewson JJ, DuPont MW, Palazzini E, Riopel LM, Ashley D, Martinez-Sandoval F: Rifaximin for the treatment of travelers' diarrhea: A randomized, double-blind clinical trial versus ciprofloxacin. Clin Infect Dis 2001;33:1807–1815.

7 Descombe JJ, Dubourg D, Picard M, Palazzine E: Pharmacokinetic study of rifaximin after oral administration in healthy volunteers. Int J Clin Pharmacol Res 1994;14:51–56.

8 Rizzello F, Gionchetti P, Venturi A, Ferretti M, Peruzzo S, Raspanti X, Picard N, Canova E, Palazzini M: Rifaximin systemic absorption in patients with ulcerative colitis. Eur J Clin Pharmacol 1998;58:91–93.

9 Gillis JC, Brogden RN: Rifaximin: A review of its antibacterial activity, pharmacokinetic properties and therapeutic potential in conditions mediated by gastrointestinal bacteria. Drugs 1995;49:467–484.

10 Haltalin KC, Nelson JD, Hinton LV, Kusmiesz HT, Sladoje M: Comparison of orally absorbable and nonabsorbable antibiotics in shigellosis. A double-blind study with ampicillin and neomycin. J Pediatr 1968;72:708–720.

11 Ericsson CD, DuPont HL, Sullivan P, Galindo E, Evans DG, Evans DJ Jr: Bicozamycin, a poorly absorbable antibiotic, effectively treats travelers' diarrhea. Ann Intern Med 1983;98:20–25.
12 DuPont HL, Ericsson CD, Mathewson JJ, de la Cabada FJ, Conrad DA: Oral aztreonam, a poorly absorbed yet effective therapy for bacterial diarrhea in US travelers to Mexico. JAMA 1992;267: 1932–1935.
13 DuPont HL, Ericsson CD, Mathewson JJ, Palazzini E, DuPont MW, Jiang Z-D, Mosavi A, De la Cabada FJ: Rifaximin: A non-absorbed antimicrobial in the therapy of travelers' diarrhea. Digestion 1998;59:708–714.
14 Amenta M, Dalle Nogare ER, Colomba D, Prestileo TS, Di Lorenzo F, Fundaro S, Colomba A, Ferrieri A: Intestinal protozoa in HIV-infected patients: Effect of rifaximin in *Cryptosporidium parvum* and *Blastocyctis hominis* infections. J Chemother 1999;11:391–395.
15 Steffen R, Sack DA, Riopel L, Jiang ZD, Sturchler M, Ericsson CD, Lowe B, Waiyaki P, White M, DuPont HL: Therapy of travelers' diarrhea with rifaximin on various continents. Am J Gastroenterol 2003;98(5):1073–1078.
16 De Leo C, Eftimiadi C, Schito GC: Rapid disappearance from intestinal tract of bacteria resistant to rifaximin. Drugs Exp Clin Res 1986;12:979–981.
17 Lucchesi M, Marchi E, Venturini AP: Antimycobacterial activity of rifaximin (L/105) in experimental tuberculosis in the Guinea-pig. Chemiotherapia 1984;3:371–372.
18 Malvisi Stracciari J, Venturini AP, Anfossi P, Marchi E, Stracciari GL: Sensitivity to rifaximin and rifampicin of *Mycobacterium tuberculosis* isolated from guinea pigs treated orally with rifaximin. Chemiotherapia 1987;6:82–84.
19 Soro O, Pesce A, Raggi M, Debbia EA, Schito GC: Selection of rifampicin-resistant *Mycobacterium tuberculosis* does not occur in the presence of low concentrations of rifaximin. Clin Microbiol Infect 1997;3:147–151.
20 Luttichau U, Arcangeli P, Sinapi S: The use of rifaximin in the treatment of acute diarrhoeal enteritis: Open study. Panminerva Med 1985;27:129–132.
21 Alvisi V, D'Ambrosi A, Loponte A, Pazzi P, Greco A, Zangirolami A, Palazzini E: Rifaximin, a rifamycin derivative for use in the treatment of intestinal bacterial infections in seriously disabled patients. J Int Med Res 1987;15:49–56.
22 Fiorentino F, Simioli F, Conte M, Postiglione A, Cinque F, Santaniello A: Open study on the antidiarrhoeal effectiveness of the L 105 compound. Chemioterapia 1984;3:132–135.
23 Lombardo S, Santangelo G: Therapeutic effectiveness of L 105, given in three pediatric formulations, as an intestinal antibacterial agent. Farmaco (Prat) 1984;39:170–175.
24 Sanfilippo A, Raciti Longo G, Raciti Longo A: Clinical experience with rifaximin in pediatric diarrhoeal syndromes. Med Praxis 1984;5:375–383.
25 Vinci M, Gatto A, Giaglio A, Raciti T, D'Avola G, Di Stefano B, Salanitri G, Di Stefano F: Double-blind clinical trial on infectious diarrhea therapy: Rifaximin versus placebo. Curr Ther Res Clin Exp 1984;36:92–99.
26 Della Marchina M, Renzi G, Palazzini E: Infectious diarrhea in the aged: Controlled clinical trial of rifaximin. Chemioterapia 1988;10:107–109.
27 De Castro R, Domenichelli V, Di Lorenzo FP, Prestipino M, Perotta ML: Rifaximin treatment for acute recurrent diarrhea in children with genitourinary disorders. Curr Ther Res Clin Exp 1999;59:746–752.
28 Alvisi A, D'Ambrosi A, Onofri W, Catellani M, Palazzini E: Treatment of secretory diarrhoeas. A double-blind trial of the effectiveness of rifaximin (L 105) and neomycin. Clin Trials J 1984;21: 215–223.
29 Stornello C, Slanitri G: Controlled trial of the clinical effectiveness of the new antidiarrheal drug rifaximin. Med Praxis 1987;8:69–78.
30 Palermo G, Di Gregorio P, Coffa G: Effectiveness of the L 105 compound in the treatment of acute diarrhoeal diseases. A short-term controlled study. Med Praxis 1984;5:147–152.
31 Mazzitelli M, Brega G, Dirani D, Andalo A: Antidiarrhoeal effectiveness and tolerance in man of a local antibiotic: Rifaximin. Comparative assessment using a control drug. Eur Rev Med Pharmacol Sci 1984;6:301–306.
32 Beseghi U, De'Angelis GL: Comparison of two non-absorbable antibiotics for treatment of bacterial enteritis in children. Eur Rev Med Pharmacol Sci 1998;3:131–136.

33 Frisari L, Viaggiano V, Pelagalli M: An open, controlled study of two non-absorbable antibiotics for the oral treatment of pediatric infectious diarrhoea. Curr Med Res Opin 1997;14:39–45.

Note Added in Proof

After the submission of this paper several publications have appeared in the literature that reinforce the role of rifaximin in the treatment of infectious diarrhea [1]. An entire issue of the Journal of Travel Medicine devoted to the use of this antibiotic in the treatment of traveler's diarrhea (TD) has been published [2–5]. In addition, a recent paper from our laboratory [6] confirmed the rifaximin efficacy also in enteroaggregative *Escherichia coli*-mediated TD. Furthermore, in a randomized, double-blind, placebo-controlled study [7] even once daily administration of the antibiotic proved to be capable of preventing TD. Finally, Lawler and Wallace [8] recently reviewed the treatment options for bacterial diarrhea and considered rifaximin a useful addition to our therapeutic armamentarium.

References

1 Ericsson CD: Travellers' diarrhoea. Int J Antimicrob Agents 2003;21(2):116–124.
2 Ericsson CD: Rifaximin: A new approach to the treatment of travelers' diarrhea. Introduction. J Travel Med 2001;8(suppl 2):S25.
3 DuPont HL: Treatment of travelers' diarrhea. J Travel Med 2001;8(suppl 2):S31–S33.
4 Steffen R: Rifaximin: A nonabsorbed antimicrobial as a new tool for treatment of travelers' diarrhea. J Travel Med 2001;8(suppl 2):S34–S39.
5 Ericsson CD: Rifaximin: A new approach to the treatment of travelers' diarrhea. Conclusion. J Travel Med 2001;8(suppl 2):S40.
6 Infante RM, Ericsson CD, Jiang ZD, Ke S, Steffen R, Riopel L, Sack DA, DuPont HL: Enteroaggregative *Escherichia coli* diarrhea in travelers: Response to rifaximin therapy. Clin Gastroenterol Hepatol 2004;2:135–138.
7 DuPont HL, Jiang ZD, Ericsson CD, de la Cabada F, Shi K, DuPont MW, Martinez-Sandoval F: Rifaximin, a nonabsorbed (<0.5%) antibiotic, prevents travelers diarrhea (TD). Gastroenterology 2004;126(suppl 2):A12.
8 Lawler JV, Wallace MR: Diagnosis and treatment of bacterial diarrhea. Curr Gastroenterol Rep 2003;5:287–294.

Charles D. Ericsson, MD
1.722 JFB
6431 Fannin St.
Houston, TX 77030 (USA)
Tel. +1 713 500 6732, Fax +1 713 500 5495, E-Mail Charles.D.Ericsson@uth.tmc.edu

This chapter should be cited as follows:

Ericsson CD, DuPont HL: Rifaximin in the Treatment of Infectious Diarrhea. Chemotherapy 2005;51(suppl 1):73–80.

Scarpignato C (ed): Rifaximin: A Poorly Absorbed Antibiotic.
Pharmacology and Clinical Use.

Antibiotic-Associated Diarrhea and Pseudomembranous Colitis: Are They Less Common with Poorly Absorbed Antimicrobials?

Christina M. Surawicz

Department of Medicine, University of Washington School of Medicine,
Seattle, Wash., USA

Abstract

Diarrhea is a well-known complication of antibiotic therapy. Rates of antibiotic-associated diarrhea (AAD) vary from 5 to 25%. Some antibiotics are more likely to cause diarrhea than others, specifically, those that are broad spectrum and those that target anaerobic flora. This paper reviews the effects of antibiotics on the fecal flora as well as host factors which contribute to AAD. Clinical features and treatment of AAD are also described. Prevention of AAD rests on wise antibiotic policies, the use of probiotics and prevention of acquisition in the hospital setting. Data from clinical trials suggest that poorly absorbed antimicrobials might have a decreased risk of causing AAD and *Clostridium difficile*-associated disease, as concluded from studies of antibiotics used for preoperative bowel decontamination and poorly absorbed antibiotics used for traveler's diarrhea. Controlled trials would prove this but are not yet available. Probiotics may be a good adjunct to poorly absorbed antibiotics to minimize the risk of diarrhea associated with antibiotics.

Introduction

Diarrhea is a well-known complication of antibiotic therapy. Rates of antibiotic-associated diarrhea (AAD) vary from 5–25% [1]. Rates of AAD vary with antibiotic as well as with the population studied. AAD occurs in up to 29% of hospitalized patients, resulting in lengthened hospital stays, increased costs of medical care, a threefold increase in mortality and a fivefold increase in the acquisition of other nosocomial infections [2–5]. Some antibiotics are more likely to cause diarrhea than others – these are broad-spectrum compared to narrow-spectrum ones, and those that target anaerobic flora compared to those that do not. In addition, multiple antibiotics are associated with an increased risk of AAD. The most severe form of AAD is due to *Clostridium difficile*, which causes colitis and pseudomembranous colitis. The first case of pseudomembranous colitis, at the time described as 'diphtheritic' colitis, was reported in 1899 [6]. A young woman developed fatal colitis after gastrointestinal tract surgery. This was clearly in the preantibiotic era. Pseudomembranous colitis as a discrete entity was widely recognized in the 1970s in association with lincomycin and clindamycin therapy, even before the pathogen *C. difficile* was recognized.

Epidemiology

Rates of AAD vary among different populations, and are probably higher for inpatients than outpatients. Two studies of adult patients in US community hospitals documented frequencies of 15 and 22%, respectively [7, 8]. In contrast, febrile neutropenic patients in another study had a frequency of AAD of 29% [9]. Rates of *C. difficile*-associated antibiotic diarrhea (CDAD) also vary – when an outbreak is documented, frequencies can be as high as 26–60% [10, 11]. Predisposing causes such as gastrointestinal tract surgery or the use of high-risk antibiotics such as clindamycin or third-generation cephalosporins can contribute to high rates as well. Other possible factors predisposing to AAD are comorbidity and altered immune status. AAD is common with HIV infection, but this may be a result of frequent antibiotic use rather than immunosuppression per se. In hospitalized patients, risk factors include prolonged hospitalization, gastrointestinal procedures such as endoscopy and enemas, and nasogastric tube feeding, though the latter is controversial [12, 13]. The lowest rates of AAD and CDAD generally occur in outpatients; perhaps they are generally more healthy and less susceptible to disruption of the normal flora (table 1) [14].

Pathophysiology and Antibiotic Risk

C. difficile overgrowth is present in only 15–25% of cases of AAD; thus, other explanations are needed to understand the pathophysiology of diarrhea. There are multiple mechanisms which can account for the diarrhea associated with antibiotics. These include altered fermentation of the flora, changes in dietary fiber and overgrowth of other potential pathogens.

Table 1. Risk factors for AAD and CDAD

Risk factor	Degree of risk	Strength of evidence
Antibiotics		
Oral antibiotics		
Clindamycin	High	Excellent
Cephalosporins	High	Excellent
Ampicillin	High	Excellent
Nonabsorbed antibiotic	Low	Minimal data to date
Parenteral antibiotics	Moderate, varies with antibiotic	Excellent
Multiple, broad-spectrum antibiotics	High	Moderate
Hospitalization	High	Excellent
Gastrointestinal tract surgery	High	Moderate
Severity of illness	High	Cofactor
HIV with immune suppression	Moderate	Unconfirmed
Gastrointestinal procedures, enemas, nasogastric tubes	Low	Not uniform
Renal failure	Low	Moderate

Overgrowth of C. difficile

Antibiotics alter the normal colonic flora, leading to loss of colonization resistance, which is the ability of the normal flora to protect against overgrowth of pathogens, especially when the anaerobic flora are depleted [15]. In CDAD, the altered colonization resistance can allow for the overgrowth of *C. difficile* in the colon. The bacteria produces two toxins which cause disease (toxin A, an enterotoxin, and toxin B, a cytotoxin). The toxins of *C. difficile* inactivate Rho proteins, which results in the loss of cytoskeletal integrity in enterocytes. Cellular damage results in fluid loss, exudation and diarrhea. The most severe form of *C. difficile* diarrhea is pseudomembranous colitis, which can cause severe colitis, toxic colon and rarely colon perforation and death.

Altered Fermentation of Colonic Carbohydrates

The fecal flora ferment unabsorbed carbohydrates with production of short-chain fatty acids (SCFAs). One likely explanation for diarrhea due to antibiotics is altered fecal flora, which results in changes in SCFA metabolism. Changes can result in acidic pH as well as osmotic changes in the lumen; either or both can contribute to the diarrhea. One study of seven patients with AAD showed reduced fecal concentration of SCFAs as well as changes in rates of production [16]. Since SCFAs stimulate salt and water absorption in the colon, a decrease in their concentration could also contribute to diarrhea.

Dietary Fiber

Dietary fiber may also play a role in AAD. Diarrhea with enteral feeding is well documented and is increased with antibiotics. Antibiotics can impair colonic fermentation of carbohydrates; studies of ampicillin documented effects on lactulose using breath hydrogen analysis and stool output measurements [17]. Lack of dietary fiber in enteral feeding can contribute to diarrhea. A study of pectin, a water-soluble fiber that stimulates epithelial growth in the colon, given to patients on enteral nutrition and antibiotics showed less diarrhea in the fiber-pectin group compared to the fiber-placebo group [18].

Overgrowth of Other Potential Pathogens

Rarely, other pathogenic bacteria have been reported to cause pseudomembranous colitis.

Klebsiella oxytoca. Two French studies of patients with acute AAD used culture of colorectal biopsy to detect *K. oxytoca*, despite negative stool culture [19, 20]. Colonoscopic findings included diffuse and focal colitis and right-sided hemorrhage colitis. The pathogenicity of these strains is still under debate.

Candida. The possible role of *Candida* as a cause of diarrhea has become more apparent lately. Early in the 1990s, two separate papers by Gupta and Ehrinpreis [21] and Danna et al. [22] documented elderly hospitalized patients with diarrhea and significant *Candida* in their stools whose diarrhea responded to antifungal therapy. Two studies of infants and children from India also suggested *Candida* as a pathogen causing diarrhea [23, 24]. However, subsequent studies in children indicated that the role of *Candida* may not be as a pathogen but as overgrowth due to the disruption of flora by antibiotic [25]. A critical literature review of *Candida-associated* diarrhea by Levine et al. [26] cast doubt on its pathogenicity, as many patients with *Candida* in their stools had had prior antibiotic therapy, but conceded that *Candida* species could cause diarrhea in selective clinical settings. Most recently, Krause et al. [27] published a large study analyzing stools from patients with AAD and controls and also concluded that elevated *Candida* counts were a result of antibiotic therapy rather than a cause of AAD, an argument bolstered by their finding of no increase in a virulence factor (SAP) in diarrhea stools.

Antibiotics and the Fecal Flora

To understand the role of antibiotics, it is important to understand their effects on the fecal flora. The normal flora consists of a complex bacterial population with 400–500 distinct species of bacteria (table 2a). More than 99% of the total organisms are accounted for by non-spore-forming anaerobic rods [28]; the four major species are *Bacteroides*, bifidobacteria, eubacteria and peptostreptococci [29].

Table 2. Normal fecal flora

a Bacteriological analysis of the normal fecal flora

Bacteria	Log 10 bacteria counts
Enterobacteria	7.4
Enterococci	5.6
Lactobacilli	6.5
Clostridia	5.4
Bacteroides	9.8
Gram-positive anaerobes (eubacteria, bifidobacteria)	10

b Most common species

Anaerobes	Aaerobes
Bacteroides	*E. coli*
Eubacteria	Enterococci
Bifidobacteria	Lactobacilli
Anaerobic cocci	

Other common species are *Escherichia coli*, *Streptococcus viridans*, *Streptococcus salivarius* and lactobacilli. Mette et al. [30] clarified the prevalence of species in fecal flora by listing the four most common anaerobes *(Bacteroides* spp., *Eubacterium* spp., *Bifidobacterium* spp. and anaerobic cocci) and three common aerobes *(E. coli* spp., *Enterococcus* spp. and *Lactobacillus* spp.) (table 2b).

The effects of antibiotics on anaerobic and aerobic flora are shown in table 3. These data are from a variety of studies of human volunteers or patients given preoperative antibiotics but receiving various antibiotics by various routes [31–44]. Variations in data can be explained by methodological differences between studies as well as variations among studied populations. Nonetheless, some trends can be observed. Antibiotics with profound effects on suppression of anaerobic flora are the same ones which have an increased incidence of *C. difficile*-associated disease: clindamycin (p.o. or i.v.), ampicillin, sulbactam and broad-spectrum cephalosporins. Broad-spectrum parenteral antibiotics (e.g. ceftriaxone) have a lower but still significant risk. Antibiotics with less anaerobic suppression (tetracycline, penicillin) appear to have a lower risk of CDAD. In one study, a cephalosporin given intravenously showed minimal anaerobic suppression; this increased when given orally [43].

Clearly, the route of administration of antibiotics can affect the rates of AAD. Rates of diarrhea are lower with intravenous than oral antibiotics.

Table 3. Antibiotic effect on suppression of normal bacterial flora of humans

	Anaerobic flora	Aerobic flora	Comment	Reference
Oral antibiotics				
Tetracycline, doxycycline	Minor (log 1–2)	no change to minor ↓	Low risk of CDAD	30, 35
Neomycin + erythromycin	Major (↓ log 5)	major (↓ log 5)		32
Kanamycin + metronidazole	Moderate (↓ log 2)	minimal		33
Neomycin + erythromycin	Moderate (log 5)	moderate (↓ log 5)		32
Penicillin	Minor ↓			
Erythromycin	Major ↓	marked ↓		35
Cephalosporins Cefoperazone	Major ↓	?		42
Clindamycin	Major ↓ (log 7) (log 4–5)	minimal to marked ↓	Flora change noted especially in PMC patients	5, 7, 30, 31, 35, 84
Ampicillin + sulbactam	Major ↓	minimal ↓	*C. difficile* correlated with abnormalities of flora	38
Ampicillin prodrugs (bacampicillin, pivampicillin)	Moderate ↓	minimal ↓	*C. difficile* correlated with abnormalities of flora	38
Parenteral antibiotics				
Imipenem/cilastatin (i.v.)	Minimal to moderate ↓	Minimal to marked ↓	Low rates of *C. difficile*	36, 41
Azlocillin	Minimal to moderate ↓	Minimal to moderate	Variability among volunteers	39
Ampicillin + sulbactam (i.v.)	Moderate ↓ (log 3)	Normal to minimal		34, 35
Temocillin (i.v.)	Marked ↓	Unknown	↓ *Enterobacter* likely low rates of *C. difficile*	37
Cephalosporins				
Cefoxitin (i.v.)	Moderate ↓	Moderate ↓		35
Cefoperazone (i.v.)	Minimal	Unknown	Asymptomatic *C. difficile* in 1 volunteer	42
Ceftriaxone (i.m.)	Minor to marked ↓	Marked ↓	2 volunteers had *C. difficile,* 1 with diarrhea	43 44
Clindamycin	Marked ↓	Minor ↓		41
Aztreonam	Minor ↓	Minor ↓		41

PMC = Pseudomembranous colitis.

Data were summarized from the references noted in the table. Some articles present disparate data. In general, a minor decrease in flora was a decrease by 1–2 logs of bacteria; a moderate decrease was a decrease by 2–4 logs, and a major decrease was a decrease by 4–5 logs.

Specific rates of diarrhea for all individual antibiotics are not available. Some reports suggest that antibiotics with biliary secretion may have higher rates of AAD. Clindamycin remains a high-risk antibiotic [31]. A recent study of an epidemic in a Veterans Affairs hospital demonstrated dramatic declines in CDAD rates when the use of clindamycin was restricted [44].

In general, these high-risk antibiotics cause less suppression of aerobic bacteria. Decreases in aerobes appear to have less effect on colonization resistance (table 3). Interestingly, colonic lavage without antibiotics decreases colonic bacterial counts by log 2 [40].

A recent prospective study of AAD and CDAD in five Swedish hospitals showed an increased risk of AAD with cephalosporins, clindamycin and broad-spectrum penicillins [42]. While CDAD is well recognized as the most common nosocomial gastrointestinal pathogen, some cases occur in the ambulatory setting. A retrospective study by Levy et al. [14] of enrollees in four community based HMOs (health maintenance organizations) showed a prevalence of 12 per 100,000 person-years. This is less than in the hospital setting, but the rate of testing for *C. difficile* is also lower – only 5% of patients with AAD were tested for *C. difficile.* In the study of Levy et al. [14], first- and third-generation cephalosporins (cephaloxin and ce-fixime) had a higher risk than other antibiotics. High rates with second- and third-generation cephalosporins have been shown by others, as well as with the use of multiple antibiotics [45–47]. It is likely that the key factor in antibiotic risk is the effect of the individual antibiotic on the colonic flora, specifically the anaerobic flora. Even metronidazole, used to treat *C. difficile*, can cause AAD and CDAD. Only vancomycin seems to have a low risk of CDAD – a single case report in a renal dialysis patient is less than convincing [48].

Nonabsorbable antibiotics are appealing because they have fewer systemic side effects and may be safer for children and pregnant women as well as in patients with renal and hepatic dysfunction. One such antibiotic, aztreonam, showed little effect on anaerobic flora in human volunteers, producing most of its effect on the aerobic flora [49, 50]. A trial showed efficacy of aztreonam for traveler's diarrhea, where most pathogens are aerobes [51]. While there are no data on rates of AAD for nonabsorbable antibiotics and *C. difficile*, these would likely be decreased. Given the preservation of the anaerobic flora, another poorly absorbed antibiotic, bicozamycin, has efficacy in traveler's diarrhea with its major effect being on fecal aerobes [52].

Rifaximin, a nonabsorbable antibiotic and a derivative of rifamycin which has been widely available in Europe since the 1980s, was shown early on to be active against anaerobic bacteria such as *Bacteroides* spp. Stool levels are high [53]. The drug has efficacy against both aerobes and anaerobes in fecal flora. It has been used in traveler's diarrhea [54], where pathogens are primarily aerobic. Its efficacy against anaerobic flora led to an in vitro study of its efficacy against

93 different strains of *C. difficile.* Seventy-four percent of the strains were susceptible to rifaximin, compared to 100% for vancomycin and metronidazole [55], suggesting a real potential use for this drug for the treatment of gastro-intestinal diseases and possibly *C. difficile.* When used as an adjunct to cefotaxime in patients undergoing colonic surgery, fewer postoperative complications occurred and intestinal function recovered more quickly [56]. However, clinical trials would be necessary before concluding that the risks of AAD and CDAD are substantially decreased with this antibiotic compared to others [57].

Rates of diarrhea also vary with host factors. Some people are more likely to develop diarrhea than others; predisposing factors are extremes of age (under 6 or over 65), severe underlying disease, chronic intestinal disorders, prior history of AAD, gastrointestinal tract surgery and nasogastric tube feeding [58]. Surgical patients are at increased risk for CDAD. In a 2-year prospective study, *C. difficile* accounted for 3% of all postoperative infections. The most commonly implicated individual antibiotics were ciprofloxacin (19%) and cefoxitin (16%). Of note, 16% of patients developed CDAD only after administration of perioperative antibiotics [59]. Factors not significantly associated with AAD are gender, antibiotic dose and inflammatory bowel disease. *C. difficile* can also be caused by nonantibiotic factors such as cancer chemotherapy, and rarely, sporadic cases do occur.

Clinical Features

Diarrhea or loose stools can start after even a few doses of antibiotics, or as long as 6 weeks after the cessation of antibiotics. Most patients develop AAD while still on antibiotics. Symptoms of AAD are watery diarrhea and cramping. Severe diarrhea with bleeding, fever and abdominal pain suggests colitis, the most severe form of AAD, which is almost always related to *C. difficile.*

Diagnosis

AAD is suspected in anyone who develops diarrhea while on antibiotics or following recent (previous 6–8 weeks) antibiotic therapy. Diarrhea that develops in hospital is almost never due to other enteric pathogens or ova and parasites, though causes in addition to antibiotics and *C. difficile* are other medications and tube feeding. Diagnosis of *C. difficile* relies on documenting *C. difficile* toxin A or B in the stool and exclusion of other causes of diarrhea. Culture positivity does not indicate disease since a carrier state can exist. Toxin B tissue culture assay is the gold standard, but it is expensive and time consuming. Thus, many hospitals are now using enzyme immunoassay tests for toxin A or toxin B or both. Fecal leukocytes are nonspecific as they indicate inflammation but not

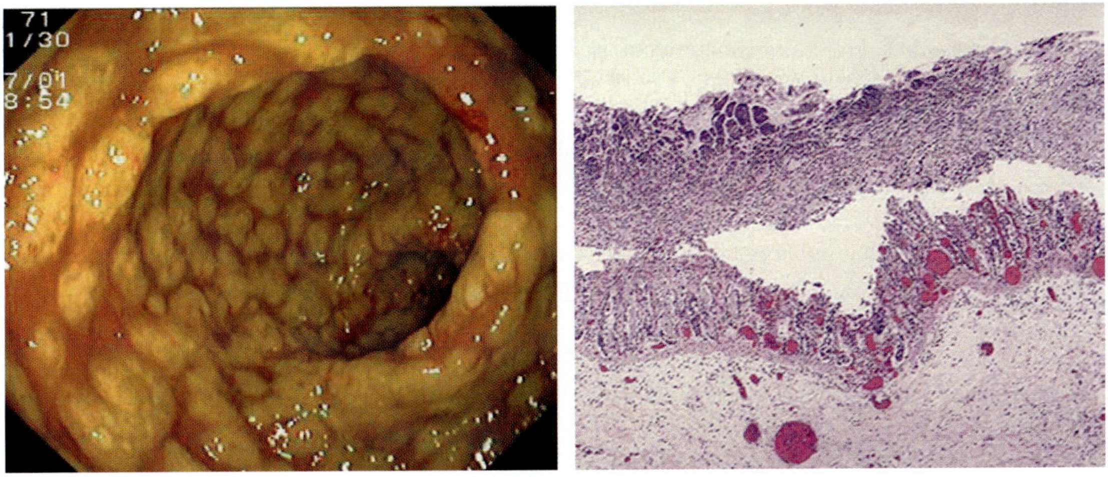

Fig. 1. Typical presentation of pseudomembranous colitis. At endoscopy (left), the mucosal surface of the colon appears hyperemic and almost completely covered by a yellow green exudate. The mucosa itself is somewhat eroded. Microscopically (right), the pseudomembrane is composed of inflammatory cells, necrotic epithelium, and mucus in which the overgrowth of microorganisms usually takes place.

a specific cause. Colonoscopy or flexible sigmoidoscopy can give an immediate diagnosis of colitis (fig. 1), but this is rarely necessary.

Treatment of AAD

When AAD is mild, the best first step is to discontinue the inciting antibiotics. Most cases will resolve spontaneously. Some advocate restriction of dietary carbohydrate as well [60]. More serious cases require specific therapy against the pathogen. Antidiarrheals and opiates should be avoided.

Treatment of CDAD

The two most frequently used antibiotics are metronidazole and vancomycin. Metronidazole is recommended as first-line therapy because of the risk of development of vancomycin-resistant enterococci with vancomycin use, as well as its much higher cost. Metronidazole and vancomycin have similar efficacy, though in one study, symptoms resolved sooner with vancomycin [61]. Metronidazole is given orally for 10 days, at a dose of 1 g per day. Vancomycin is given orally for

10 days; doses vary from 500 mg/day to 2 g/day. For mild to moderately severe CDAD, low-dose vancomycin is as effective as high-dose vancomycin. Vancomycin use is generally restricted to patients who cannot take metronidazole (allergy, intolerant to side effects, pregnancy) or in those in whom metronidazole has failed. Other antibiotics have been used. One study showed similar cure rates for vancomycin (94%), metronidazole (94%), teicoplanin (96%) and fusidic acid (93%) [62].

Rifaximin is a derivative of rifamycin SV. The drug is not absorbed in the gastrointestinal tract and has activity against both Gram-positive and Gram-negative aerobic and anaerobic bacteria by inhibiting bacterial RNA synthesis. Active drug reaches the intestinal lumen. Rifaximin is widely used in Europe, and clinical trials have shown its efficacy in infectious diarrhea in children and adults, colonic diverticular disease, *H. pylori* eradication and treatment of hepatic encephalopathy [57]. It has also been shown to be effective in the treatment of traveler's diarrhea [63]. The antibiotic is active against a variety of intestinal pathogens in vitro, including *Camplyobacter jejuni*, *Yersinia* spp. and *C. difficile.* In one study, 56 *C. difficile* strains were tested, and 34 strains (60.7%) were sensitive to rifaximin, compared to 27 strains (48.2%) with the same concentrations of rifampicin [64]. In the previously cited study, the efficacy of rifaximin against 74% of 93 *C. difficile* strains isolated from patients in Italian hospitals [55] led to a clinical trial that compared treatment of 20 patients with *C. difficile* pseudomembranous colitis using rifaximin, 200 mg thrice daily orally for 10 days, with vancomycin, 500 mg twice daily orally for 10 days. All 10 patients treated with vancomycin were cured, but there was 1 treatment failure in the rifaximin group. Thus, overall efficacy was 100% for vancomycin and 90% for rifaximin in this small trial. However, the time to disappearance of *Clostridium* toxins was more rapid in the vancomycin group (4.8 ± 1.8 days) compared to the rifaximin group (8.1 ± 1.8 days) [65]. The authors conclude that rifaximin can be used as a replacement for vancomycin when the use of the latter is not possible.

Recurrent CDAD is a particularly difficult problem which occurs in up to 20% of patients. Most patients will need repeated antibiotic treatment with metronidazole or vancomycin. Treatment strategies include pulsing or tapering antibiotics and adding probiotic agents, such as *Lactobacillus GG* or the non-pathogenic yeast *Saccharomyces boulardii* [66].

Prevention of AAD and CDAD

The cornerstone of prevention of AAD and *C. difficile* disease is wise antibiotic use policies. Restricting the use of high-risk antibiotics such as clindamycin has been shown to control hospital epidemics of *C. difficile.* In hospitals, hand washing and enteric precautions can minimize person-to-person transmission of *C. difficile.*

As diarrhea is a known and common complication of antibiotic therapy, many approaches have been used for prevention. The use of probiotics administered with the antibiotic is appealing. A probiotic is a live microbial food supplement that beneficially affects the host animal, improving its microbial balance [67]. Certain probiotics can reduce the risk and duration of diarrhea [68]. Agents used in prevention of AAD include lactobacilli, such as *Lactobacillus GG*, *Streptococcus faecium*, bifidobacteria and the yeast *S. boulardii.*

Lactobacilli used have included a commercial mixture *of Lactobacillus acidophilus* and *Lactobacillus bulgaricus* (Lactinex®) and *Lactobacillus GG.* decreased AAD in adults receiving amoxicillin (3.3%) compared to placebo (21%), but the difference was not statistically significant [69]. A study in children receiving amoxicillin failed to demonstrate a significant decrease in AAD with this probiotic mixture [70]. Variability in lots may explain differences in efficacy in many trials [71]. *Lactobacillus GG* may have a better efficacy than this probiotic mixture in the prevention of AAD. Adults taking erythromycin and children taking oral amoxicillin had fewer diarrhea stools with *Lactobacillus GG* compared to placebo [72, 73]. In a controlled trial, prophylactic *Lactobacillus GG* also decreased AAD when given with antibiotics to children with respiratory infections [74]. In a recent study *of Lactobacillus GG* added to a week of standard *anti-H. pylori* triple antibiotic therapy, diarrhea was decreased compared to the placebo group, as was the symptom of bloating [75].

Bifidobacteria are part of the normal flora. Recent interest in this organism resulted from studies of its use in acute diarrhea in hospitalized infants. *S. faecium* (SF68) is a nonpathogenic nontoxigenic *Streptococcus*, available in some European countries as Bioflorin®, which has been shown to decrease AAD compared to placebo in two separate studies in adults [76, 77]. Its efficacy appears to be limited based on data from these two studies.

S. boulardii is a nonpathogenic yeast with proven efficacy in the prevention of AAD in multiple trials in adults and children [7, 8, 78]. The yeast may compensate for changes in microbial fermentation in response to antibiotic therapy [78]. Its use to prevent AAD in at-risk patients should be a good adjunct to other methods such as limiting *C. difficile* overgrowth [1].

Prevention of acquisition of *C. difficile* in a hospital setting includes careful attention to hand washing, disposable gloves, wise antibiotic policies and enteric precautions.

Conclusion

Data from a variety of clinical trials does suggest that poorly absorbed antimicrobials have a decreased risk of causing AAD and CDAD. These trials include studies of such antibiotics for preoperative bowel decontamination for gastrointestinal tract surgery as well as studies of antibiotics used for traveler's diarrhea (aztreonam, bicozamycin and rifaximin). Such antibiotics are appealing because systemic side effects are decreased. Their efficacy in traveler's diarrhea is a result of efficacy against aerobic pathogens. Rifaximin shows significant suppression of anaerobes, but its efficacy against many strains of *C. difficile* may offset its risk of *C. difficile* diarrhea and in fact decrease it. The use of probiotics as an adjunct to poorly absorbed antibiotics would be an interesting area for future study of minimizing the risk of diarrhea.

One of the leaders in the field, Carl Erik Nord, stated that 'ecological effects are difficult to predict and clinical studies of new antibiotics should include investigations of their impact on the normal human intestinal flora' [41]. Nonetheless, the risk of CDAD may be difficult to predict accurately as other factors besides antibiotics contribute to this risk.

Acknowledgements

The author is grateful to Dr. Lynne McFarland for critical review of the manuscript and to Susan Sperline for expert manuscript preparation.

References

1 Bergogne-Berezin E: Treatment and prevention of antibiotic associated diarrhea. Int J Antimicrob Agents 2000;16:521–526.

2 Bartlett JG: Antibiotic-associated diarrhea. Clin Infect Dis 1992;15:573–581.

3 McFarland LV: Diarrhea acquired in the hospital; in Giannella RA (ed): Acute Infectious Diarrhea. Philadelphia, W.B. Saunders, 1993, pp 563–577.

4 Znidi N, Ponce de Leon S, Oritz RM, et al: Hospital-acquired diarrhea in adults: A prospective case-controlled study in Mexico. Infect Control Hosp Epidemiol 1991;12:349–355.

5 Lima N, Guerrant RL, Kaiser DL, Germanson T, Farr BM: A retrospective cohort study of nosocomial diarrhea as a risk factor for nosocomial infection. J Infect Dis 1990;161:948–952.

6 Finney JMT: Gastro-enterostomy for cicatrizing ulcer of the pylorus. Johns Hopkins Med J 1893; 4;53–55.

7 Surawicz CM, Elmer GW, Speelman P, McFarland LV, Chinn J, Van Belle G: Prevention of antibiotic-associated diarrhea by *Saccharomyces boulardii.* A prospective study. Gastroenterology 1989;96: 981–998.

8 McFarland LV, Surawicz CM, Greenberg RN, Elmer GW, Moyer KA, Melcher SA, Bowen KE, Cox JL: Prevention of ß-lactam-associated diarrhea by *Saccharomyces boulardii* compared with placebo. Am J Gastroenterol 1995;90:439–448.

9 Winston DJ, Winston GH, Bruckner DA, Champlin RE: Beta-lactam antibiotic therapy in febrile granulocytopenic patietns. Ann Intern Med 1991;115:849–859.
10 McFarland LV, Stamm WE: Nosocomial *Clostridium difficile* infection (letter). N Engl J Med 1989;321:190.
11 Knobel H, Salvado M, Plass E, Orfila A, Llorach I, Diez A: Nosocomial epidemic outbreak of diarrhea from *Clostridium difficile.* Comparative study of diarrhea associated with the use of antibiotics (in Spanish). Med Clin (Barc) 1994;102:165–168.
12 Barbut F, Petits JC: Epidemiology of *Clostridium difficile-associated* infections. Clin Microbiol Infect 2001;7:405–410.
13 Buchner AM, Sonnenberg A: Medical diagnoses and procedures associated with *Clostridium difficile* colitis. Am J Gastroenterology 2001;96:766–772.
14 Levy DG, Stergachis A, McFarland LV, Van-Vorst K, Graham DJ, Johnson ES, Park B-J, Shatin D, Clouse JC, Elmer GW: Antibiotics and *Clostridium difficile* diarrhea in the ambulatory care setting. Clin Ther 2000;22:91–102.
15 Van der Waaij D: Colonization resistance of the digestive tract – mechanism and clinical consequences. Nahrung 1987;81:507–517.
16 Clausen MR, Bonnen H, Tvede M, Mortensen PB: Colonic fermentation to short-chain fatty acids is decreased in antibiotic-associated diarrhea. Gastroenterology 1991;101:1497–1504.
17 Rao SS, Edwards CA, Austen CJ, Bruce C, Read NW: Impaired colonic fermentation of carbohydrate after ampicillin. Gastroenterology 1988;94:928–932.
18 Schultz AA, Ashby-Hughes B, Taylor R, Gillis DE, Willkins M: Effects of pectin on diarrhea in critically ill tube-fed patients receiving antibiotics. Am J Crit Care 2000;9:430–411.
19 Benoit R, Dorval D, Loulergue J, Bacq Y, Oliver JM, Audurier A, Metman EH: Post-antibiotic diarrheas: Role of *Klebsiella oxytoca* (in French). Gastroenterol Clin Biol 1992;16:860–864.
20 Bellaiche G, Le Pennec MP, Coudat L, Ley G, Slama JL: Value of proctosigmoidoscopy with bacteriological culture of colonic biopsies in the etiological diagnosis of post-antibiotic acute diarrhea in adults. Prospective study in 24 patients. Pathol Biol 1997;45:70–715.
21 Gupta TP, Ehrinpreis MN: Candida-associated diarrhea in hospitalized patients. Gastroenterology 1990;98:780–785.
22 Danna PL, Urban C, Bellin E, Rahal JJ: Role of candida in pathogenesis of antibiotic-associated diarrhoea in elderly inpatients. Lancet 1991;337:511–514.
23 Chaudhury A, Nath G, Shukla B, Panda S, Singh TB: Diarrhoea associated with *Candida* spp.: Incidence and seasonal variation. J Diarrhoeal Dis Res 1996;14:110–112.
24 Ponnuvel KM, Rajkumar R, Menon T, Sankaranarayanan VS: Role of *Candida* in indirect pathogenesis of antibiotic associated diarrhoea in infants. Mycopathologia 1996;135:145–147.
25 Forbes D, Ee L, Camer-Pesci P, Ward PB: Faecal candida and diarrhoea. Arch Dis Child 2001;84: 328–331.
26 Levine J, Dykoski RK, Janoff EN: Candida-associated diarrhea: A syndrome in search of credibility. Clin Infect Dis 1995;21:881–886.
27 Krause R, Schwab E, Bachhiesl D, Daxbock F, Wenisch C, Krejs GJ, Reisinger EC: Role of *Candida* in antibiotic-associated diarrhea. J Infect Dis 2001;184:1065–1069.
28 Hill MJ, Drasar BS: The normal colonic bacterial flora. Gut 1975;16:318–323.
29 Peach S, Fernandez F, Johnson K, Drasar S: The non-sporing anaerobic bacteria in human faeces. J Med Microbiol 1974;7:213–221.
30 Mette U, Werner H, Krasemann C, Ungerechts J: The effect of antimicrobial agents on human intestinal flora, with particular reference to *Bacteroides* species. Infection 1980;8(suppl 2):S215–S218.
31 Marr JJ, Sans MD, Tedesco FJ: Bacterial studies of clindamycin-associated colitis. A preliminary report. Gastroenterology 1975;69:362–358.
32 Bartlett JG, Condon RE, Gorbach SL, Clarke JS, Nichols RL, Ochi S: Veterans Administration Cooperative Study on Bowel Preparation for Elective Colorectal Operations: Impact of oral antibiotic regimen on colonic flora, wound irrigation cultures and bacteriology of septic complications. Ann Surg 1978;188:249–254.
33 Vergnes D, Moatti N, Monrozies X, Lazorthes F, Enjalbert L: Pre-operative colonic preparation using kanamycin and metronidazole: Qualitative and quantitative effects on the bacterial flora of the intestine. J Antimicrob Chemother 1980;6:709–716.

34 Krager L, Liljeqvist L, Malmborg AS, Nord CE, Pieper R: Effects of ampicillin plus sulbactam on bowel flora in patients undergoing colorectal surgery. Antimicrob Agents Chemother 1982;22: 208–212.
35 Nord CE, Heimdahl A, Kager L, Malmborg AS: The impact of different antimicrobial agents on the normal gastrointestinal microflora of humans. Rev Infect Dis 1984;6(suppl 1):S270–S275.
36 Nord CE, Kager L, Philipson A, Stiernstedt G: Effect of impipenem/cilastatin on the colonic microflora. Rev Infect Dis 1985;7(suppl 3):S432–S434.
37 Mittermayer HW: Influence of temocillin on human bowel flora. Drugs 1985;29(suppl 5): 43–48.
38 Sjovall J, Huitfeldt B, Magni L, Nord CE: Effect of beta-lactam prodrugs on human intestinal microflora. Scand J Infect Dis Suppl 1986;49:73–84.
39 Nord CE, Bergman T, Aase S: Impact of azlocillin on the colon microflora. Scand J Infect Dis 1986;18:163–166.
40 Van den Bogaard AE, Weidema WF, van Boven CP, van der Waay D: Recolonization and colonization resistance of the large bowel after three methods of preoperative preparation of the gastrointestinal tract for elective colorectal surgery. J Hyg (Lond) 1986;97:49–59.
41 Nord CE, Kager L, Malmborg AS: Effects of antimicrobial prophylaxis on colonization resistance. J Hosp Infect 1988;11(suppl A):259–264.
42 Wistrom J, Norrby SR, Myhre EB, Eriksson S, Granstrom G, Lagergren L, Englund G, Nord CE, Svenungsson B: Frequency of antibiotic-associated diarrhoea in 2462 antibiotic-treated hospitalized patients: A prospective study. J Antimicrob Chemother 2001;47:43–50.
43 Silva M, Cornick NA, Gorbach SL: Suppression of colonic microflora by cefoperazone and evaluation of the drug as potential prophylaxis in bowel surgery. Antimicrob Agents Chemother 1989; 33:835–848.
44 Climo MW, Israel DS, Wong ES,Williams D, Coudron P, Markowitz SM: Hospital-wide restriction of clindamycin: Effect on the incidence of *Clostridium difficile-associated* diarrhea and cost. Ann Intern Med 1998;128:989–995.
45 Welling GW, Meijer-Severs GJ, Helmus G, van Santen E, Tonk RH, de Vries-Hospers HG, van der Waaij D: The effect of ceftriaxone on the anaerobic bacterial flora and the bacterial enzymatic activity in the intestinal tract. Infection 1991;19:313–316.
46 Cavallaro V, Catania V, Bonaccorso R, Maz-zone S, Seciale A, Di Marco R, Blandino G, Caccamo F: Effect of a broad-spectrum cephalosporin on the oral and intestinal microflora in patients undergoing colorectal surgery. J Chemother 1992;4:82–87.
47 Nelson DE, Auerbach SB, Baltch AL, Desjardin E, Beck-Sague C, Rheal C, Smith RP, Jar-vis WR: Epidemic *Clostridium difficile-associated* diarrhea: Role of second- and third-generation cephalosporins. Infect Control Hosp Epidemiol 1994;15:88–94.
48 Hecht JR, Olinger EJ: *Clostridium difficile* colitis secondary to intravenous vancomycin. Dig Dis Sci 1989;34:148–149.
49 Swabb EA, Sugerman A, Stern M: Oral bio-availability of the monobactam aztreonam (SQ 26, 776) in healthy subjects. Antimicrob Agents Chemother 1983;23:548–550.
50 De Vries-Hospers HG, Welling GW, Swabb EA, Van der Waaij D: Selective decontamination of the digestive tract with aztreonam: A study of 10 healthy volunteers. J Infect Dis 1984;150:636–642.
51 DuPont HL, Ericsson CD, Mathewson JJ, de la Cabada FJ, Conrad DA: Oral aztreonam, a poorly absorbed yet effective therapy for bacterial diarrhea in US travelers to Mexico. JAMA 1992; 267:1932–1935.
52 Ericsson CD, DuPont HL, Sullivan P, Galindo E, Evans DG, Evans DJ: Bicozamycin, a poorly absorbable antibiotic, effectively treats traveler's diarrhea. Ann Intern Med 1983;98:20–25.
53 Jiang ZD, Ke S, Palazzini E, Riopel L, DuPont H: In vitro activity and fecal concentration of rifaximin after oral administration. Antimicrob Agents Chemother 2000;44:2205–2206.
54 Steffen R: Rifaximin: A nonabsorbed antimicrobial as a new tool for treatment of travelers' diarrhea. J Travel Med 2001;8(suppl 2):S34–S39.
55 Marchese A, Salerno A, Pesce A, Debbia EA, Schito GC: In vitro activity of rifaximin, metronidazole and vancomycin against *Clostridium difficile* and the rate of selection of spontaneously

resistant mutants against representative anaerobic and aerobic bacteria, including ammonia-producing species. Chemotherapy 2000;46:253–266.
56 Bresadola F, Intini S, Anania G, Noce L, Ce-dolini C, DeAnna D, Ferrieri A: Chemotherapeutic prophylaxis in the preparation of the large intestine for surgical interventions: Rifaximin p.o. vs. cephalosporin i. v. (in Italian). Ann Ital Chir 1992;63:201–207.
57 Gillis JC, Brogden RN: Rifaximin. A review of its antibacterial activity, pharmacokinetic properties and therapeutic potential in conditions mediated by gastrointestinal bacteria. Drugs 1995;49: 467–484.
58 McFarland LV: Epidemiology, risk factors and treatments for antibiotic-associated diarrhea. Dig Dis 1998;16:292–307.
59 Crabtree TD, Pelletier SJ, Gleason TG, Pruett TL, Sawyer RG: Clinical characteristics and antibiotic utilization in surgical patients with *Clostridium difficile-associated* diarrhea. Am Surg 1999; 65:507–511.
60 Hogenauer C, Hammer HF, Krejs GJ, Reisinger EC: Mechanisms and management of antibiotic-associated diarrhea. Clin Infect Dis 1998;27:702–710.
61 Wilcox MH, Howe R: Diarrhoea caused by *Clostridium difficile:* Response time for treatment with metronidazole and vancomycin. J Antimicrob Chemother 1995;36:673–679.
62 Wenisch C, Parschalk B, Hasenhundl M, Hirschel AM, Graninger W: Comparison of vancomycin, teicoplanin, metronidazole, and fusidicacid for the treatment of *Clostridium difficile-associated* diarrhea. Clin Infect Dis 1996;22:813–818.
63 DuPont HL, Ericsson CD, Mathewson JJ, Plalzzini E, DuPont MW, Jiang ZD, Mosavi A, de la Cabada FJ: Rifaximin: A nonabsorbed antimicrobial in the therapy of travelers' diarrhea. Digestion 1998;59:708–714.
64 Ripa S, Mignini F, Prenna M, Falconi E: In vitro antibacterial activity of rifaximin against *Clostridium difficile, Campylobacter jejuni* and *Yersinia* spp. Drugs Exp Clin Res 1987;13: 483–488.
65 Boero M, Berti E, Morgando A, et al: Terapia della colite da *Clostridium difficile:* Risultati diuno studio randomizzato aperto rifaximina vs. vancomicina. Microbiol Med 1990;5:74–77.
66 McFarland LV, Surawicz CM, Elmer GE: Breaking the cycle: Treatment strategies for 163 cases of recurrent *Clostridium difficile* disease cases. Am J Gastroenterol 2002;97:1769–1775.
67 Fuller R: Probiotics in human medicine. Gut 1991;32:439–442.
68 Reid G: Probiotics in the treatment of diarrheal diseases. Curr Infect Dis Rep 2000;2:78.
69 Gotz V, Romankiewicz JA, Moss J, Murray HW: Prophylaxis against ampicillin-associated diarrhea with a *Lactobacillus* preparation. Am J Hosp Pharm 1979;36:754–757.
70 Tankanow RM, Ross MB, Ertel IJ, Dickinson DG, McCormick LS, Garfinkel JF: A double-blind, placebo-controlled study of the efficacy of Lactinex in the prophylaxis of amoxicillin-induced diarrhea. DICP 1990;24:382–384.
71 Clements ML, Levine MM, Ristaino PA, Daya VE, Hughes TP: Exogenous lactobacilli fed to man – their fate and ability to prevent diarrehal disease. Prog Food Nutr Sci 1983;7:29–37.
72 Siitonen S, Vapatalo H, Salminen S, Gordin A, Saxelin M, Wikberg R, Kirkkola AL: Effect of *Lactobacillus GG* yoghurt in prevention of antibiotic assoicated diarrhoea. Ann Med 1990;22: 57–59.
73 Contardi I: Batterioterapia orale quale prevenzione della diarrea da antibiotici en età pediatrica. Clin Ter 1991;136:409–413.
74 Arvola T, Laiho K, Torkkeli S, Mykkanen H, Salminen S, Maunula L, Isolauri E: Prophylactic *Lactobacillus GG* reduces antibiotic-associated diarrhea in children with respiratory infections: A randomized study. Pediatrics 1999;104:e64.
75 Armuzzi A, Cremonini F, Ojetti V, Bartolozzi F,Canducci F, Candelli M, Santarelli L, Cammarota G, De Lorenzo A, Pola P, Gasbarrini G, Gasbarrini A: Effect of *Lactobacillus GG* supplementation on antibiotic-associated gas trointestinal side effects during *Helicobacter pylori* eradication therapy: A pilot study. Digestion 2001;63:1–7.
76 Borgia M, Sepe N, Brancato V, Borgia R: A controlled clinical study on *Streptococcus faecium* preparation for the prevention of side reactions during long-term treatments. Curr Ther Res 1982; 31:265–271.

77 Wunderlich PF, Braun L, Fumagalli I, D'Apuzzo V, Heim F, Karly M, Lodi R, Politta G, Vonbank F, Zeltner L: Double-blind report on the efficacy of lactic-acid-producing *Enterococcus* SF68 in the prevention of antibiotic-associated diarrhoea and in the treatment of acute diarrhoea. J Int Med Res 1989;17:333–338.
78 Breves G, Faul K, Schroder B, Holst H, Caspary WF, Stein J: Application of the colon-simulation technique for studying the effects of *Saccharomyces boulardii* on basic parameters of porcine cecal microbial metabolism disturbed by clindamycin. Digestion 2000;61:193–200.

Christina M. Surawicz, MD, FACP, FACG
Harborview Medical Center
325 Ninth Avenue, Box 359773
Seattle, WA 98104 (USA)
Tel. +1 206 341 4634, Fax +1 206 731 8698, E-Mail surawicz@u.washington.edu

This chapter should be cited as follows:

Surawicz CM: Antibiotic-Associated Diarrhea and Pseudomembranous Colitis: Are They Less Common with Poorly Absorbed Antimicrobials? Chemotherapy 2005;51(suppl 1):81–89.

Scarpignato C (ed): Rifaximin: A Poorly Absorbed Antibiotic.
Pharmacology and Clinical Use.

Management of Hepatic Encephalopathy: Role of Rifaximin

Maria Luisa Zeneroli[a], *Rossella Avallone*[b], *Lorenzo Corsi*[b], *Ivo Venturini*[a], *Claudia Baraldi*[a], *Mario Baraldi*[b]

Departments of [a]Medicine and Medical Specialities and [b]Pharmaceutical Sciences, University of Modena and Reggio Emilia, Modena, Italy

Abstract

Hepatic encephalopathy (HE) is a neuropsychiatric syndrome, which develops in patients with acute or chronic liver failure. It is widely accepted to be due to impairment of hepatic clearance of toxic products from the gut such as ammonia. Accumulation of ammonia induces a glutamate neurotoxicity leading to an increased tone of the γ-aminobutyric acid A (GABA-A) receptor system in the brain which results in HE. Factors either increasing the ammonia levels (protein load, constipation, sepsis, or gastrointestinal bleeding) or potentiating the functional activity of the GABAergic system [natural benzodiaze-pine-like compounds (NBZDs) or exogenous benzodiazepines] may act as precipitating factors of HE. NBZDs are present in trace amounts in the blood of normal subjects and have been found to be increased in the blood of patients with liver cirrhosis, with or without HE. These compounds may derive either from the diet since they have been found in plants, vegetables and animals or from gut bacteria. The observation that intestinal bacterial flora is involved in the production of both primary agent of HE (ammonia) and precipitating factors (NBZDs) suggests that the use of nonabsorbable antibiotics such as rifaximin may be useful in preventing episodes of HE in patients with liver cirrhosis.

Introduction

Hepatic encephalopathy (HE) is a neuropsychiatric syndrome characterized by a general depression of the central nervous system, which occurs in fulminant hepatic failure or as a complication of liver cirrhosis. The neurological symptoms of HE range from minimal abnormalities of intellectual functions to deep coma [1]. From a pathogenetic point of view, HE is considered secondary to the accumulation of toxic products such as ammonia in extracellular fluids. These toxins, which increase in blood during severe hepatocellular disease and portal-systemic shunting because of the decreased clearance capacity by the liver, have been suggested to play a key role in HE. There are, however, other compounds, such as benzodiazepines [either natural benzodiazepine-like compounds (NBZDs) and the exogenously administered drugs] that are involved in HE and are today considered as precipitating factors.

Ammonia

There have been debates and controversies for decades about ammonia, the first toxin claimed to be the primary agent of HE [1–4], but it is now recognized as the major factor of this syndrome [5, 6]. Ammonia toxicity does not only seem to be related to an altered brain metabolism, but more specifically to its ability to damage astrocytic cells by a glutamate-related neurotoxicity [7–9], which in turn may alter the entire γ-aminobutyric acid A (GABA-A) receptor system [10]. Moreover, ammonia has been shown to induce an increased production of neurosteroids that exert a positive modulatory effect on the GABA-A receptors [11] and this phenomenon has been ascribed to the upregulation of peripheral benzodiazepine receptors present in HE [12, 13]. These complex metabolic cerebral events, which affect both astrocytes and neurons, result in an imbalance in the functional activity of excitatory and inhibitory receptor systems leading to a prevalence of the latter thanks to an increased tone of the GABA-A receptor system [14, 15]. This is represented by a large supramolecular entity [16], which includes GABA receptors, benzodiazepine recognition sites, chloride ionophores and endogenous modulators. The plasticity of GABA-A receptors, that is up- and downregulation in the number of receptors, is regulated by the levels of neurotransmitters at the synaptic level. In the case of HE, the upregulation of GABA-A receptors, interpreted as an expression of a denervation supersensitivity phenomenon [14] with a consequent increase in GABAergic tone [14–17], is explained by a decreased presence of GABA at the neuronal level [18] rather than by an increased presence of GABA in blood and brain (gut-derived hypothesis) [17]. Indeed, studies performed in animal models of encephalopathy have shown that the mild stage of encephalopathy is characterized by a 45–50% increase in the number of both low and high affinity GABA receptors without changes in the affinity constants [14, 19] and also by an increased number of benzodiazepine receptors of the central type [20]. These findings have recently been confirmed in humans by in vivo studies using positron emission tomography [21] and ^{1}H magnetic resonance spectroscopy [22] in which an increased presence of central-type benzodiazepine receptors in the brain of patients with recurrent HE and a decreased cortical GABA level were demonstrated. These alterations seem to explain the supersensitivity to the administration of tranquillizers and in particular of benzodiazepines in patients with acute or chronic liver diseases. This phenomenon, originally attributed to an altered metabolism of benzodiazepines in such patients, is now recognized to be mainly due to an increased central nervous system sensitivity to this class of drugs [23, 24].

Ammonia must be regarded as the main pathogenetic factor of HE but a variety of other events may precipitate the syndrome in patients with severe liver disease. Indeed, there are precipitating events which act by inducing an increased concentration of ammonia in brain tissues (diuretic therapy, hypokalemia, hyperazotemia, constipation, protein overload, sepsis) [1] and factors which enhance the latent but already present increased tone of the GABAergic system in the brain (NBZDs or exogenous benzodiazepines) [2].

Natural Benzodiazepines

Commercial benzodiazepines are widely used drugs for the treatment of anxiety and sleep disturbances. NBZDs such as diazepam and nordiazepam and other unknown benzodiazepine-like compounds are naturally present in several plants and vegetables [25–28], in different animal species and in humans [29–31]. Moreover, both plasma and brain contain other compounds with benzodiazepine-like activity called 'endozepines' apparently produced in mammalian cells [32, 33]. The observation that NBZDs are present in human brain samples stored since 1940 [30], when benzodiazepines were not yet synthesized, clearly indicates that NBZDs do not derive from environmental pollution by synthetic benzodiazepines, which entered the market only in 1959. Several attempts to find out the endogenous biosynthetic pathways of NBZD production have been made [31–34]. However, an endogenous biochemical pathway of NBZDs has not yet been identified in mammalian cells [33] while it has been found that microorganisms like *Streptomyces* and *Penicillium* can synthesize molecules like anthramy-cin and cyclopeptine, respectively, both containing the basic 1,4-benzodiazepine structure [35]. Moreover, evidence has been provided that some gut bacteria, such as *Acinetobacter lwoffi*, can produce precursors of benzodiazepine receptor ligands [36]. Since NBZDs have been found in food [25–28, 37], it could be speculated that at least part of these compounds found in the human body could be of alimentary source.

NBZDs are present in trace amounts in the blood of normal subjects but they may rise severalfold in the blood of patients with liver cirrhosis, with or without encephalopathy [2, 38]. Increased levels of these compounds are inconstantly

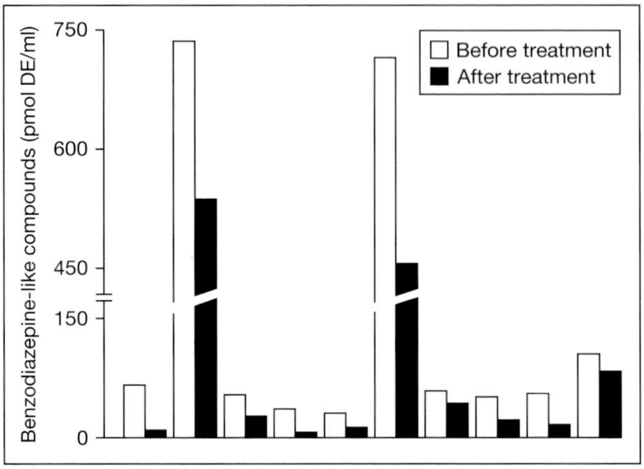

Fig. 1. Serum concentrations of benzodiazepine-like compounds in patients with cirrhosis of the liver before and after treatment with rifaximin (800 mg/day) lasting 7 days [normal values: 9.5 ± 2.9 pmol diazepam equivalents (DE)/ml, mean ± SEM]. Each couple of columns refers to a single patient. One-way ANOVA showed a significant difference in the values before and after treatment ($p < 0.05$) (from Zeneroli et al. [39]).

present in cirrhotic patients. A significant albeit week correlation [38] between circulating NBZDs in patients and the degree of HE does exist, suggesting a pathogenetic role of NBZDs in HE. In a large number of patients we [2] found, however, that NBZD levels correlate with the severity of the liver dysfunction but not with the degrees of HE. It is, therefore, likely that NBZDs represent an occasional precipitating agent of the syndrome rather than a 'true' pathogenetic factor.

Although food does contain NBZDs, it is unlikely that the minute amounts of dietary pharmacologically active substances (in the range of nanograms of diazepam equivalent/gram) cause any appreciable pharmacological effect [37]. However, it should be taken into account that in normal subjects benzodiazepines have a low clearance rate so that a chronic intake of even small amounts of NBZDs could lead to their accumulation in blood and brain, thus exerting a dietary influence on brain function and behavior. This phenomenon could be magnified in cirrhotic patients whose liver displays reduced clearance capabilities. Since food can only partially contribute to the increased NBZD levels in blood and brain of cirrhotic patients, it has been suggested that bacterial flora could also contribute to NBDZ formation [31, 36].

In order to ascertain whether bacterial flora is implicated in the synthesis of these compounds, we measured serum NBZD levels in patients with liver cirrhosis before and after the reduction of bacterial flora with rifaximin, a poorly absorbed antibiotic and found – after treatment – a 40% decrease (fig. 1)

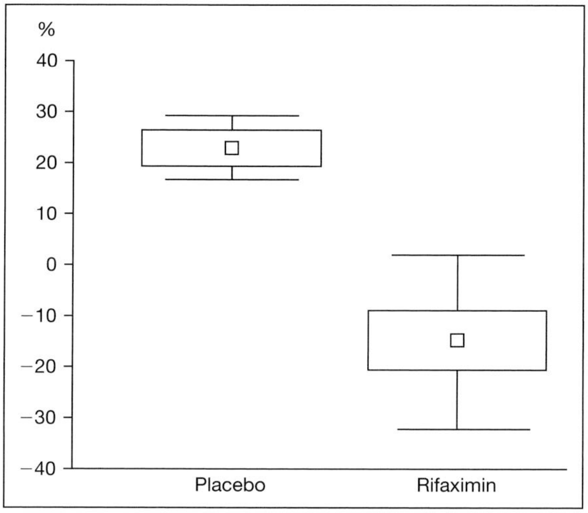

Fig. 2. Percent variation of beta rhythm in cirrhotic patients after a 1-week period of treatment with rifaximin (200–400 mg t.i.d.) or placebo. The relative beta power of the EEG decreased in the rifaximin-treated group (Wilcoxon paired test: $Z = 2.1$, $p = 0.03$), but not in the placebo-treated group ($Z = 1.07$, p = nonsignificant) (from Del Piccolo et al. [40]).

[39]. Our results are in line with the finding of Del Piccolo et al. [40], who observed that the EEG beta activity, which is well known to be increased by benzodiazepines, is significantly reduced in patients with cirrhosis and HE treated with rifaximin (fig. 2). The results of both studies are consistent with the hypothesis that the intestinal bacterial flora is at least partially involved in the production of NBZDs.

Rifaximin in the Management of HE

Both dietary and endogenous ammoniagenic substrates are removed from the intestinal lumen by the osmotic cathartic action of nonabsorbable disaccharides such as lactulose and lactitol. These compounds are currently the main therapeutic agents for chronic HE. The efficacy of oral lactulose for the treatment of HE has been established in controlled trials [41–43]. Besides having a cathartic effect, lactulose lowers the colonic pH as a result of the production of organic acids by bacterial fermentation. The decrease in pH creates an environment that is hostile to the survival of urease-producing intestinal bacteria and may promote the growth of non-urease-producing lactobacilli, resulting in a reduced production of ammonia in the colonic lumen.

Table 1. Controlled clinical trials with rifaximin in the treatment of HE

Year	Authors	Ref.	Comparative agent (study design)	Duration of treatment	Evaluation criteria	Overall assessment
1984	De Marco et al.	49	Paromomycin (open)	6–12 days	NH_3, state of consciousness, intellectual functions,behavior, neurological symptoms	E:Rif ≅ Par T: Rif ≥ Par
1985	Testa et al.	50	Paromomycin (open)	5 days	Antibacterial assays in vitro, NH_3, number connection test	E: Rif ≥ Par T: Rif ≅ Par
1991	Di Piazza et al.	51	Neomycin (double-blind)	7 days	Flapping tremor, bradylalia, patient self-evaluation, visual evoked potential reaction, trial making test	E: Rif ≥ Neo T: Rif ≅ Neo
1991	Pedretti et al.	52	Neomycin (double-blind)	21 days	NH_3, mental status, Reitan test, asterixis, EEG, PSE sum, PSE index	E: Rif ≥ Neo T: Rif ≥ Neo
1992	Parini et al.	44	Paromomycin (open)	10 days	NH_3, state of consciousness, intellectual functions, behavior	E: Rif ≅ Par T: Rif ≅ Par
1992	Festi et al.	53	Neomycin (open)	21 days	NH_3, asterixis, Reitan test, EEG	E: Rif ≅ Neo T: Rif ≅ Neo
			Lactulose (open)	21 days	NH_3, asterixis, Reitan test, EEG	E: Rif. ≅ Lac T: Rif ≥ Lac
1993	Massa et al.	54	Lactulose (double-blind)	15 days	Mental status, 'A' cancellation test, Reitan test, EEG, HE severity	E: Rif ≥ Lac T: Rif > Lac
1993	Fera et al.	55	Lactulose (double-blind)	14 consecutive days each month for 3 months	Mental status, asterixis, cancellation test, Reitan test, EEG, NH_3, PSE severity	E: Rif > Lac T: Rif > Lac

1993	Bucci and Palmieri	56	Lactulose (double-blind)	15 days	Mental status, asterixis, cancellation test, Reitan test, EEG, NH_3	E: Rif > Lac T: Rif > Lac
1997	Miglio et al.	58	Neomycin (double-blind)	14 consecutive days each month for 6 months	Disturbances in speech, memory, behavior and mood, gait, writing, asterixis, NH_3, Reitan test	E: Rif ≅ Neo T: Rif ≥ Neo
2000	Williams et al.	59	3 different rifaximin dose regimens: 200 mg × 3 400 mg × 3 800 mg × 3 (double-blind)	7 days	HE index, mental status, asterixis, Reitan test, EEG, NH_3	E: Rif 800 mg × 3 ≥ other doses No clear dose response explained by the short treatment period T: good for all doses
2003	Loguercio et al.	61	Rif + sorbitol Rif + lactitol Lactitol (double-blind)	14 consecutive days each month for 3 months	Mental status, asterixis, blood NH_3, number connection test	E: Rif + Lat = Rif+Sor >Lat T: Rif + Lat = Rif + Sor = Lat
2003	Mas et al.	62	Lactitol (double-blind)	5–10 days	HE index, mental status, asterixis, NH_3, number connection test, EEG	E:Rif ≥ Lat T:Rif = Lat

E = Efficacy; T = tolerability; Rif = rifaximin; PSE = portal systemic encephalopathy; Par = paromomycin; Neo = neomycin; Lac = lactulose; Lat = lactitol; Sor = sorbitol.

Antibiotics with activity against urease-producing bacteria, such as neomycin [42], paromomycin [44] or metronidazole [45], also reduce the production of intestinal ammonia and have proved to be of value. Vancomycin has also been used in patients with lactulose-resistant chronic encephalopathy [46]. The efficacy of neomycin is similar to that of lactulose [42]. However, a small percentage of this drug is absorbed from the gastrointestinal tract and may cause ototoxic and nephrotoxic effects, especially with continuous use over several months [47]. This drug should be used with particular caution by patients with renal insufficiency. The efficacy of metronidazole for 1 week is similar to that of neomycin [45], although the occurrence of gastrointestinal disturbance and other systemic side effects limit the use of this agent for longer periods.

Rifaximin is a synthetic rifamycin derivative, which acts by inhibiting bacterial ribonucleic acid (RNA) synthesis [48]. It is virtually unabsorbed after oral administration and is, therefore, used primarily to treat gastrointestinal infections. Rifaximin possesses a broad spectrum of antimicrobial activity, covering Gram-positive and Gram-negative bacteria, both arerobic and anaerobic [49]. Several studies [44, 49–62] have shown that in patients with HE rifaximin displays an efficacy similar to that of lactulose and neomycin (table 1). A recently published study [62] compared the efficacy and safety of rifaximin to that of lactitol. This large prospective, randomized, double-blind, double-dummy, controlled trial confirmed that this rifamycin derivative is as effective as lactitol in the treatment of grade I–III HE. Rifaximin, however, was significantly more effective in reducing plasma ammonia levels.

Altogether, these data clearly show that rifaximin represents a good alternative to nonabsorbable disaccharides and may actually be effective in the management of patients resistant to their administration. Taking into account that circulating NBDZs are significantly reduced during administration of this antibiotic [39], cyclic administration of rifaximin – by preventing blood accumulation of both pathogenetic (e.g. ammonia) and precipitating (e.g. NBDZs) factors – might be capable of reducing the number of acute episodes of HE.

References

1 Conn HO, Bircher J: Hepatic Encephalopathy: Syndromes and Therapies. Bloomington, Medi-Ed Press, 1994.

2 Avallone R, Zeneroli ML, Venturini I, Corsi L, Schreier P, Kleinschnitz M, Ferrarese C, Farina F, Baraldi C, Pecora N, Frigo M, Baraldi M: Endogenous benzodiazepine-like compounds and diazepam binding inhibitor in serum of liver cirrhosis patients with and without encephalopathy. Gut 1998;42:860–867.

3 Zeneroli ML, Ventura E, Baraldi M, Penne A, Messori E, Zieve L: Visual evoked potentials in encephalopathy induced by galactosamine, ammonia, dimethyldisulfide and octanoic acid. Hepatology 1982;2:532–538.

4 Baraldi M, Pinelli G, Ricci P, Zeneroli ML: Toxins in hepatic encephalopathy: The role of the synergistic effect of ammonia, mercaptans and short chain fatty acids. Arch Toxicol 1984;7: 103–105.
5 Wang V, Saab S: Ammonia levels and the severity of hepatic encephalopathy. Am J Med 2003;114: 237–238.
6 Ong JP, Aggarwal A, Krieger D, Easley KA, Karafa MT, Van Lente F, Arroliga AC, Mullen KD: Correlation between ammonia levels and the severity of hepatic encephalopathy. Am J Med 2003; 114:188–193.
7 Moroni F, Lombardi G, Moneti G, Cortesini C: The release and neosynthesis of glutamic acid are increased in experimental models of hepatic encephalopathy. J Neurochem 1983;40:850–854.
8 Ferenci P, Pappas SC, Munson PJ, Jones AE: Changes in glutamate receptors on synaptic membranes associated with hepatic encephalopathy or hyperammonemia in the rabbit. Hepatology 1984;4:25–29.
9 Butterworth RF, Lavoie J, Peterson C, Cotman CW, Szerb J: Excitatory amino acids and hepatic encephalopathy; in Pomier Larargue G, Butterworth RF (eds): Hepatic Encephalopathy: Pathophysiology and Treatment. Clifton, Humana Press, 1989, pp 417–433.
10 Baraldi M: Supersensitivity of GABA-A receptors in hepatic encephalopathy. Neurochem Res1990;15:153–160.
11 Norenberg MD, Itzhak Y, Bender S: The peripheral benzodiazepine receptor and neurosteroids in hepatic encephalopathy. Adv Exp Med Biol 1997;420:95–111.
12 Zanoli P, Giacobazzi A, Vaccari G, Zeneroli ML, Baraldi M: Up-regulation of peripheral benzodiazepine receptors in brain areas of rats with galactosamine-induced hepatic encephalopathy; in Bengtsson F, Jeppson B (eds): Progress in Hepatic Encephalopathy. Miami, CRC Press, 1991, pp 161–168.
13 Lavoie J, Pomier Layrargues G, Butterworth RF: Increased densities of peripheral-type benzodiazepine receptors in brain autopsy samples from cirrhotic patients with hepatic encephalopathy. Hepatology 1990;11:874–882.
14 Baraldi M, Zeneroli ML: Experimental hepatic encephalopathy: Changes in the binding of gamma-aminobutyric acid. Science 1982;216:427–429.
15 Basile AS, Gammal SH, Jones EA, Skolnick P: GABA-A receptor complex in an experimental model of hepatic encephalopathy: Evidence for elevated levels of an endogenous benzodiazepine receptor complex ligand. J Neurochem 1989;53:1057–1063.
16 Baraldi M, Guidotti A, Schwartz JP, Costa E: GABA receptors in clonal cell lines: A model for study of benzodiazepine action at molecular level. Science 1979;205:821–823.
17 Schafer DF, Jones EA: Hepatic encephalopathy and the gamma-aminobutyric-acid neurotransmitter system. Lancet 1982;ii:18–20.
18 Zeneroli ML, Iuliano E, Racagni C, Baraldi M: Metabolism of gamma-aminobutyric acid and brain uptake in galactosamine induced hepatic encephalopathy. J Neurochem 1982;33:1219–1222.
19 Zeneroli ML, Baraldi M, Ventura E, Vezzelli C, Tofanetti O, Germini M, Casciarri I: Alterations of GABA-A and dopamine D2 brain receptors in dogs with portal-systemic encephalopathy. Life Sci 1991;48:37–50.
20 Baraldi M, Zeneroli ML, Ventura E, Penne A, Pinelli G, Ricci P, Santi M: Supersensitivity of benzodiazepine receptor in hepatic encephalopathy due to fulminant hepatic failure in the rat: Reversal by a benzodiazepine antagonist. Clin Sci 1984;67:167–175.
21 MacDonald GA, Frey KA, Agranoff BW, Minoshima S, Koeppe RA, Kuhl DE, Shulkin BL, Lucey MR: Cerebral benzodiazepine receptor binding in vivo in patients with recurrent hepatic encephalopathy. Hepatology 1998;26:277–282.
22 Behar KL, Rothman DL, Petersen KF, Hooten M, Delaney R, Petroff OA, Shulman GI, Navarro V, Petrakis IL, Charney DS, Krystal JH: Preliminary evidence of low cortical GABA levels in localized ^{1}H-MR spectra of alcohol-dependent and hepatic encephalopathy patients. Am J Psychiatry 1999;156:952–954.
23 Branch RA, Morgan MH, James J, Read AE: Intravenous administration of diazepam in patients with chronic liver disease. Gut 1976;17:975–983.
24 Bakti G, Fisch HU, Karlaganis G, Bircher J: Mechanism of the excessive sedative response of cirrhotics to benzodiazepine: Model experiments with triazolam. Hepatology 1987;7:629–638.

25 Wildmann J, Vetter W, Ranadaler UB, Schmidt K, Maurer R, Möhler H: Occurrence of pharmacologically active BZD in trace amounts in wheat and potato. Biochem Pharmacol 1988;37:3549–3559.
26 Medina JH, Pena C, Levi de Stein M, Wolfman C, Paladini AC: Benzodiazepine-like molecules as well as other ligands for the brain benzodiazepine receptors are relatively common constituents of plants. Biochem Biophys Res Commun 1989;165:547–553.
27 Avallone R, Zanoli P, Corsi L, Cannazza G, Baraldi M: Benzodiazepine-like compounds and GABA in flower heads of *Matricaria chamomilla.* Phytother Res 1996;10:177–179.
28 Avallone R, Corsi L, Zanoli P, Di Bella M, Monzani A, Venturini I, Zeneroli ML, Baraldi M: Sostanze ad attività benzodiazepino-simili in alimenti e in droghe vegetali: implicazioni fisiologiche e patologiche. Acta Phytother 1997;3:42–50.
29 Sangameswaran L, De Blas AL: Demonstration of the benzodiazepine-like molecules in the mammalian brain with a monoclonal antibody to benzodiazepines. Proc Natl Acad Sci USA 1985;82: 5560–5564.
30 De Blas AL, Park D, Friedrich P: Endogenous benzodiazepine-like molecules in human, rat and bovine brains studied with a monoclonal antibody to benzodiazepines. Brain Res 1987;413: 275–284.
31 Unseld E, Klotz U: Benzodiazepines: Are they of natural origin? Pharmacol Res 1989;6:1–3.
32 Olasmaa M, Rothstein JD, Guidotti A, Weber PJ, Paul SM, Spector S, Zeneroli ML, Baraldi M, Costa E: Endogenous benzodiazepine in human and animal hepatic encephalopathy. J Neurochem 1990;55:2015–2023.
33 Rothstein JD: Benzodiazepine-receptor ligands and hepatic encephalopathy: A causal relationship? Hepatology 1994;19:248–250.
34 Leimgruber W, Batcho AD, Schenker F: The structure of anthramycin. J Am Chem Soc 1965;87: 5793–5795.
35 Luckner M, Nover L: Biosynthesis of the benzodiazepine and quinoline alkaloids of *Penicillum cyclopium* and *Penicillum viridatum;* in Mothes K, Kurt H (eds): Biochemistry: Physiology of Alkaloids. 4th Int Symp. Berlin, AkademieVerlag, 1969, pp 525–533.
36 Yurdaydin C, Walsh TJ, Howard DE, Ha J, Li Y, Jones EA, Basile AS: Gut bacteria provide precursors of benzodiazepine receptor ligands in a rat model of hepatic encephalopathy. Brain Res 1995;679:42–48.
37 Avallone R, Corsi L, Zeneroli ML, Baraldi M: Presence of benzodiazepine-like molecules in food and their implication in the nutrition of cirrhotic patients. Inn Food Sci Technol 2001;23:193–198.
38 Basile AS, Harrison PM, Hughes RD, Gu ZQ, Pannell L, McKinney A, Jones EA, Williams R: Relationship between plasma benzodiazepine receptor ligand concentrations and severity of hepatic encephalopathy. Hepatology 1994;19:112–121.
39 Zeneroli ML, Venturini I, Stefanelli S, Farina F, Cosenza R, Miglioli L, Minelli E, Amedei R, Ferrieri A, Avallone R, Baraldi M: Antibacterial activity of rifaximin reduces the levels of benzodiazepine-like compounds in patients with liver cirrhosis. Pharmacol Res 1997;35:557–560.
40 Del Piccolo F, Amodio P, Mapelli D, Montagnese S, Pellegrini A, Valenti P, Ferrieri A, Gatta A: Rifaximin reduces EEG relative beta power in patients with minimal hepatic en cephalopathy: Preliminary findings; in Jones EA, Mejer AJ, Chamuleau RAFM (eds): Encephalopathy and Nitrogen Metabolism in Liver Failure. Dordrecht, Kluwer Academic Publishers, 2003, chap 35, pp 361–367.
41 Bircher J, Muller J, Guggenheim P, Haemmerli UP: Treatment of chronic portal-systemic encephalopathy with lactulose. Lancet 1966;1:890–892.
42 Conn HO, Leevy CM, Vlahcevic ZR, Rodgers JB, Maddrey WC, Seeff L, Levy LL: Comparison of lactulose and neomycin in the treatment of chronic portal-systemic encephalopathy. A double blind controlled trial. Gastroenterology 1977;72:573–583.
43 Lanthier PL, Morgan MY: Lactitol in the treatment of chronic hepatic encephalopathy: An open comparison with lactulose. Gut 1985;26:415–420.
44 Parini P, Cipolla A, Ronchi M, Salzetta A, Mazzella G, Roda E: Effect of rifaximin and paromomycin in the treatment of portal-systemic encephalopathy. Curr Ther Res 1992;52:34–39.
45 Morgan MH, Read AE, Speller DCE: Treatment of hepatic encephalopathy with metronidazole. Gut 1982;23:1–7.
46 Tarao K, Ikeda T, Hayashi K, Sakurai I: A Successful use of vancomycin hydrochloride in the treatment of lactulose-resistant chronic hepatic encephalopathy. J Gastroenterol Hepatol 1989;4:284–286.

47 Berk DP, Chalmers T: Deafness complicating antibiotic therapy of hepatic encephalopathy. Ann Intern Med 1970;73:393–396.
48 Gillis JC, Brogden RN: Rifaximin: A review of its antibacterial activity, pharmacokinetic properties and therapeutic potential in conditions mediated by gastrointestinal bacteria. Drugs 1995;49: 467–484.
49 De Marco F, Santamaria Amato P, D'Arienzo A: Rifaximin in collateral treatment of portal-systemic encephalopathy: A preliminary report. Curr Ther Res 1984;36:668–674.
50 Testa R, Eftimiadi C, Sukkar GS, De Leo C, Rovida S, Schito GC, Celle G: A non-absorbable rifamycin for treatment of hepatic encephalopathy. Drugs Exp Clin Res 1985;11:387–392.
51 Di Piazza S, Filippazzo GM, Valenza LM, Morello S, Pastore L, Conti A, Cottone S, Pagliaro L: Rifaximin versus neomycin in the treatment of portosystemic encephalopathy. Ital J Gastroenterol 1991;23:403–407.
52 Pedretti G, Calzetti C, Missale G, Fiaccadori F: Rifaximin versus neomycin on hyperammoniemia in chronic portal systemic encephalopathy of cirrhotics. A double-blind, randomized trial. Ital J Gastroenterol 1991;23:175–178.
53 Festi D, Mazzella G, Parini P, Ronchi M, Cipolla A, Orsini M, Sangermano A, Bazzoli F, Aldini R, Roda E: Treatment of hepatic encephalopathy with non-absorbable antibiotics. Ital J Gastroenterol 1992;24:14–16.
54 Massa MD, Vallerino MD, Dodero MD: Treatment of hepatic encephalopathy with rifaximin: Double blind, double dummy study versus lactulose. Eur J Clin Res 1993;4:7–1 8.
55 Fera G, AgostinacchioF, Nigro M, Schiraldi O, Ferrieri A: Rifaximin in the treatment of hepatic encephalopathy. Eur J Clin Res 1993;4:57–66.
56 Bucci L, Palmieri GC: Double-blind, double- dummy comparison between treatment with rifaximin and lactulose in patients with medium to severe degree hepatic encephalopathy. Curr Med Res Opin 1993;13:109–118.
57 PuxedduA, Quartini M, Massimetti A, Ferrieri A: Rifaximin in the treatment of chronic hepatic encephalopathy. Curr Med Res Opin 1995;13:274–281.
58 Miglio F, Valpiani D, Rossellini SR, Ferrieri A: Rifaximin, a non-absorbable rifamycin, for the treatment of hepatic encephalopathy. A double-blind, randomised trial. Curr Med Res Opin 1997; 13:593–601.
59 Williams R, James OF, Warnes TW, Morgan MY: Evaluation of the efficacy and safety of rifaximin in the treatment of hepatic encephalopathy: A double-blind, randomized, dose-finding multicentre study. Eur J Gastroenterol Hepatol 2000;12:203–208.
60 Lata J, Hulek P, Fejfar T, Spicak J, Drastich P, Marecek Z, Bruha R, Husova L, Senkyrik M: Rifaximin in the treatment of hepatic encephalopathy. Vnitr Lek 2002;6:578–582.
61 Loguercio C, Federico A, De Girolamo V, Ferrieri A, Del Vecchio Blanco C: Cyclic treatment of chronic hepatic encephalopathy with rifaximin. Minerva Gastroenterol Dietol 2003;49:53–62
62 Mas A, Rodes J, Sunyer L, Rodrigo L, Planas R, Vargas V, Castells L, Rodriguez-Martinez D, Fernandez-Rodriguez C, Coll I, Pardo A: Comparison of rifaximin and lactitol in the treatment of acute hepatic encephalopathy: Results of a randomized, double-blind, double-dummy, controlled clinical trial. J Hepatol 2003;38:51–58.

Note Added in Proof

After the submission of the manuscript three interesting papers [1–3] dealing with the management of hepatic encephalopathy have been published. A Cochrane systematic review [1] evaluating 30 randomized controlled trials did conclude that antibiotics appear to be superior to nonabsorbable disaccharides in improving symptoms of portal systemic encephalopathy. The authors also emphasized that there is insufficient high-quality evidence to support the use of lactulose or lactitol. A combination of a disaccharide and an antibiotic has been suggested, but not consistently demonstrated to be beneficial [2]. Finally, the use of probiotics has been proposed [3], whose administration could actually follow that of antibiotics.

References

1 Als-Nielsen B, Gluud LL, Gluud C: Non-absorbable disaccharides for hepatic encephalopathy: Systematic review of randomised trials. BMJ 2004;328:1046–1050.

2 Dasarathy S: Role of gut bacteria in the therapy of hepatic encephalopathy with lactulose and antibiotics. Indian J Gastroenterol 2003;22(suppl 2):S50–S53.

3 Solga SF, Diehl AM: Gut flora-based therapy in liver disease? The liver cares about the gut. Hepatology 2004;39:1197–1200.

Prof. Maria Luisa Zeneroli, MD
Cattedra e Divisione di Medicina Interna II
Dipartimento di Medicina e Specialità Mediche, Università di Modena e Reggio Emilia
Via del Pozzo 71, IT–41100 Modena (Italy)
Tel. +39 059 4222150, Fax +39 059 4224363, E-Mail zeneroli.marialuisa@unimore.it

This chapter should be cited as follows:

Zeneroli ML, Avallone R, Corsi L, Venturini I, Baraldi C, Baraldi M: Management of Hepatic Encephalopathy: Role of Rifaximin. Chemotherapy 2005;51(suppl 1):90–95.

Scarpignato C (ed): Rifaximin: A Poorly Absorbed Antibiotic.
Pharmacology and Clinical Use.

Management of Inflammatory Bowel Disease: Does Rifaximin Offer Any Promise?

Paolo Gionchetti, Fernando Rizzello, Claudia Morselli, Rossella Romagnoli, Massimo Campieri

IBD Unit, Department of Internal Medicine and Gastroenterology,
University of Bologna, Italy

Abstract

An increasing number of both clinical and laboratory-derived observations support the importance of luminal components in driving the inflammatory response in ulcerative colitis and Crohn's disease. Although its role is unclear, antibiotic therapy is commonly used in clinical practice for the treatment of moderately to severely active ulcerative colitis. Metronidazole and/or ciprofloxacin are currently employed in active Crohn's disease, particularly in patients with colonic involvement and with perianal disease. Rifaximin, a rifamycin-derived antibiotic, is characterized by a wide range of antibacterial activity and a very low systemic absorption. Some preliminary data show its efficacy in severe active ulcerative colitis, pouchitis and prevention of postoperative recurrence in Crohn's disease.

Role of Intestinal Microflora in Inflammatory Bowel Disease

Although the pathogenesis of inflammatory bowel disease (IBD) remains unclear, increasing evidence suggests that the enteric microflora plays a central role in this process. The distal ileum and the colon are the areas with the highest bacterial concentrations and represent the sites of inflammation in IBD; similarly pouchitis appears to be associated with bacterial overgrowth and dysbiosis.

Recent experimental data, coming particularly from animal models of IBD, are consistent with the hypothesis that gut flora and bacterial products are implicated in the initiation and/or perpetuation of chronic intestinal inflammation. Purified bacterial products can initiate and perpetuate experimental colitis [1, 2].

The leading hypothesis for the development of chronic intestinal inflammation is that an abnormal immune response to normal flora might be crucial. This loss of tolerance might be due to a lack of regulatory mediators or cells, or a breakdown in barrier function which makes possible the access of inflammatory bacterial products to the local immune system, thereby overwhelming the normal regulation [3]. These possibilities were supported by data obtained from several studies in IBD patients, reporting an important role for T cells in the proliferative response to intestinal flora [3], T cell-mediated immune responses to different autologous and heterologous species of bacteria from intestinal flora regulated by a complex network of T cell specificity [4], and enhanced IgG levels against cytoplasmic proteins from commensal bacteria in active IBD. In patients with Crohn's disease (CD) diversion of the fecal stream determines a decrease in disease activity, with disease recurrence occurring after restoration of the fecal stream [5]. Moreover, studies have demonstrated the ability of luminal contents, presumably dominated by bacteria or their products, to trigger postoperative recurrence in the terminal ileum within a few days, providing further evidence of the role of enteric microflora. In fact, D'Haens et al. [6] showed that the exposure of the mucosa of the excluded normal ileal loop to autologous fecal material in CD quickly (8 days) activates the mucosal immune system: biopsy specimens showed morphological evidence of focal inflammation with recruitment of inflammatory cells and differentiation of mononuclear cells into functional macrophages and epithelioid cells. Another study has tested the effect of the ultrafiltrated ileal effluent when infused into defunctioned colon; no signs of mucosal lesions were found, suggesting that the intact bacteria and large dietary particles may be responsible for the recurrence of inflammation. The most compelling evidence, however, comes from studies conducted in animal models of colitis; spontaneous colitis that consistently develops in many transgenic and knockout mutant murine models of colitis may not occur when these lines are maintained in a germ-free environment [7].

Taken together these experimental and clinical observations support the hypothesis that there is no gut inflammation without bacteria, and that the manipulation of enteric microflora may represent a possible therapeutic approach in IBD.

For many years, investigators have tried to find out whether a specific pathogen could determine IBD. For instance, much attention has been paid to the role of *Mycobacteria* at the onset of CD [8] and more recently it has been suggested that a particular subtype of *Escherichia coli* could play a pathogenic role in CD [9]. The presence of *Shigella* or *Shigella*-like toxin, *Salmonella* and *Yersinia* has been investigated as a possible cause of ulcerative colitis (UC), whereas *Clostridium difficile* toxin has been associated with disease exacerbation [10]; a similar role has been suggested for *Salmonella* infection perhaps associated with a diminished protective activity of the mucus [11]. More recently, high serum antibody titers to the outer membrane protein of *Bacteroides vulgatus* were found in patients with UC [12], but all these results have been rather inconclusive. Since *E. coli* is the predominant aerobic Gram-negative species of the normal intestinal flora, much more attention has been paid to a possible role of its subtypes. Besides commensal bacteria, certain specific strains possess virulent properties and cause disease in humans; the diarrheagenic subtypes of *E. coli* belong to this latter group, showing properties such as adherence to the gut mucosa, production of enterotoxins and cytotoxins and tissue invasion [13].

The presence of *E. coli* in patients with UC has been investigated, and it has been reported that *E. coli* could be detected only in a small proportion of tissue samples [14, 15]. Studies on mucosal adhesion of pathogenic bacteria in UC are controversial. A significantly enhanced adhesion of isolates of *E. coli* from stool specimens and rectal biopsies from UC patients to buccal epithelial cells was found in comparison with patients with infectious diarrhea or normal controls. The adhesive properties were similar to those of pathogenic intestinal *E. coli,* suggesting that virulent *E. coli* strains might participate in the pathogenesis of UC [16, 17]. Another study reported adherence of only the DAEC and EAggEC *E. coli* subtypes to rectal mucosa; however, no differences in adhesion could be found between UC patients and controls [18]. Adherence of a different species (EHEC) has also been described [19]. Using a hybridization in situ technique, a significantly higher number of bacteria was found within the mucus layer and not adherent to the surface of the epithelium in UC patients compared to controls, independently of the degree of inflammation. The bacteria belong, most likely, to a variety of species regarding the broad specificity of the probe used in this study [20]. In summary, incomplete information and controversies exist about the role, the adherent properties, and the subtypes of *E. coli* which might be important in the pathogenesis of IBD.

An alternative hypothesis suggests that alteration in normal intestinal ecology can cause inflammation through impairment of epithelial cell metabolism. Colonic anaerobic bacteria are able to break down the ingested carbohydrates and proteins through the process of fermentation into short-chain fatty acids, which are the main source of energy for colonocytes [21]. It has been postulated that a deficiency of this energetic support might lead to the onset of colitis [22]. Furthermore, in patients with active UC there is an overproduction of hydrogen sulfide, a metabolite very toxic for the intestinal mucosa, which seems to be related to an excess of sulfate-reducing bacteria (*Desulfibrio desulfuricans*) in fecal samples [23, 24]. This theory is supported by the evidence that administration of sulfated polysaccharides (carrageenan) in guinea pigs induces a chronic colonic inflammation whose features are similar to human UC [25] and that treatment with 5-ASA is able to reduce fecal concentration of sulfide [26]. It is, therefore, evident that some bacteria do locate in the mucus and might possibly act by degrading its protective structure, leading as a consequence to mucosal invasion.

Therefore, the unresolved question remains of whether chronic, recurring inflammation is the result of a persistent infection with a specific pathogen, an exaggerated exposure to resident normal luminal bacteria products because of increased intestinal permeability or alteration of mucus composition, or an abnormally aggressive immune response to luminal components.

Antibiotic Treatment in IBD

Leaving from these data, few clinical trials have been performed using antibiotic therapy in UC and CD with contradictory results.

Antibiotics in UC

Only few trials with antibacterial agents have been carried out in IBD and the results are controversial.

Dickinson et al. [27], in 1985, published a double-blind controlled trial on the use of oral vancomycin as an adjunctive therapy in acute exacerbations of idiopathic colitis. No significant difference was found between the two treatment groups with only a trend in favor of a superior efficacy of vancomycin. It is important to underline that 7 of the 40 patients enrolled had colonic CD and that none of them had *C. difficile* infection that could explain the action of vancomycin. Subsequently, intravenous metronidazole, in addition to steroids, was effective similar to placebo in inducing remission [28].

In 1990, Burke et al. [29] published a double-blind, placebo-controlled trial on the use of oral tobramycin in acute UC. Eighty-four patients were randomized to receive steroid plus tobramycin or placebo. After 1 week of treatment, 74% of patients in the tobramycin treatment group versus 43% in the placebo group ($p < 0.003$) achieved a complete remission. Subsequently, tobramycin and metronidazole were associated with a standard steroid treatment in severely acute UC. At the end, no difference was found between the two groups [30].

Ciprofloxacin has been tested in a randomized, placebo-controlled study; 70 patients with mildly to moderately active UC were randomized to receive ciprofloxacin 250 mg b.i.d. or placebo for 14 days. At the end of the study, 70.5% of patients in the ciprofloxacin group versus 72% in the placebo group showed an improvement [31]. Nevertheless, in a more recent randomized, placebo-controlled trial, ciprofloxacin was administered for 6 months to patients with active UC poorly responding to conventional therapy with steroids and mesalazine. At the end of the study, the treatment failure rate was 21% in the ciprofloxacin-treated group and 44% in the placebo group ($p < 0.002$). Also endoscopic and histological evaluation showed a better improvement in the ciprofloxacin group [32].

Based on the experimental observation of a beneficial effect of intracolonic amoxicillin-clavulanic acid in a rat model of colitis, Casellas et al. [33] used an enteric-coated amoxicillin-clavulanic acid (1 g amoxicillin plus 250 mg clavulanic acid, t.i.d.) in active UC. They also evaluated the release of inflammatory mediators (IL-8, TXB2, PGE2) in rectal dialysates. After short-term treatment, this formulation decreased intraluminal release of IL-8 and other inflammatory mediators and led to an improvement of patients with active UC.

Antibiotics in CD

Metronidazole has been the mostly investigated agent. In 1978, Blichfeldt et al. [34] performed the first controlled study of metronidazole in CD. They did not find a difference between metronidazole and placebo-treated patients but a positive trend in favor of metronidazole was observed when the colon was involved. In the National Cooperative Swedish study, metronidazole was compared to sulfasalazine; no significant difference was found between the two groups; however, in the crossover section of the study, metronidazole was effective in patients not responding to sulfasalazine [35].

Metronidazole was used as single therapy or associated with cotrimoxazole compared to placebo in patients with a symptomatic relapse of CD. At the end of the 4 weeks of treatment there was no difference in response among the three groups [36]. In a Canadian study, two different dosages of metronidazole (10 and 20 mg/kg/daily) were used versus placebo in patients with active CD; no difference was found between the two groups, but in the metronidazole-treated group there was a high rate of dropout because of side effects or intolerance [37].

An antibiotic association was used in an Italian randomized controlled study in which metronidazole 250 mg 4 times daily plus ciprofloxacin 500 mg twice daily were compared to a standard steroid treatment. No differences were found and it was concluded that the antibiotic association could be an alternative to steroid treatment in acute phases of CD [38].

Ciprofloxacin has an excellent activity against enteric pathogens and Gram-negative Enterobacteriaceae associated with immunosuppressive properties. Ciprofloxacin 1 g/daily was compared to mesalazine 4 g/daily in a controlled study in mildly to moderately active CD. After 6 weeks an equivalence in efficacy was registered, offering an alternative treatment in active CD [39].

In a small study ciprofloxacin was shown to be effective in association with standard treatment in patients with resistant disease [40]. The results of this study were challenged by a controlled study in which ciprofloxacin (1 g/day) was associated with budesonide (9 mg/day) in ileocolic active CD. No difference was found compared to placebo, but surprisingly the overall response in both groups was lower than that reported in previous studies with budesonide [41].

A lot of studies have tried to evaluate the efficacy of antimycobacterial drugs in patients with CD, investigating the possibility that a strain of *Mycobacterium* might be an etiological agent in CD. Borgaonkar et al. [42] evaluated all randomized controlled trials in which antimycobacterial therapy was compared with placebo, suggesting an efficacy of antimycobacterial therapy only in few patients. However, the investigator emphasized that because of the small number of studies included in the meta-analysis, the data were not conclusive and a high rate of side effects was registered.

Metronidazole at the dose of 20 mg/kg/day was also tested by Rutgeerts et al. [43] in the prevention of postoperative recurrence. Sixty patients were randomized to receive metronidazole or placebo for 12 weeks. At the end of the treatment, endoscopic relapse was evaluated by the Rutgeerts score. Metronidazole significantly reduced the incidence of severe endoscopic relapse (grade 3 or 4) but was complicated by a high incidence of side effects. Recently, ornidazole, another nitroimidazole derivative, was proposed in the prevention of postoperative recurrence in order to reduce the incidence of side effects. After 12 months, ornidazole was significantly more effective than placebo in the prevention of recurrence [44].

Rifaximin in the Treatment of IBD

Rifaximin is a rifamycin-derived antibiotic [45] with (1) a large antimicrobial spectrum covering most Gram-positive and Gram-negative bacteria, including aerobes and anaerobes and (2) poor absorption after oral administration and complete fecal excretion as unchanged drug.

Rifaximin has revealed as excellent safety profile: in clinical trials adverse reactions were observed in less than 2% of patients; most of the side effects were of gastrointestinal type or origin (such as nausea, vomiting, flatulence/meteorism, abdominal pain/cramp) while a mild to moderate urticarioid rash was infrequent [45].

A first open, uncontrolled study [46], performed in 12 patients with active IBD refractory to standard treatment who all had positive stool culture, suggested that adding rifaximin (800 mg daily) could be beneficial. A further small but controlled investigation performed in our unit [47] evaluated the efficacy and systemic absorption of rifaximin in patients with moderately to severely active UC refractory to steroid treatment. Patients were eligible if they had no response to intravenous corticosteroid therapy (methylprednisolone 1 mg/kg/day)

Table 1. Rifaximin vs. placebo in severe UC: outcome after 10 days of therapy (from Gionchetti et al. [47])

	Rifaximin			Placebo		
	Before	After	p	Before	After	p
Stool frequency	6.3 ± 2.5	4.2 ± 2.5	<0.02	6.3 ± 2.8	5.2 ± 2.5	NS
Rectal bleeding	1.41 ± 0.51	1.0 ± 0.0	<0.05	1.43 ± 0.51	1.29 ± 0.49	NS
Fever	36.6 ± 0.3	36.5 ± 0.18	0.07	36.7 ± 0.4	36.9 ± 1.0	NS
Sigmoidoscopic score	2.58 ± 0.51	1.83 ± 0.83	<0.01	2.14 ± 0.36	1.57 ± 0.85	0.06
Clinical activity	2.21 ± 0.43	1.57 ± 0.65	<0.05	2.42 ± 0.51	1.83 ± 0.83	<0.05

after 7–10 days. Twenty-eight patients were randomized to receive rifaximin 400 mg b.i.d. or placebo for 10 days as an add-on medication to standard steroid treatment. Clinical and endoscopic evaluation were performed before and after the treatment, and stool frequency, consistency and presence of blood were also recorded. Plasma and urine samples were collected before and after the treatment to determine the systemic absorption of rifaximin. Although there was no significant difference in clinical efficacy between the two treatments, only rifaximin determined a significant improvement of stool frequency, rectal bleeding and sigmoidoscopic score (table 1) [47]. The cumulative excretion of rifaximin in 24-hour urine after 10 days was 64,617 ng, confirming the poor systemic absorption also in presence of colonic inflammation [47]. The efficacy of this rifamycin derivative as add-on medication in patients with mild to moderate UC was recently confirmed in another open-label study [48], where the clinical activity index decreased by 30% after 4 weeks of treatment.

In patients, who experienced a clinical exacerbation of UC and who had a past history of serious adverse reactions to steroids, the antibiotic (400 mg b.i.d. for 4 weeks) was added to mesalazine (2.4 g daily) treatment [49]. In 7 out of 10 patients (i.e. 70%) a clinical remission was achieved without corticoid use, thus showing that rifaximin displays a steroid-sparing effect.

Rifaximin, at a very high dosage (2 g/day), was also used in association with ciprofloxacin 1 g/day in the therapy of chronic, treatment-resistant pouchitis [50]. This 15-day regimen induced a clinical, endoscopic and histological remission in 89% of treated patients with no side effects (fig. 1). Microbiological results have shown a significant decrease in the fecal concentration of most of the colonic bacterial species (table 2), suggesting the need for an antibiotic association in the case of refractory pouchitis to determine a wide antibacterial activity against either Gram-positive or Gram-negative bacteria, both anaerobes and aerobes. Pharmacokinetic data confirmed again the very limited excretion

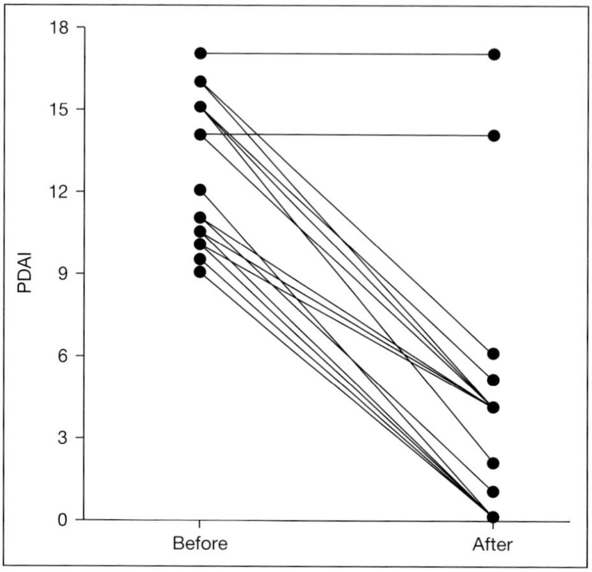

Fig. 1. Pouchitis Disease Activity Index (PDAI) score changes before and after antibiotic therapy in patients with chronic, treatment-resistant pouchitis (from Gionchetti et al. [50]).

Table 2. Bacterial counts in fecal samples of patients with active chronic pouchitis before and after combined antibiotic treatment (from Gionchetti et al. [50])

Bacterial species	Bacterial count (log 10 CFU/g fecal dry weight)	
	Basal values	Values after antibiotic treatment
Total anaerobes	7.12 ± 2.03	5.17 ± 2.33**
Total aerobes	7.34 ± 1.49	5.37 ± 2.55**
Enterococci	6.14 ± 1.66	3.99 ± 2.39**
Coliforms	4.03 ± 2.56	3.57 ± 2.36
Bifidobacteria	3.82 ± 1.89	2.78 ± 1.38*
Lactobacilli	4.03 ± 2.03	2.89 ± 1.56**
Clostridium perfringens	3.67 ± 1.71	2.97 ± 1.69
Bacteroides	2.77 ± 1.70	2.17 ± 0.68*

Data are expressed as mean ± SEM. * $p < 0.05$; ** $p < 0.01$.

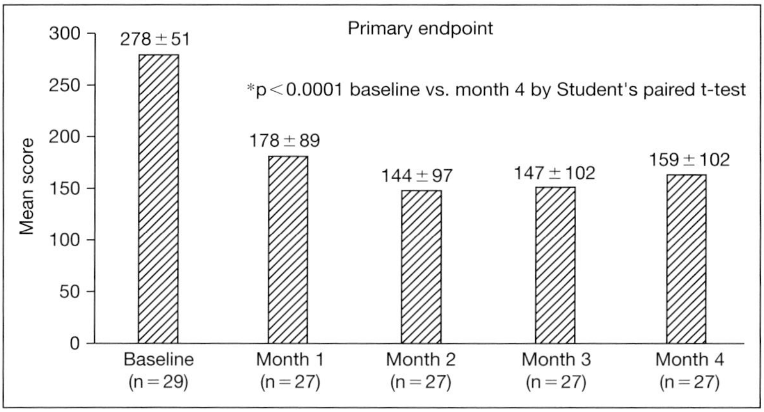

Fig. 2. Effect of rifaximin treatment on CDAI in patients with mildly to moderately active CD (from Shafran et al. [52]).

of unchanged rifaximin in the 24-hour urine samples (24.563 ng/ml, range 0–134.181) [50].

More recently, Campieri et al. [51] performed a randomized trial to evaluate the efficacy in the prevention of postoperative recurrence with rifaximin 1.8 g daily for 3 months followed by a probiotic preparation (VSL#3) 6 g daily for 9 months versus mesalazine 4 g daily for 12 months in 40 patients after curative resection for CD. After 3 months of treatment, patients on rifaximin had a significantly lower incidence of severe endoscopic recurrence compared to those on mesalazine [2/20 (10%) vs. 8/20 (40%)]. This difference was maintained since the end of the study using probiotics [4/20 (20%) vs. 8/20 (40%)].

In conclusion, the results of this pilot study suggest the efficacy of the sequential combination of rifaximin and the highly concentrated probiotic preparation VSL#3 in the prevention of severe endoscopic recurrence of CD after surgical resection [51].

Finally, Shafran et al. [52] presented recently an open-label study on the efficacy and safety of rifaximin 600 mg/day for 16 weeks in the treatment of mildly to moderately active CD. At the end of the study, 59% of patients were in remission (as defined by a Crohn's Disease Activity Index, CDAI, <150) with a significant reduction of the mean CDAI score compared to baseline ($p < 0.0001$) (fig. 2). Only one nonserious drug-related adverse event was reported, confirming the safety of the drug.

All these data, taken together suggest that this antibiotic is clinically useful in most cases of active intestinal inflammation.

References

1 Sartor RB: Enteric microflora in IBD: Pathogens or commensal? Inflamm Bowel Dis 1997;3: 230–235.

2 Simon GL, Gorbach SL: Intestinal flora in health and disease. Gastroenterology 1984;86: 174–193.

3 Duchman R, Kaiser I, Hermann E, Mayet W, Ewe K, Meyer zum Buschenfelde KH: Tolerance exists towards resident intestinal flora but is broken in active inflammatory bowel disease (IBD). Clin Exp Immunol 1995;102:448–455.

4 Duchmann R, May E, Heike M, Knolle P, Neurath M, Meyer zum Buschenfelde KH: T cell specificity and cross-reactivity towards enterobacteria, Bacteroides, Bifidobacterium and antigens from resident intestinal flora in humans. Gut 1999;44:812–818.

5 Rutgeerts P, Goboes K, Peeters M, Hiele M, Penninckx F, Aerts R, Kerremans R, Vantrappen G: Effect of faecal stream diversion on recurrence of Crohn's disease in the neoterminal ileum. Lancet 1991;338:771–774.

6 D'Haens GR, Goboes K, Peeters M, Penninckx F, Rutgeerts P: Early lesions of recurrent Crohn's disease caused by infusion of intestinal contents in excluded ileum. Gastroenterology 1998;114: 262–267.

7 Duchmann R, Schmitt E, Knolle P, Meyer zum Buschenfelde KH, Neurath M: Tolerance towards resident intestinal flora in mice is abrogated in experimental colitis and restored by treatment with interleukin-10 or antibodies to interleukin-12. Eur J Immunol 1996;26:934–938.

8 Sanderson JD, Moss MT, Tizard ML, Hermon-Taylor J: *Mycobacterium paratuberculosis* found in Crohn's disease DNA in Crohn's disease tissue. Gut 1992;33:890–896.

9 Darfeuille-Michaud A, Neut C, Barnich N, Lederman E, Di Martino P, Desreumaux P, Gambiez L, Joly B, Cortot A, Colombel JF: Presence of adherent *Escherichia coli* strains in ileal mucosa of patients with Crohn's disease. Gastroenterology 1998;115:1405–1413.

10 Sartor RB, Rath HC, Sellon RK: Microbial factors in chronic intestinal inflammation. Curr Opin Gastoenterol 1996;12:327–333.

11 Rhodes JM: Unifying hypothesis for inflammatory bowel disease and associated colon cancer: Sticking the pieces together with sugar. Lancet 1996;347:40–44.

12 Bamba T, Matsuda H, Endo M, Fujiyama Y: The pathogenetic role of *Bacteroides vulgatus* in patients with ulcerative colitis. J Gastroenterol 1995;30:45–47.

13 Nataro JP, Kaper JB: Diarrheagenic *Escherichia coli.* Clin Microbiol Rev 1998;11:142–201.

14 Walmsey RS, Anthony A, Sim R, Pounder RE, Wakefield AJ: Absence *of Escherichia coli, Listeria monocytogenes* and *Klebsiella pneumoniae* antigens within inflammatory bowel disease tissues. J Clin Pathol 1988;51:657–661.

15 Kallinowski F, Wassmer A, Hofmann MA, Harmsen D, Heesemann J, Karch H, Herfarth C, Buhr HJ: Frequency of enteropathogenic bacteria in surgically treated chronic inflammatory bowel disease. Hepatogastroenterology 1998;45:1552–1558.

16 Burke DA, Axon ATR: Ulcerative colitis and *Escherichia coli* with adhesive properties. J Clin Pathol 1987;40:782–786.

17 Burke DA, Axon ATR: Adhesive *Escherichia coli* in inflammatory bowel disease and infective diarrhea. BMJ 1988;297:102–104.

18 Schultsz C, Moussa M, van Ketel H, Tytgat GN, Dankert J: Frequency of pathogenic and enteroadherent *Escherichia coli* in patients with inflammatory bowel disease and controls. J Clin Pathol 1997;50:573–579.

19 von Wulffen H, Russmann H, Karch H, Karch H, Meyer T, Bitzan M, Kohrt TC, Aleksic S: Verocytoxin-producing *Escherichia coli* O2:H5 isolated from patients with ulcerative colitis. Lancet 1989;i:1449–1450.

20 Schultsz C, van den Berg FM, ten Kate FW, Tytgat GN, Dankert J: The intestinal mucus layer from patients with inflammatory bowel disease harbours numbers of bacteria compared with controls. Gastroenterology 1999;117:1089–1097.

21 Cummings JH: Short chain fatty acids in the human colon. Gut 1981;22:763–779.

22 Roedinger WEW: The colonic epithelium in ulcerative colitis: An energy deficient disease? Lancet 1980;ii:712–715.

23 Pitcher MC, Beatty ER, Cummings JH: The contribution of sulphate reducing bacteria and 5-aminosalicylic acid to faecal sulphide in patients with ulcerative colitis. Gut 2000;46:64–72.
24 Pitcher MCL, Cummings JH: Hydrogen sulphide: A bacterial toxin in ulcerative colitis? Gut 1996;39:1–4.
25 Marcus R, Watt J: Ulcerative colitis in laboratory animals induced by pepsin inhibitors. Gastroenterology 1974;67:473–483.
26 Pitcher MCL, Beatty ER, Cummings JH: Salicylates inhibit bacterial sulphide production within the colonic lumen in ulcerative colitis. Gut 1995;37:A15.
27 Dickinson RJ, O'Connor HJ, Pinder I, Hamilton I, Johnston D, Axon AT: Double-blind controlled trial of oral vancomycin as adjunctive treatment in acute exacerbations of idiopathic colitis. Gut 1985;26:1380–1384.
28 Chapman RW, Selby WS, Jewell DP: Controlled trial of intravenous metronidazole as adjunct to corticosteroids in severe ulcerative colitis. Gut 1986;27:1210–1212.
29 Burke DA, Axon ATR, Clayden SA, Dixon MF, Johnston D, Lacey RW: The efficacy of tobramycin in the treatment of ulcerative colitis. Aliment Pharmacol Ther 1990;4:123–129.
30 Mantzaris GJ, Hatzis A, Kontogiannis P, Triadaphyllou G: Intravenous tobramycin and metronidazole as an adjunct to corticosteroids in acute, severe ulcerative colitis. Am J Gastroenterol 1994;89:43–46.
31 Mantzaris GJ, Archavlis E, Christoforidis P, Kourtessas D, Amberiadis P, Florakis N, Petraki K, Spiliadi C, Triantafyllou G: A prospective randomised controlled trial of oral ciprofloxacin in acute ulcerative colitis. Am J Gastroenterol 1997;92:454–456.
32 Turunen UM, Farkkila MA, Hakala K, Seppala K, Sivonen A, Ogren M, Vuoristo M, Valtonen VV, Miettinen TA: Long-term treatment of ulcerative colitis with ciprofloxacin: A prospective, double-blind, placebo-controlled study. Gastroenterology 1998;115:1072–1078.
33 Casellas F, Borruel N, Papo M, Guarner F, Antolin M, Videla S, Malagelada JR: Anti-inflammatory effects of enterically coated amoxicillin-clavulanic acid in ulcerative colitis. Inflamm Bowel Dis 1998;4:1–5.
34 Blichfeldt P, Blomhoff JP, Myhre E, Gjone E: Metronidazole in Crohn's disease. A double-blind cross-over clinical trial. Scand J Gastroenterol 1978;13:123–127.
35 Ursing B, Alm T, Barany F, Bergelin I, Ganrot-Norlin K, Hoevels J, Huitfeldt B, Jarnerot G, Krause U, Krook A, Lindstrom B, Nordle O, Rosen A: A comparative study of metronidazole and sulfasalazine for active Crohn's disease: The cooperative Crohn's disease study in Sweden. II. Result. Gastroenterology 1982;83:550–562.
36 Ambrose NS, Allan RN, Keighley MR, Burdon DW, Youngs D, Lennard-Jones JE: Antibiotic therapy for treatment in relapse of intestinal Crohn's disease. A prospective randomized study. Dis Colon Rectum 1985;28:81–85.
37 Sutherland LR, Singleton J, Sessions J, Hanauer S, Krawitt E, Rankin G, Summers R, Mekhjian H, Greenberg N, Kelly M: Double-blind, placebo-controlled trial of metronidazole in Crohn's disease. Gut 1991;32:1071–1075.
38 Prantera C, Zannoni F, Scribano ML, Berto E, Andreoli A, Kohn A, Luzzi C: An antibiotic regimen for the treatment of active Crohn's disease: A randomized controlled clinical trial of metronidazole plus ciprofloxacin. Am J Gastroenterol 1996;91:328–332.
39 Colombel JF, Lemann M, Cassagnou M, Bouhnik Y, Duclols B, Dupas JL, Notteghem B, Mary JY: A controlled trial comparing ciprofloxacin with mesalazine for the treatment of active Crohn's disease. Am J Gastroenterol 1999;94:674–678.
40 Arnold GL, Beaves MR, Prydun VO, Mook WJ: Preliminary study of ciprofloxacin in active Crohn's disease. Inflamm Bowel Dis 2002;8:10–15.
41 Steinhart AH, Feagan BG, Wong CJ, Vandervoort M, Mikolainins S, Croitoru K, Seidmand E, Leddin DJ, Bitton A, Drouin E, Cohen A, Greemberg GR: Combined budesonide and antibiotic therapy for active Crohn's disease: A randomized controlled trial. Gastroenterology 2002;123:33–40.
42 Borgaonkar MR, MacIntosh DG, Fardy JM: A meta-analysis of antimycobacterial therapy for Crohn's disease. Am J Gastroenterol 2000;95:725–729.
43 Rutgeerts P, Hiele M, Geboes K, Peeters M, Penninckx F, Aerts R, Kerremans R: Controlled trial of metronidazole treatment for prevention of Crohn's recurrence after ileal resection. Gastroenterology 1995;108:1617–1621.

44 Rutgeerts P, D'Haens G, Baert F, et al: Nitroimidazol antibiotics are efficacious for prophylaxis of postoperative recurrence of Crohn's disease: A placebo controlled trial. Gastroenterology 1999; 116:A808.
45 Gillis JC, Brogden RN: Rifaximin. A review of its antibacterial activity, pharmacokinetic properties and therapeutic potential in conditions mediated by gastrointestinal bacteria. Drugs 1995;49:467–484.
46 Pinto A, Borrutto G, Deall'Anna A, Turco L, Ferrieri A: An open, uncontrolled trial of oral rifaximin, a non-absorbable antibiotic, in inflammatory bowel disease refractory to conventional therapy. Eur J Clin Res 1997;9:217–224.
47 Gionchetti P, Rizzello F, Ferrieri A, Venturi A, Brignola C, Ferretti M, Peruzzo S, Miglioli M, Campieri M: Rifaximin in patients with moderate or severe ulcerative colitis refractory to steroid-treatment: A double-blind, placebo-controlled trial. Dig Dis Sci 1999;44:1220–1221.
48 Lukas M, Konecny M, Zboril V: Rifaximin in patients with mild to moderate activity of ulcerative colitis: An open label study. Gastroenterology 2002;122(suppl 1):A434.
49 Guslandi M, Giollo P, Testoni PA: Corticosteroid-sparing effect of rifaximin, a nonabsorbable oral antibiotic in active ulcerative colitis: Preliminary clinical experience. Curr Ther Res 2004;65: 292–296.
50 Gionchetti P, Rizzello F, Venturi A, Ugolini F, Rossi M, Brigidi P, Johansson R, Ferrieri A, Poggioli G, Campieri M: Antibiotic combination therapy in patients with chronic, treatment-resistant pouchitis. Aliment Pharmacol Ther 1999;13:713–718.
51 Campieri M, Rizzello F, Venturi A, Poggioli G, Ugolini F, Helwig U, Amadini C, Romboli E, Gionchetti P: Combination of antibiotic and probiotic treatment is efficacious in prophylax is of post-operative recurrence of Crohn's disease: A randomized controlled study versus mesalazine. Gastroenterology 2000;118(suppl 1):A781.
52 Shafran I, Dondelinger PJ, Johnson LK, et al: Efficacy and tolerability of rifaximin, a nonabsorbed, gut-selective, oral antibiotic in the treatment of active Crohn's disease: Results of an open-label study. Am J Gastroenterol 2003;98(9 suppl):S250.

Paolo Gionchetti, MD
Department of Internal Medicine and Gastroenterology
University of Bologna, O.P.S. Orsola-Malpighi
Via Massarenti 9, IT–40138 Bologna (Italy)
Tel. +39 051 636 4122, Fax +39 051 392 538, E-Mail paolo@med.unibo.it

This chapter should be cited as follows:

Gionchetti P, Rizzello F, Morselli C, Romagnoli R, Campieri M: Management of Inflammatory Bowel Disease: Does Rifaximin Offer Any Promise? Chemotherapy 2005;51(suppl 1):96–102.

Scarpignato C (ed): Rifaximin: A Poorly Absorbed Antibiotic.
Pharmacology and Clinical Use.

Treatment of Small Intestine Bacterial Overgrowth and Related Symptoms by Rifaximin

Michele Di Stefano, Gino Roberto Corazza

Gastroenterology Unit, IRCCS 'S. Matteo' Hospital,
University of Pavia, Pavia, Italy

Abstract

The treatment of small intestine bacterial overgrowth should address different aims: the removal of the predisposing condition, guarantee of adequate nutritional support to reintegrate both caloric and vitamin requirements and, obviously, suppression of the contaminating bacterial flora, which represents the major goal. The polymicrobic nature of contaminating flora suggests the administration of wide-spectrum antibiotics, but until now there has been no conclusive information on the most effective therapeutic approach. In this paper, the efficacy of the different therapeutic approaches used is reviewed.

Introduction

The treatment of small intestine bacterial overgrowth (SIBO) is a clinical challenge for physicians, as data contained in the peer review literature do not offer conclusive information on the most effective therapeutic approach. In this paper, available data were reviewed in order to suggest some indications.

Clinical and Pathophysiological Aspects

SIBO is due to the presence of more than 10^6 colony-forming units per milliliter of intestinal aspirate and/or colonic-type species [1]. Although asymptomatic cases, mostly among the elderly [2], have been described, the condition is generally accompanied by malabsorption and the consequent clinical syndrome is characterized by major symptoms, such as diarrhea, steatorrhea and weight loss, together with abdominal pain, bloating and flatulence. Therefore, an impairment of the nutritional status is frequently present and several nutritional defects have been described [3–9].

Malabsorption in SIBO is considered the consequence of abnormalities occurring mainly in the intraluminal environment; in fact, the excessive number of intraluminal bacteria interfere with the absorption process. However, in some cases, the presence of bacterial species capable of more aggressive adhesion to small bowel epithelium is probably the cause of direct damage to the absorptive surface, in particular in the blind loop syndrome [10, 11].

Generally, it is not easy to determine how important the role of the predisposing condition and that of bacterial overgrowth are in the pathogenesis of malabsorption. In fact, conditions like gastrectomy, ileocolonic fistula and short bowel may be causes of malabsorption regardless of the concomitant presence of bacterial overgrowth. The pathophysiological role of bacteria lies in their ability to metabolize nutritional substances, such as carbohydrates, lipids and proteins, normally absorbed at the level of the small bowel. This concerns two different problems. The first is the nutritional defect, due to the lack of caloric substrates available for absorption. The second is a series of effects due to the products of bacterial metabolism, such as increased carbohydrate fermentation [12], which is responsible for the presence of symptoms like flatulence, bloating, abdominal colicky pain and abdominal distention; increased levels of short-chain fatty acids, which trigger the irritation of the colonic wall, acidification of both the bowel lumen and feces and, finally, diarrhea accompanied by abdominal pain, and reduced mucosal disaccharidase activity, due to its inactivation by proteases secreted by anaerobic bacteria [13].

Aims of Treatment

The aims of the treatment of SIBO are listed in table 1. First, physicians should take into consideration the possibility of eliminating the predisposing condition. The importance of the role of these conditions (table 2) was shown by the demonstration of the presence of SIBO in around three-quarters of patients with malabsorption symptoms associated with a predisposing condition [14]. However, elimination of such conditions is not always possible. In patients who have undergone surgical reconstruction with loss of the gastric acid barrier or ileocecal valve, complete recovery from this syndrome is never possible and bacterial overgrowth will always represent a clinical problem to be taken into consideration. On the other hand, in patients with stenosing or fistulizing Crohn's disease, the timing of surgery is subject to complex evaluation

Table 1. Aims of the treatment of SIBO

Nutritional support
Minerals
Vitamins
Caloric requirements
Removal of predisposing conditions
Surgery
Prokinetics (?)
Suppression of contaminating flora
Antibiotics
Probiotics (?)

Table 2. Conditions predisposing to SIBO

Anatomical defects
Blind loops
Strictures
Fistulae
Diverticula
Gastric resections
Ileocolonic resections
Functional defects
Impaired motility causing intestinal stasis
Ageing
Reduced gastric acid secretion
Reduced activity of intestinal immune system

and, therefore, relapsing symptoms of SIBO syndrome often have to be dealt with.

Moreover, adequate nutritional support is mandatory. The aim of this therapeutic measure should be the reintegration of both caloric and vitamin requirements, often defective in these patients. The nutritional defect is caused both by the predisposing condition and by the malabsorption syndrome.

Finally, suppression of the contaminating bacterial flora represents the major aim of treatment for SIBO.

Therapeutic Approaches

Prokinetics

In some patients SIBO is caused by intestinal stasis secondary to motility defects, and the restoration of normal intestinal motility may represent an effective approach. Prokinetic agents have been shown to improve intestinal motility [15, 16], and the use of this therapeutic approach has been shown to be effective: in patients with scleroderma, low-dose octreotide proved to be useful in the reduction of bacterial overgrowth [17]. Unfortunately, cisapride was recently removed from the market due to cardiotoxicity, and, apart from an erythromycin analog without antibiotic effects which showed no effects in rats [18], no other drugs have been tested. Consequently, the role of these agents in the treatment of SIBO still needs to be explored.

Antibiotics

The polymicrobic nature of contaminating flora makes the use of wide-spectrum antibiotics mandatory [19, 20]. The choice of the drug is frequently empirical because small bowel aspiration and culture are impractical and, if performed, will show with certainty multiple organisms with different antibiotic sensitivity. However, the reason why we need to use wide-spectrum antibiotics lies on a still lacking information: we do not know which organisms should be eliminated to achieve the improvement of symptoms [19]. Several antibiotics have been shown to be effective (table 3). However, as can be clearly seen from this table, available data are based very frequently on the description of single cases. Although anaerobes are responsible for the main metabolic alterations, tetracyclines [21–23] have been used for a long time and with satisfactory results, in spite of their poor activity against these bacteria [3, 20, 24]. A rapid improvement of symptoms was evident in most cases after a single therapeutic course of 10–14 days at a dose of 250 mg four times a day [3]. Aerobe suppression induced by tetracyclines probably render the intraluminal microclimate unfavorable to anaerobes, due to the increased bioavailability of oxygen [19]. However, it was recently reported that about 60% of patients do not respond to this treatment [25]. Metronidazole [3, 23], ampicillin [26] and erythromycin [27] have been used as an alternative to tetracycline, while other drugs active against anaerobes, such as lincomycin [23, 28, 29] and chloramphenicol [3, 22], are no longer employed due to the high risk of severe side effects. Neomycin was shown to be of little efficacy when used alone in this condition [29]. Scanty information is available on cotrimoxazole, which was shown to be effective at a low dosage in a case report [30].

If contaminating flora is sensitive to the administered antibiotic, in most patients, a single course of 7–10 days of therapy is able to induce an improvement of symptoms [31]; however, a quick relapse of symptoms is often evident, but it can be treated with the same antibiotics [3, 27]. In these cases, good results can be achieved with intermittent antibiotic treatment [3].

In a recent study, the bacterial populations contaminating the upper gut in SIBO patients and their antibiotic susceptibility were determined. Amoxicillin-clavulanic acid and cefoxitin were effective against <90% of

Table 3. Antibiotic regimens used in SIBO

Drug	Dose	n	Predisposing conditions	Responders
Tetracycline				
Kahn et al., 1966 [21]	250 mg q.i.d.	4	Scleroderma	75%
Goldstein et al., 1961 [22]	250 mg q.i.d.	1	Billroth II	+
Gorbach and Tabaqchali, 1969 [28]	250 mg q.i.d.	1	Ileocolonic anastomosis in Crohn's disease	–
Bjorneklett et al., 1983 [23]	NA	3	Small bowel diverticulosis	100%
Di Stefano et al., 2000 [42]	333 mg t.i.d.	11	GI surgery, intestinal stasis	27%
Chloramphenicol				
Goldstein et al., 1961 [22]	500 mg q.i.d.	1	Billroth II	+
Lincomycin				
Bjorneklett et al., 1983 [23]	NA	1	Radiation fibrosis	–
Gorbach and Tabaqchali, 1969 [28]	500 mg t.i.d.	2	Small bowel diverticulosis	50%
Ampicillin				
Goldstein et al., 1970 [26]	250 mg q.i.d.	1	Diabetic autonomic neuropathy	+
Metronidazole				
Bjorneklett et al., 1983 [23]	NA	6	Radiation fibrosis, small bowel diverticulosis	83%
Cotrimoxazole				
Elsborg, 1977 [30]	400 mg b.i.d.	1	Small bowel diverticulosis	+
Norfloxacin				
Attar et al., 1999 [45]	400 mg b.i.d.	10	GI surgery or intestinal stasis	30%
Amoxicillin-clavulanic acid				
Attar et al., 1999 [45]	500 mg t.i.d.	10	GI surgery or intestinal stasis	50%
Rifaximin				
Trespi and Ferrieri, 1999 [43]	400 mg t.i.d.	8	Chronic pancreatitis and Billroth II	100%
Di Stefano et al., 2000 [42]	400 mg t.i.d.	10	GI surgery or intestinal stasis	70%

NA = Not applicable; GI = gastrointestinal; + = positive effect of therapy; – = no effect of therapy.

anaerobic strains, while aminopenicillins, cephalosporins and cotrimoxazole were effective against the microaerophilic population. Erythromycin, clindamycin and rifampicin were ineffective. Data on metronidazole and fluoroquinolones are not available [32].

Rifaximin, a nonabsorbable derivative of rifamycin, has shown promising bactericidal action against both aerobes and anaerobes, such as bacterioides, lactobacilli and clostridia [33, 34]. The development of resistance to this antibiotic can occur, but resistant strains rapidly disappear from the intestine thus allowing cyclic administration of rifaximin. Controlled clinical trials showed efficacy of rifaximin in adult and pediatric patients with infectious diarrhea [36, 37], hepatic encephalopathy [38], post-surgical complications [39] and colonic diverticulosis [40]. Only recently was the efficacy of rifaximin in the treatment of SIBO demonstrated [41–43].

The most important evidence is probably offered by a recent double-blind, randomized trial which showed a better therapeutic effect of rifaximin in comparison to tetracycline in a cohort of SIBO syndrome patients [42]; in particular, rifaximin administration produced a significant reduction of breath hydrogen levels in fasting conditions, peak of hydrogen excretion and cumulative breath hydrogen excretion after an oral dose of 50 g of glucose (fig. 1). Normalization of the test results was evident in 70% of the sample studied.

A significant improvement of symptom severity and the absence of side effects was also evident after rifaximin administration but not after tetracycline, reinforcing, therefore, the validity of the therapeutic approach adopted. Rifaximin has proved to be effective in the treatment of gas-related symptoms; in fact, in a recent paper, it was reported that a 7-day course of therapy significantly improved the severity of symptoms in a cohort of patients suffering from functional abdominal complaints (pain, bloating, flatulence) [44]. This effect should also be important in patients with SIBO syndrome; it would probably become more evident if courses of therapy longer than 1 week are prescribed, in view of the interference with the therapeutic efficacy due to the presence of predisposing conditions. A correlation between variation in breath H_2 excretion and variation in the number of flatus episodes was actually found in the abovementioned study (fig. 2).

Another recent controlled trial showed a good therapeutic effect of both amoxicillin-clavulanic acid and norfloxacin in SIBO patients [45]. However, a rapid relapse of diarrhea just few days after the withdrawal of antibiotics was evident. In this paper, the efficacy of probiotics in SIBO patients was also evaluated, but no significant effect was described. While on the one hand these results confirm the frequent need of several courses of antibiotic therapy in SIBO patients, on the other they support the idea that rifaximin may represent a good choice on the basis of its excellent tolerability.

In our opinion, the pivotal topic of the treatment of SIBO syndrome is probably represented by the careful evaluation of clinical polymorphism in these patients; the presence of several predisposing conditions, very different with respect to both pathophysiological and clinical aspects, may modify the clinical response of individual patients, thus affecting the overall efficacy of the therapeutic programs. Preliminary results, in fact, have shown that patients with

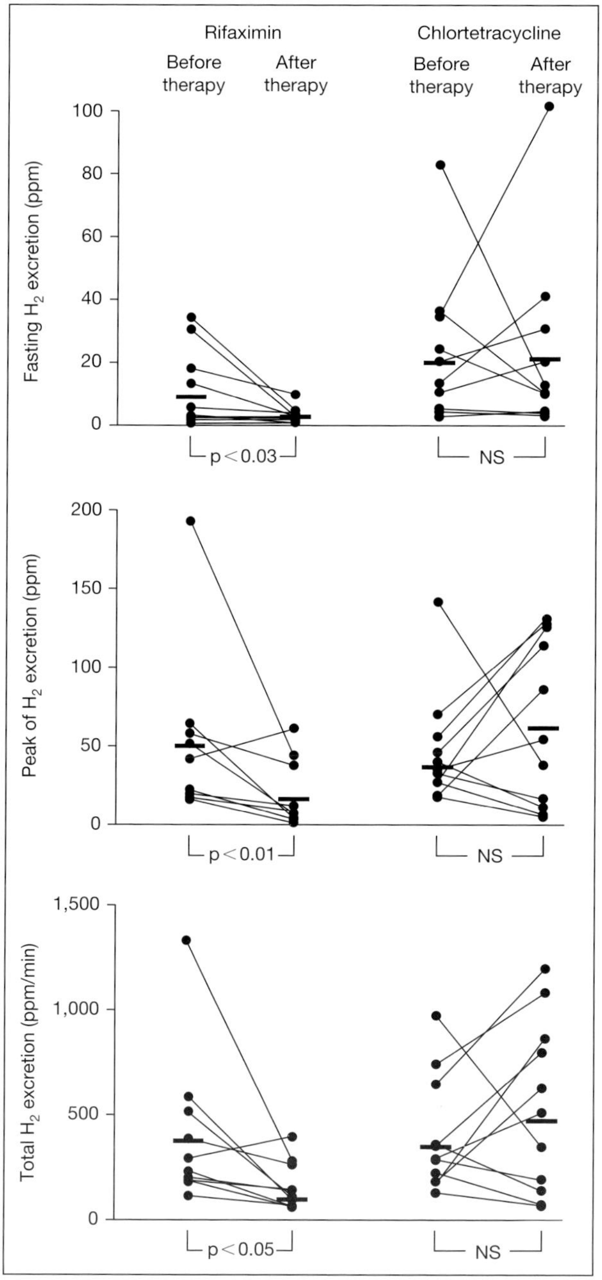

Fig. 1. Fasting, peak and total breath H_2 excretion before and after rifaximin or chlortetracycline therapy in two groups of patients with SIBO (from Di Stefano et al. [42]). NS = Not significant.

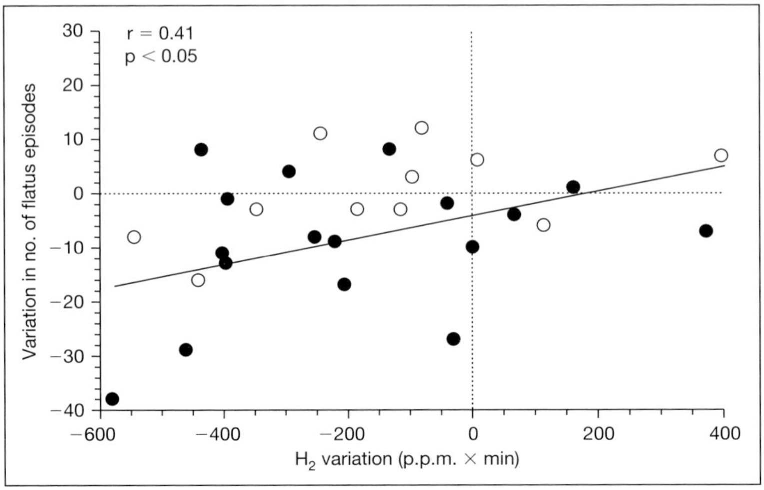

Fig. 2. Correlation between variation in breath H_2 excretion and variation in the number of flatus episodes recorded before and after therapy. Black circles indicate rifaximin-treated patients, white circles indicate charcoal-treated patients. Patients with score >0 were considered (from Di Stefano et al. [44]).

SIBO and blind loop syndrome display a better clinical response after metronidazole therapy than after rifaximin, likely due to a lower drug concentration at the level of the blind loop [46]. It is, therefore, possible that in future the study of subgroups of patients will give us more informations and will clarify several still nonstandardized issues such as the optimal dosage and duration of therapy. Moreover, the availability of nonabsorbable antibiotics in clinical practice will represent an improvement of the current therapeutic strategies.

References

1 Donaldson RM Jr: Normal bacterial populations of the intestine and their relation to intestinal function. N Engl J Med 1964;270:938–945.
2 Saltzman JR, Kowdley KV, Pedrosa MC, Sepe T, Golner B, Perrone G, Russell RM: Bacterial overgrowth without clinical malabsorption in elderly hypochlorhydric subjects. Gastroenterology 1994;106:615–623.
3 King CE, Toskes PP: Small intestine bacterial overgrowth. Gastroenterology 1979;76:1035–1055.
4 Jones EA, Craigie A, Tavill AS, Franglen G, Rosenoer VM: Protein metabolism in the intestinal stagnant loop syndrome. Gut 1968;9:466–469.
5 Rutgeerts L, Mainguet P, Tytgat G, Eggermont E: Enterokinase in contaminated small-bowel syndrome. Digestion 1974;10:249–254.
6 Su J, Smith MB, Rerknimitr R, Morrow D: Small intestine bacterial overgrowth presenting as protein-losing enteropathy. Dig Dis Sci 1998;43:679–681.
7 Schjonsby H, Hofstad T: The uptake of vitamin B_{12} by the sediment of jejunal contents in patients with blind loop syndrome. Scand J Gastroenterol 1975;10:305–309.

8 Brandt LJ, Bernstein LH, Wagle A: Production of vitamin B_{12} analogues in patients with small bowel bacterial overgrowth. Ann Intern Med 1977;87:546–551.
9 Di Stefano M, Veneto G, Malservisi S, Corazza GR: Small bowel bacterial overgrowth and metabolic osteopathy. Dig Dis Sci 2001;46:1077–1082.
10 Schiffer LM, Faloon WW, Chodos RB: Malabsorption syndrome associated with intestinal diverticulosis. Gastroenterology 1962;42:63–68.
11 Ament ME, Shimoda SS, Saunders DR, Rubin CE: Pathogenesis of steatorrhea in three cases of small intestinal stasis syndrome. Gastroenterology 1972;63:728–747.
12 Strocchi A, Levitt MD: Intestinal gas; in Sleisenger MH, Fordtran JS (eds): Gastrointestinal Disease. Philadelphia, Saunders, 1993, pp 1035–1042.
13 Riepe S, Goldstein J, Alpers DH: Effect of secreted *Bacteroides* proteases on human intestinal brush border hydrolases. J Clin Invest 1980;66:314–322.
14 Corazza GR, Menozzi MG, Strocchi A, Rasciti L, Vaira D, Lecchini R, Avanzini P, Chezzi C, Gasbarrini G: The diagnosis of small bowel bacterial overgrowth. Gastroenterology 1990;98: 302–309.
15 Camilleri M, Malagelada JR, Abell TL, Brown ML, Hench V, Zinsmeister AR: Effect of six weeks of treatment with cisapride in gastroparesis with intestinal pseudoobstruction. Gastroenterology 1989;96:704–712.
16 Kaye SA, Lim SG, Taylor M, Patel S, Gillespie S, Black CM: Small bowel bacterial overgrowth in systemic sclerosis: Detection using direct and indirect methods and treatment outcome. Br J Rheumatol 1995;34:265–269.
17 Soudah HC, Hasler WL, Owyang C: Effect of octreotide on intestinal motility and bacterial overgrowth in scleroderma. N Engl J Med 1991;325:1461–1467.
18 Nieuwenhuijs VB, van Duijvenbode-Beumer H, Verheen A, Visser MR, Vrhoef J, Gooszen HG, Akkermans LMA: The effects of ABT-229 and octreotide on interdigestive small bowel motility, bacterial overgrowth and bacterial translocation in rats. Eur J Clin Invest 1999;29:33–40.
19 Banwell JG, Kistel LA, Giannella RA, Weber FL, Lieber A, Powell DE: Small intestine bacterial overgrowth syndrome. Gastroenterology 1981;80:834–845.
20 Sherwood WC, Goldstein F, Haurani FI, et al: Studies of the small intestinal bacterial flora and of intestinal absorption in pernicious anemia. Am J Dig Dis 1964;9:416–425.
21 Kahn IJ, Jeffries GH, Sleisenger MH: Malabsorption in intestinal scleroderma: Correction by antibiotics. N Engl J Med 1966;274:1339–1344.
22 Goldstein F, Wirts CW, Kramer S: The relationship of afferent loop stasis and bacterial flora to the production of postgastrectomy steatorrhea. Gastroenterology 1961;40:47–54.
23 Bjorneklett A, Fausa O, Midtvedt T: Bacterial overgrowth in jejunal and ileal disease. Scand J Gastroenterol 1983;18:289–298.
24 Bjorneklett A, Hoverstad T, Hovig T: Bacterial overgrowth. Scand J Gastroenterol 1985;109: 123–132.
25 Toskes PP, Kumar A: Enteric bacterial flora and bacterial overgrowth syndrome; in Feldman M, Sleisenger MH, Scharschmidt BF (eds): Sleisenger & Fordtran's Gastrointestinal and Liver Disease: Pathophysiology, Diagnosis, Management. Philadelphia, WB Saunders, 1998, pp 1523–1535.
26 Goldstein F, Wirts CW, Kowlessar OD: Diabetic diarrhea and steatorrhea. Ann Intern Med 1970;72:215–218.
27 Donaldson RM: Small bowel bacterial over growth. Adv Intern Med 1970;16:191–212.
28 Gorbach SL, Tabaqchali S: Bacteria, bile and the small bowel. Gut 1969;10:963–972.
29 Joiner KA, Gorbach SL: Antimicrobial therapy of digestive diseases. Clin Gastroenterol 1979;8: 3–35.
30 Elsborg L: Malabsorption in small intestinal diverticulosis treated with a low dosage sulphonamide-trimethoprim. Dan Med Bull 1977;24:33–35.
31 Tabaqchali S: The pathophysiological role of small intestinal bacterial flora. Scand J Gastroenterol Suppl 1970;6:139–163.
32 Bouhnik Y, Alain S, Attar A, Flourie B, Raskine L, Sanson-Le Pors MJ, Rambaud JC: Bacterial population contaminating the upper gut in patients with small intestinal bacterial over growth syndrome. Am J Gastroenterol 1999;94:1327–1331.
33 Vinci M, Gatto A, Gilgio A, et al: Double-blind clinical trial on infectious diarrhoea therapy: Rifaximin versus placebo. Curr Ther Res 1984;36:92–99.

34 Lamanna A, Orsi A: In vitro activity of rifaximin and rifampicin against some anaerobic bacteria. Chemioterapia 1984;6:365–367.
35 DeLeo C, Eftimiadi C, Schito GC: Rapid disappearance from the intestinal tract of bacteria resistant to rifaximin. Drugs Exp Clin Res 1986;12:979–981.
36 Alvisi V, D'Ambrosi A, Onofri W, Castellani M: Treatment of secretory diarrhoeas. A double-blind trial of the effectiveness of rifaximin (L/105) and neomycin. Clin Trials J 1984;21:215–223.
37 Palermo G, Di Gregorio P, Coffa G: Effectiveness of the L 105 compound in the treatment of acute diarrhoeal diseases. A short-term controlled study. Med Praxis 1984;5:147–152.
38 Eftimiadi C, DeLeo C, Schito GC: Treatment of hepatic encephalopathy with L/105, a new non-absorbable rifamycin. Drugs Exp Clin Res 1984;10:691–696.
39 Gruttaduria G, LaBarbera F, Cutaia G, Salanitri G: Prevention of infection in colonic surgery by rifaximin. A controlled prospective randomized trial. Eur Rev Med Pharmacol Sci 1987;9:101–105.
40 Papi C, Ciacco A, Koch M, Capurso L: Efficacy of rifaximin on symptoms of uncomplicated diverticular disease of the colon. A pilot multicentre open trial. Diverticular Disease Study Group. Ital J Gastroenterol 1992;24:452–456.
41 Corazza GR, Ventrucci M, Strocchi A, Sorge M, Pranzo L, Pezzilli R, Gasbarrini G: Treatment of small intestine bacterial overgrowth with rifaximin, a non-absorbable rifamycin. J Int Med Res 1988;16:312–316.
42 Di Stefano M, Malservisi S, Veneto G, Ferrieri A, Corazza GR: Rifaximin versus chlortetracycline in the short-term treatment of small intestine bacterial overgrowth. Aliment Pharmacol Ther 2000;14:551–556.
43 Trespi E, Ferrieri A: Intestinal bacterial overgrowth during chronic pancreatitis. Curr Med Res Opin 1999;15:47–52.
44 Di Stefano M, Strocchi A, Malservisi S, Veneto G, Ferrieri A, Corazza GR: Non-absorbable antibiotics for managing intestinal production and gas-related symptoms. Aliment Pharmacol Ther 2000;14:1001–1008.
45 Attar A, Flourie B, Rambaud JC, Franchisseur C, Ruszniewski P, Bouhnik Y: Antibiotic efficacy in small intestinal bacterial overgrowth-related chronic diarrhea: A crossover, randomized trial. Gastroenterology 1999;117:794–797.
46 Di Stefano M, Pezzimenti D, Veneto G, Missanelli A, Corazza GR: Absorbable vs. non-absorbable antibiotics in the therapy of small intestine bacterial overgrowth (SIBO) in patients with blind loop syndrome. Dig Liver Dis 2001;33:A93.

Note Added in Proof

While this review was being typeset, some papers of interest were published. The efficacy of rifaximin in relieving functional symptoms such as bloating and flatulence was recently confirmed in a randomized, double-blind, placebo controlled trial [1]. In a cohort of 145 patients with Crohn's disease the presence of SIBO was found by hydrogen breath test after glucose administration in 20% of patients [2]. Both metronidazole and ciprofloxacin proved to be effective in the management of bacterial overgrowth and breath hydrogen excretion normalized in 86% and 100% of patients, respectively. In metronidazole group, 1 patient out of 15 withdrew after two days because of nausea and, together with the other 2 patients resistant to metronidazole, was successfully treated with ciprofloxacin. After a 1-year period of follow-up, only 1 patient presented a recurrence of bacterial overgrowth. This study suggests, therefore, that ciprofloxacin is more effective than norfloxacin in the treatment of SIBO and confirms that side effects represent a major problem for the therapy with metronidazole. Moreover, in 50 consecutive patients with various malabsorption syndromes, 42% of jejunal aspirates showed a bacterial count greater than 10^5 CFU/ml. *Streptococcus* species and *Escherichia coli* were the commonest Gram positive and negative isolated bacteria, respectively, and proved to be more sensitive to quinolones than to tetracycline, ampicillin, erythromycin and cotrimoxazole [3]. Unfortunately, no data are available on rifaximin. Finally, the effect of probiotics on SIBO-related diarrhea was investigated in another paper. Two different *Lactobacillus* strains, namely *L. casei* and *L. acidophilus* strains Cerela, were administered and results were compared to placebo. A short-term improvement of the number of bowel movements and breath hydrogen excretion was achieved by probiotic treatment, suggesting that probiotics may represent an important therapeutic option in the treatment of SIBO provided prolonged courses are adopted [4].

References

1 Sharara AI, Aoun E, Mounzer R, Sidani S, El Hajj I: Rifaximin in abdominal bloating and flatulence trial (RAFT): A randomized double-blinded, placebo-controlled trial. Am J Gastroenterol 2004;99(suppl):S281.

2 Castiglione F, Rispo A, Di Girolamo E, Cozzolino A, Manguso F, Grassia R, Mazzacca G: Antibiotic treatment of small bowel bacterial overgrowth in patients with Crohn's disease. Aliment Pharmacol Ther 2003;18:1107–1112.

3 Ghoshal U, Ghoshal UC, Ranjan P, Naik SR, Ayyagari A: Spectrum and antibiotic sensitivity of bacteria contaminating the upper gut in patients with malabsorption syndrome from the tropic. BMC Gastroenterology 2003;3:9.

4 Gaon D, Garmendia C, Murrielo NO, de Cucco Games A, Cerchio A, Quintas R, Gonzalez SN, Oliver G: Effect of Lactobacillus strains (*L. casei* and *L. acidophilus* strains cerela) on bacterial overgrowth-related chronic diarrhea. Medicina (B Aires) 2002;62:159–163.

Prof. Gino Roberto Corazza, MD
Gastroenterology Unit, IRCCS 'S. Matteo' Hospital, University of Pavia
P.le C. Golgi 5, IT–27100 Pavia (Italy)
Tel. +39 0382 502973, Fax +39 0382 502618, E-Mail gr.corazza@smatteo.pv.it

This chapter should be cited as follows:

Di Stefano M, Corazza GR: Treatment of Small Intestine Bacterial Overgrowth and Related Symptoms by Rifaximin. Chemotherapy 2005;51(suppl 1):103–109.

Scarpignato C (ed): Rifaximin: A Poorly Absorbed Antibiotic.
Pharmacology and Clinical Use.

Management of Diverticular Disease: Is There Room for Rifaximin?

Claudio Papi, Maurizio Koch, Lucio Capurso

Department of Gastroenterology and Internal Medicine, S. Filippo Neri Hospital, Rome, Italy

Abstract

Treatment of symptomatic diverticular disease of the colon is aimed at the relief of symptoms and the prevention of major complications. The efficacy of fiber supplementation and of anticholinergic and spasmolytic agents remains controversial. Antibiotics are commonly used in the treatment of inflammatory complications of diverticular disease. Data from open labelled and randomized controlled trials do suggest the efficacy of rifaximin in obtaining symptomatic relief in patients with diverticular disease. Approximately 30% therapeutic gain compared to fiber supplementation only can be expected after one year of intermittent treatment with rifaximin. Considering the safety and tolerability of rifaximin, this drug can be recommended for patients with symptomatic uncomplicated diverticular disease.

Introduction

Diverticular disease of the colon is extremely common in developed countries and its prevalence is correlated with advancing age [1]. Estimates based on necroscopy or radiologic findings indicate that it occurs in about 10% of people in the United States, the United Kingdom and Australia [2] and that it is currently found in one third to one half of all autopsies of people over 60 years of age [3]. In North America, diverticular disease is estimated to occur in one third of all individuals above 45 years of age and two thirds of individuals above 85 years of age [4].

The different prevalence rates in various geographic areas and ethnic groups have been confirmed by several reports; the high prevalence of diverticular disease in developed western countries is in contrast with the rarity with which the disease is observed in less industrialized countries and in Japan

[4–6]. This led to the hypothesis that the high frequency of diverticular disease in western societies results from a low fiber consumption by an aging population [3, 4]. The dietary fiber hypothesis is largely supported by epidemiological observations [4, 5, 7–9] and case-control studies [10–12]. Recently, a prospective cohort study of 43,881 male health professionals 40–75 years of age demonstrated that dietary fiber consumption was inversely associated with the risk of developing diverticular disease and this association was particularly strong for cellulose [13]. In more recent years, with increasing globalization, factors previously uncommon in developing countries, such as the availability of highly processed foods, may be operating to cause a similar prevalence of diverticular disease in these populations as in European and American populations [14].

The majority of patients harboring colonic diverticula remain asymptomatic throughout their life (asymptomatic diverticular disease); only 20% will develop symptoms and signs of illness [15]. Symptomatic diverticular disease is further subdivided into painful diverticular disease (symptomatic diverticular disease with no inflammation) and diverticulitis (symptomatic diverticular disease with inflammation). Diverticulitis is further subdivided into uncomplicated and complicated diverticulitis [16].

Treatment of Diverticular Disease of the Colon

The vast majority of patients with colonic diverticula will remain entirely asymptomatic. There are no data to support any therapeutic recommendations or routine follow-up in this large population, although it is reasonable to recommend a diet high in fruit and vegetable fiber.

Treatment of symptomatic diverticular disease is aimed at the relief of symptoms and the prevention of major complications. The efficacy of fiber supplementation in the treatment of painful diverticular disease remains controversial. Some controlled clinical trials have shown a benefit of high-fiber diets for symptomatic relief [17–20], but other studies failed to show positive results [21–23]. Despite these conflicting data, bran and bulking agents are commonly used in the treatment of symptomatic diverticular disease. The high intraluminal colonic pressure is of critical importance in the formation of diverticula, and this formed the basis for the high-fiber diet recommended to individuals with symptomatic diverticular disease [5]. Recent American College of Gastroenterology Guidelines [24] recommended a high-fiber diet for patients with symptomatic diverticular disease of the colon; some amelioration of symptoms can be expected, and other potential health benefits of fiber should be considered.

The observed hypermotility of the sigmoid colon in many symptomatic patients provides the rationale for using anticholinergic drugs and spasmolytic agents [25]. However, the efficacy of these agents has never been clearly documented in randomized controlled trials [3, 24].

Antibiotics are commonly used in the treatment of inflammatory complications of diverticular disease [3, 24]. In painful diverticular disease, when inflammation is excluded by definition, there is no rationale for using antibiotics. In a subset of patients with more severe symptoms, when an inflammatory component may be clinically suspected, a short course of antibiotics may be advisable [15].

However, some observations suggest a possible role of gut microflora in determining symptoms related to diverticular disease. Bacterial metabolism is the major source of intestinal gas such as H_2, CO_2 and CH_4 via carbohydrate fermentation [26]. Excessive production of bowel gas can play a role in determining abdominal symptoms such as bloating, pain and discomfort [27]; these symptoms, although nonspecific, are commonly observed in patients with diverticular disease of the colon. Antimicrobial drugs have been shown to reduce colonic H_2 production [28, 29] and gas-related symptoms [30]. Interactions between dietary fiber, bacterial metabolism and colonic functions are complex and not fully elucidated. It is well known that fiber increases stool bulk and affects colonic transit time in several ways: by water holding, by proliferation of bacteria and by the products of bacterial fermentation [31]. It has been assumed since the earliest times that fiber exerts its effect on bowel habits by virtue of retaining water in the gut and stimulating peristalsis through increased bulk [32]. However, water holding is an in vitro property of fiber which is inversely related to fecal bulking and colonic transit time in vivo [33]. This is not surprising, because virtually all fiber is broken down in the gut by intestinal bacteria [32]. Moreover, water holding can be equated with the solubility of fiber, and soluble fiber is more rapidly degraded by gut microflora [32]. This view is supported by a study in humans in which it was shown that antimicrobial therapy causes a rise in mean fecal weight in subjects with a constant fiber intake, probably due to the reduction of bacterial mass and bacterial degradation of fiber [34]. Therefore, a role of antibiotics in diverticular disease symptoms may be suggested, with respect to both bacterial gas production and fiber degradation.

Rifaximin in Diverticular Disease of the Colon

Rifaximin is a semisynthetic rifamycin derivate that acts by inhibiting bacterial ribonucleic acid synthesis [35]. In vitro data indicate a good antibacterial activity against Gram-positive organisms and less activity against

Gram-negative organisms; conflicting data exist for activity against bacteroides [35]. Rifaximin is virtually unabsorbed after oral administration; thus, it is used primarily to treat local conditions within the gastrointestinal tract [35]. Rifaximin has been successfully used in the treatment of infectious diarrheas [36, 37], including travelers' diarrhea [38], and it has been shown to be at least as effective as neomycin in the treatment of portosystemic encephalopathy [39, 40]. Furthermore, rifaximin has been shown to be effective in the treatment of intestinal bacterial overgrowth [41] and in the prophylaxis of postoperative complications following colorectal surgery [42].

Several clinical observations suggest a role of rifaximin in the management of symptomatic uncomplicated diverticular disease of the colon.

In a pilot multicenter open trial [43], 217 patients with symptomatic uncomplicated diverticular disease were treated with glucomannan 2 g/day or with glucomannan plus rifaximin 400 mg twice a day for 7 days each month. Clinical evaluation was performed at admission and at 2-month intervals for 12 months; a symptom score including 8 clinical variables was used as a measure of the therapeutic effect. After 12 months of treatment, a significant reduction of the symptom score was observed in patients treated with glucomannan plus rifaximin compared to patients treated with glucomannan only (63.9 vs. 47.6%; $p < 0.001$). At the end of the study period, 58% of patients treated with rifaximin and glucomannan were symptom free compared to 24% of patients treated with glucomannan only ($p < 0.001$).

Similar results were obtained in a large prospective open trial including 968 outpatients with symptomatic diverticular disease [44]. Patients were randomly assigned to receive fiber supplementation (glucomannan 4 g/day) or fiber supplementation plus rifaximin (400 mg twice a day for 7 days every month) for 12 months. After 12 months, 56.5% of patients in the rifaximin group were symptom free compared to 29.2% of patients in the fiber supplementation only group ($p < 0.001$).

In a multicenter double-blind placebo-controlled trial [45], 168 outpatients with symptomatic uncomplicated diverticular disease were randomly assigned to receive fiber supplementation (glucomannan 2 g/day) plus rifaximin (400 mg twice a day for 7 days every month for 12 months), or fiber supplementation plus placebo. A symptom score including 6 clinical indications (upper abdominal pain/discomfort, bloating, lower abdominal pain/discomfort, tenesmus, diarrhea and abdominal tenderness) was calculated to assess the clinical response. Both treatments were shown to be effective in reducing the score after the first 3 months of treatment; however, patients treated with rifaximin showed a significantly greater reduction in the score compared to patients treated with placebo at 6, 9 and 12 months (fig. 1). Symptoms such as abdominal pain, abdominal tenderness and bloating appeared to be particularly affected by

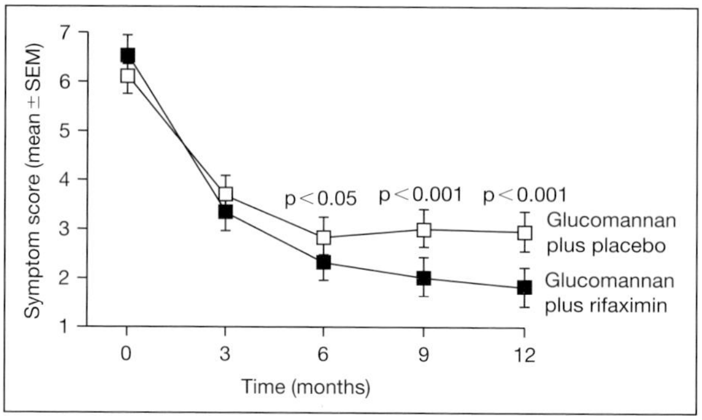

Fig. 1. Global symptom score in patients treated with glucomannan plus rifaximin and in patients treated with glucomannan plus placebo (from Papi et al. [45]).

rifaximin treatment. After 12 months of treatment, 68.9% of patients in the rifaximin group were symptom free compared to 39.5% in the placebo group [absolute benefit increase 29.7%, 95% confidence interval (CI) 15.3–44.1%]. Long-term intermittent rifaximin administration appears to be safe; no relevant side effects were reported in any of these trials [42–44].

Open-labeled and randomized controlled trial data support some evidence for the efficacy of intermittent long-term administration of rifaximin in patients with symptomatic diverticular disease. A therapeutic gain of approximately 30% compared to fiber supplementation only can be expected with respect to obtaining symptomatic relief after 1 year of treatment (table 1). Considering the safety and tolerability of rifaximin, this drug can be recommended for patients with symptomatic uncomplicated diverticular disease.

Although there is some evidence for the efficacy of long-term treatment with rifaximin for symptomatic relief in patients with uncomplicated diverticular disease, an unresolved issue is whether rifaximin can prevent major inflammatory complications of diverticular disease. In the two prospective open trials discussed above, the occurrence rate of complications in 12 months was lower in patients treated with glucomannan plus rifaximin compared to patients treated with glucomannan only: 2.7 versus 0.9% [43] and 3.2 versus 1.3% [44]. This observation was not confirmed in the double-blind placebo-controlled trial [45] in which no difference in the 1-year complication rate was observed between the rifaximin and placebo groups. However, in all the studies, the number of patients suffering complications in a 12-month period was too small to detect any statistically significant difference between the two treatment groups (table 1). In a retrospective study of 505 patients admitted to hospital for a major complication of diverticular disease of the colon (occlusion, perforation, fistula or bleeding) and discharged after conservative management, long-term

Table 1. Studies addressing rifaximin for the treatment of symptomatic diverticular disease

Author	Patients	Study design	Treatment	Study period months	Asymptomatic patients, %	RD, % (95% CI)	Complica-tions, %	RD, % (95% CI)
Papi et al. 1992 [43]	217	Open	Glucomannan 2 g	12	24	34.3 (22.0–46.5)	2.7	−1.8 (−5.3 to 1.7)
			Glucomannan 2 g + rifaximin[1]		58		0.9	
Latella et al. 2003 [44]	968	Open	Glucomannan 4 g	12	29	27.0 (20.9–33.1)	3.2	−1.8 (−3.8 to 0.1)
			Glucomannan 4 g + rifaximin[1]		56		1.3	
Papi et al. 1995 [45]	168	RCT	Glucomannan 2 g + placebo	12	39	29.7 (15.3–44.1)	2.3	0 (−4.6 to 4.6)
			Glucomannan 2 g + rifaximin[1]		69		2.3	

RD = Rate difference; RCT = randomized controlled trials. [1]Rifaximin 400 mg twice a day for 7 days each month for 12 months.

treatment with poorly absorbable antibiotics (neomycin plus bacitracin, paromomycin or rifaximin) reduced by 50% the relative risk of readmission for complications compared to no antibiotic treatment [46].

Conclusions

There is some evidence that long-term cyclic administration of rifaximin combined with fiber supplementation is effective for inducing symptomatic relief in patients with uncomplicated diverticular disease of the colon. A therapeutic gain of approximately 30% compared to fiber supplementation only can be expected. The drug is well tolerated and no relevant side effects have been reported. Symptoms attributed to diverticula (abdominal pain or discomfort, bloating, disturbance of bowel habits) are nonspecific symptoms and are also features of irritable bowel syndrome. It has been suggested that irritable bowel syndrome and diverticular disease of the colon may coexist in many people and when bowel symptoms occur with diverticulosis coli, they may be due to a coexistent irritable bowel rather to the diverticula themselves [47, 48]. This hypothesis is supported by the fact that many patients with symptomatic diverticular disease show colonic motility patterns similar to those with irritable bowel syndrome [25], and patients with asymptomatic disease have colonic myoelectric activity similar to that of normals [49]. A fundamental issue is that treatment with rifaximin may be related to colonic symptoms rather than to diverticula per se; this would suggest the inclusion, in future studies, of an additional arm of patients with symptoms of irritable bowel syndrome but not diverticula.

No definitive conclusions can be drawn concerning a possible role of rifaximin in preventing major complications of diverticular disease. Double-blind placebo-controlled trials with an adequate sample size are needed. However, such trials are difficult to perform considering the requirement of a large number of patients. Assuming a baseline risk of complications of diverticular disease of 5% per year [2], a randomized controlled trial able to detect a 50% risk reduction in complications should include 1,600 patients per treatment group considering a power of 80% ($1 - \beta$) and an α error of 5%.

References

1 Parks TG: Natural history of diverticular disease of the colon. Clin Gastroenterol 1975;4:53–69.
2 Naitove A, Almy TP: Diverticular disease of the colon; in Sleisenger MH, Fordtran JS (eds): Gastrointestinal Disease: Pathophysiology, Diagnosis, Management, ed 4. Philadelphia, WB Saunders, 1989, pp 1419–1434.
3 Almy TP, Howell DA: Diverticular disease of the colon. N Engl J Med 1980;302:324–331.
4 Roberts PL, Veidenheimer MC: Diverticular disease of the colon; in Bayless TM (ed): Current Therapy in Gastroenterology and Liver Disease. Toronto, BC Decker, 1990, vol 3, pp 416–419.

5 Painter NS, Burkitt DP: Diverticular disease of the colon, a 20th century problem. Clin Gastroenterol 1975;4:3–21.
6 Narasaka T, Watanabe H, Yamagata S, Munakata A, Tajima T, Matatsunaga F: Statistical analysis of diverticulosis of the colon. Tohoku J Exp Med 1975;115:271–275.
7 Kyle J, Adesola AD, Tinckler LF, De Beaux J: Incidence of diverticulitis. Scand J Gastroenterol 1967;2:44–47.
8 Painter NS: The high fiber diet in the treatment of diverticular disease of the colon. Postgrad Med J 1974;50:629–635.
9 Burkitt DP: Dietary fiber and 'pressure diseases'. J R Coll Physicians Lond 1975;9:138–147.
10 Manousos O, Day NE, Tzonou A, Papadimitriou C, Kapetanakis A, Polychronopoulou-Trichopoulou A, Trichopoulou D: Diet and other factors in the aetiology of diverticulosis: An epidemiological study in Greece. Gut 1985;26:544–549.
11 Brodribb AJM, Humphreys DM: Diverticular disease: Three studies. I. Relation to other disorders and fibre intake. Br Med J 1976;i:424–430.
12 Gear JSS, Ware A, Fursdon P, Mann JI, Nolan DJ, Brodribb AJ, Vessey MP: Symptomless diverticular disease and intake of dietary fibre. Lancet 1979;i:511–514.
13 Aldoori WH, Giovannucci EL, Rockett HRH, Sampson L, Rimm EB, Willet WC: A prospective study of dietary fiber types and symptomatic diverticular disease in men. J Nutr 1998;128:717–719.
14 Chia JG, Wilde CC, Ngoi SS, Goh PM, Ong CL: Trends of diverticular disease of the large bowel in a newly developed country. Dis Colon Rectum 1991;34:498–501.
15 Torsoli A, Inoue M, Manousos O, Smith A, Van Steensel CJ: Diverticular disease of the colon: Data relevant to treatment. Gastroenterol Int 1991;4:3–20.
16 Farrell RJ, Farrell JJ, Morrin MM: Diverticular disease in the elderly. Gastroenterol Clin North Am 2001;30:475–496.
17 Brodribb AJM: Treatment of symptomatic diverticular disease with a high-fibre diet. Lancet 1977;i:664–666.
18 Ornstein MH, Littlewood ER, Baird IM, Fowler J, Cox AG: Are fibre supplements really necessary in diverticular disease of the colon? A controlled trial. Br Med J (Clin Res Ed) 1981;282:1629–1630.
19 Weinreich J: The treatment of diverticular disease. Scand J Gastroenterol Suppl 1982;79:128–129.
20 Ewerth S, Ahlberg J, Holmstrom B, Persson U, Uden R: Influence on symptoms and transit time of Vi-SiblinR in diverticular disease. Acta Chir Scand Suppl 1980;500:40–59.
21 Solotof JI, Gudmand Hoyer E, Kreg B, Kristensen E, Wolff HR: A double blind trial of wheat bran on symptoms of irritable bowel syndrome. Lancet 1976;i:270–272.
22 Hodgson WJB: The placebo effect: Is it important in diverticular disease? Am J Gastroenterol 1977;67:157–162.
23 Longstreth GF, Fox DD, Youkeles L, Forsythe AB, Wolochow DA: Psyllium therapy in the irritable bowel syndrome. Ann Intern Med 1981;95:53–56.
24 Stollman NH, Raskin JB: Diagnosis and management of diverticular disease of the colon in adults. Am J Gastroenterol 1999;94:3110–3121.
25 Ritchie L: Similarity of bowel distension characteristics in the irritable bowel syndrome and diverticulosis. Gut 1977;18:990.
26 Levitt MD, Bond JH: Volume, composition and source of intestinal gas. Gastroenterology 1970;59:921–929.
27 Strocchi A, Levitt MD: Intestinal gas; in Sleisenger MH, Fordtran JS (eds): Gastrointestinal Disease: Pathophysiology, Diagnosis, Management, ed 5. Philadelphia, Saunders, 1993, pp 1035–1042.
28 Bjorneklett A, Midvedt T: Influence of three antimicrobial agents – penicillin, metronidazole and doxycyclin – on the intestinal microflora of healthy humans. Scand J Gastroenterol 1988;94: 928–932.
29 Rao SC, Edwards CA, Austen CJ, Bruce C, Read NW: Impaired colonic fermentation of carbohydrate after ampicillin. Gastroenterology 1988;94:928–932.
30 Di Stefano M, Strocchi A, Malservisi S, Veneto G, Ferrieri A, Corazza GR: Non-absorbable antibiotics for managing intestinal gas production and gas-related symptoms. Aliment Pharmacol Ther 2000;14:1001–1008.
31 Stephen AM, Cummings JH: Mechanism of action of dietary fiber in the human colon. Nature 1980;284:283–284.

32 MacFarlane GT, Cummings JH: The colonic flora, fermentation and large bowel digestive function; in Phillips SF, Pemberton JH, Shorter RG (eds): The Large Intestine: Physiology, Pathophysiology and Disease. New York, Raven, 1991, pp 51–92.
33 Stephen AM, Cummings JH: Water holding by dietary fibre in vitro and its relationship to fecal output in man. Gut 1979;20:722–729.
34 Kurpad AV, Shetty PS: Effects of antimicrobial therapy on fecal bulking. Gut 1986;27:55–58.
35 Gillis JC, Brogden RN: Rifaximin. A review of its antibacterial activity, pharmacokinetic properties and therapeutic potential in conditions mediated by gatrointestinal bacteria. Drugs 1995;49:467–484.
36 Vinci M, Gatto A, Giglio A, Raciti T, D'Avola G, Di Stefano B, Salanitri G, Di Stefano F: Double blind clinical trial on infectious diarrhoea therapy: Rifaximin versus placebo. Curr Ther Res 1984;36:92–99.
37 Alvisi V, D'Ambrosi A, Loponte A, Pazzi P, Greco A, Zangirolami A, Palazzini E: Rifaximin, a rifamycin derivative for use in the treatment of intestinal bacterial infections in seriously disabled patients. J Int Med Res 1987;15:49–56.
38 DuPont HL, Jiang ZD, Ericsson CD, Adachi JA, Mathewson JJ, DuPont MW, Palazzini E, Riopel LM, Ashley D, Martinez-Sandoval F: Rifaximin versus ciprofloxacin for the treatment of traveler's diarrhea: A randomized, double-blind clinical trial. Clin Infect Dis 2001;1:1807–1815.
39 Cottone M, Pagliaro L: Rifaximin versus neomycin in the treatment of portosystemic encephalopathy. Ital J Gastroenterol 1991;23:403–407.
40 Pedretti G, Calzetti C, Missale G, Ficcadori F: Rifaximin versus neomycin on hyperammoniemia in chronic portal systemic encephalopathy of cirrhotics. A double blind randomizedtrial. Ital J Gastroenterol 1991;23:175–178.
41 Di Stefano M, Malservisi S, Veneto G, Ferrieri A, Corazza GR: Rifaximin versus chlortetracycline in the short term treatment of small intestine bacterial overgrowth. Aliment Pharmacol Ther 2000;14: 551–556.
42 Gruttaduria G, La Barbera F, Gutaia G, Salanitri G: Prevention of infection of colonic surgery by rifaximin. A controlled, prospective randomized trial. Eur Rev Med Pharmacol Sci 1987;9:101–105.
43 Papi C, Ciaco A, Koch M, Capurso L, Camarri E, Ferrieri A, Guardascione F, Miglio F, Minoli G, Terruzzi V, Parodi MC, Riegler G, Russo A: Efficacy of rifaximin on symptoms of uncomplicated diverticular disease of the colon. A pilot multicentre open trial. Ital J Gastroenterol 1992;24:452–456.
44 Latella G, Pimpo MT, Sottili S, Zippi M, Viscido A, Chiaramonte M, Frieri G: Rifaximin improves symptoms of acquired uncomplicated diverticular disease of the colon. Int J Colorectal Dis 2003; 18:55–62.
45 Papi C, Ciaco A, Koch M, Capurso L, Diverticular Disease Study Group: Efficacy of rifaximin in the treatment of symptomatic diverticular disease of the colon. A multicentre double-blind placebo-controlled trial. Aliment Pharmacol Ther 1995;9:33–39.
46 Porta E, Germano A, Ferrieri A, Koch M: The natural history of diverticular disease of the colon: A role for antibiotics in preventing complications? A retrospective study. Eur Rev Med Pharmacol Sci 1994;16:33–39.
47 Thompson WG, Patel DG, Tao N, Nair RC: Does uncomplicated diverticular disease produce symptoms? Dig Dis Sci 1982;27:605–608.
48 Thompson WG, Patel DG: Clinical picture of diverticular disease of the colon. Clin Gastroenterol 1986;4:903–916.
49 Gold MH, Carlson GM, Mathias JR: Colonic myoelectric activity in diverticulosis. Gastroenterology 1979;76:1139.

Claudio Papi, MD
Unità Operativa di Gastroenterologia, Ospedale S. Filippo Neri
via Martinotti 20, IT–00135 Roma (Italy)
Tel. +39 06 33062245, Fax +39 06 33062641, E-Mail c.papi@tin.it

This chapter should be cited as follows:

Papi C, Koch M, Capurso L: Management of Diverticular Disease: Is There Room for Rifaximin? Chemotherapy 2005;51(suppl 1):110–114.

Scarpignato C (ed): Rifaximin: A Poorly Absorbed Antibiotic.
Pharmacology and Clinical Use.

Mechanical and Antibacterial Bowel Preparation in Colon and Rectal Surgery

Ronald Lee Nichols, Ella U. Choe, Christopher B. Weldon

Department of Surgery, Tulane University School of Medicine,
Tulane University Health Sciences Center, New Orleans, La., USA

Abstract

Colorectal surgery performed prior to 1970 was fraught with postoperative infectious complications which occurred in more than 30–50% of all operations. Diversion of the fecal stream appeared mandatory when operating on an urgent or emergent basis, thereby requiring the performance of multiple, staged operations instead of a single surgery encompassing resection and primary anastomosis as is performed commonly today. Multiple studies conducted in the early 1970s determined that anaerobic colonic microflora were causative agents in postoperative infections in colon and rectal surgery, and these studies initiated the development of effective oral preoperative antibiotic prophylaxis in combination with preoperative mechanical bowel preparation. This dual-tier regimen significantly reduced the incidence of postoperative infectious complications, thus allowing most uncomplicated colon and rectal surgeries to be performed in a single stage without the need for the diversion of the fecal stream and multiple operations. Therefore, a preoperative mechanical and antibacterial bowel regimen serves as the cornerstone of modern elective colorectal surgery, and these regimens now comprise three therapeutic directives. The first step is preoperative mechanical cleansing of the bowel, which is then followed by preoperative oral antibiotic prophylaxis. Finally, perioperative parenteral antibiotics directed against aerobic and anaerobic colonic microflora are utilized.

Introduction

The advent of this new century marked the 30-year anniversary of a revolution in colon and rectal surgery – preoperative bowel sterilization, resulting in a significant decrease in infectious complications and the commonplace practice of single-stage operations. The past three decades have produced a plethora of clinical trials that clearly show that preoperative bowel preparation is an advantageous therapeutic endeavor in a surgeon's armamentarium. For decades, medical science has recognized and understood the important symbiotic relationship of the enormous reservoir of aerobic and anaerobic bacteria that inhabit the distal ileum and colon from infancy [1]. Furthermore, the intestinal epithelium and mucous membrane, which serve as a vital shield against these microbes, have also been recognized as a vital component of the human body's defense against these microbes [2]. Should this defensive mechanism break down secondary to disease or traumatic processes – iatrogenic or otherwise – local or systemic spread of these microorganisms could result in a significant clinical infection. Accordingly, therapeutic directives targeted at diminishing this bacterial load for elective surgical intervention have been attempted for over 100 years [3]. These efforts have culminated in a standard three-tier regimen practiced widely in the United States [4], which includes (1) preoperative mechanical cleansing to reduce the fecal load and facilitate the efficacy of the orally administered antibiotics, (2) preoperative oral antimicrobial bactericidal therapy targeting both aerobic and anaerobic species, and (3) perioperative parenteral antimicrobial therapy. This therapeutic attack has resulted in a dramatic fall in the incidence of infectious postoperative complications in colon and rectal surgery.

Mechanical Preparation

Mechanical cleansing of the colonic lumen before elective colon resection is a time-tested procedure that, when done appropriately, reduces total fecal mass, thus facilitating operative manipulation of the colon and enhancing the action of oral antibiotics. Vigorous mechanical cleansing alone, however, whether it includes lavage or follows the classic approach (dietary restriction, enemas and cathartics), does not significantly reduce the number of microorganisms in the residual colonic material [5] or mucosal-associated bacteria [6, 7].

Today, approaches to mechanical cleansing vary considerably. The historically touted 5-day preoperative preparation has been abandoned due to the risk of inducing severe metabolic abnormalities. Modern approaches fall into two general categories: (1) whole-gut lavage with polyethylene glycol-electrolyte solution or sodium phosphate on the day before operation, and (2) dietary restriction and cathartics for a 2-day period [4]. These two procedures may also be combined (table 1). Though these techniques are considered safer, complications arising from their use have been reported [8].

Table 1. Alternate approaches to bowel preparation in patients undergoing elective resection of the large bowel

Environment	Approach 1, home or outpatient	Approach 2, home or outpatient
Diet	Clear liquids beginning at 6.00 a.m. the day prior to surgery	Clear liquids beginning at 5.00 p.m. 2 days prior to surgery
Preoperative mechanical bowel preparation	Polyethylene glycol-electrolyte solution lavage – 4 liters p.o. over 3–4 h starting at 6.00 a.m. on the day prior to surgery	Sodium phosphate[1] prep of 45 ml p.o. at 6.00 p.m. 2 days prior to surgery and 6.00 a.m. the day prior to surgery
Enemas	None	None
Preoperative oral antibiotic bowel preparation	1 g of erythromycin base and 1 g of neomycin SO_4 p.o. at 1.00, 2.00 and 11.00 p.m. on the day prior to surgery (surgery at 8.00 a.m.)	1 g of erythromycin base and 1 g of neomycin SO_4 p.o. at 1.00, 2.00 and 11.00 p.m. the day prior to surgery (surgery at 8.00 a.m.)
Perioperative parenteral antibiotics	Yes: with appropriate aerobic and anaerobic antimicrobial coverage with a single dose within 30 min of incision	Yes: with appropriate aerobic and anaerobic antimicrobial coverage with a single dose within 30 min of incision

[1]Sodium phosphate is contraindicated as an oral mechanical bowel preparation in patients with renal or cardiac disease [8].

Three separate reports in the literature some 12 years apart document the North American perspective of 100% compliance with preoperative mechanical bowel cleansing [4, 9, 10]. The first study is a 1990 survey of 372 clinically active, board-certified colon and rectal surgeons in the United States and Canada [10]. The authors reported that every surgeon surveyed employed some form of mechanical cleansing in addition to antibiotics in preparing for elective colon resection. Fifty-eight percent of those surgeons who responded to the survey used lavage with polyethylene glycol-electrolyte solution, while 36% of surgeons used a more traditional approach that included dietary restriction, cathartics and enemas. The remaining 6% of surgeons used either preoperative lavage with mannitol or whole-gut lavage. More recently, 808 board-certified North American colorectal surgeons were surveyed for their current bowel preparation practices before elective procedures [4]. Of the 471 surgeons who responded to the survey (58%), all used some form of mechanical preparation. Oral polyethylene glycol-electrolyte solution was the most frequently reported mechanical preparation employed (70.9% of the respondents), while oral sodium phosphate solution with or without bisacodyl was the next most prevalent mechanical bowel preparation method used (28.4%). The 'traditional' method of dietary restriction, cathartics and enemas was the regimen employed least often (28.4%). Finally, the extensive literature review of Zmora et al. [9] confirmed the continued need for preoperative mechanical bowel preparations, even in light of recent reports to the contrary [11, 12]. However, these commonplace North American practice guidelines are not uniform to all surgeons worldwide.

Multiple studies have been performed that investigated the necessity of performing mechanical cleansing before elective colon resection [11–17]. Two found no differences in the rates of anastomotic dehiscence or infectious complications between patients who received mechanical cleansing and those who did not [13, 14]. These investigators relied on intravenous antibiotics for preoperative intestinal antisepsis and did not employ oral regimens. Another similarly designed Brazilian study showed a higher wound infection rate in the group of patients receiving mechanical cleansing [15]. The authors suggested that 'mechanical bowel preparation is unnecessary and may be harmful in terms of preventing wound infection and anastomotic dehiscence in patients undergoing elective colorectal surgery' [15]. It must be stressed that these three studies did not employ oral antibiotics in their bowel preparation regimens. Furthermore, four recent prospective studies [11, 12, 16, 17] documented that mechanical bowel preparations are not needed, on the basis of low anastomotic leakage rates (0–5%), low postoperative infection rates (5–6%) and equivalent total hospital stays.

Antibiotic Preparation

All surgeons employ antibiotics in preparing patients for an elective colon resection. As noted earlier, it is agreed that the antibiotics used should be bactericidal to both aerobic and anaerobic species, but what constitutes the ideal antibiotic regimen is a topic of considerable debate. Advocates of the oral administration of antibiotics typically emphasize the importance of reducing the number of microorganisms in the colonic lumen and mucosa before opening the colon, whereas advocates of parenteral administration emphasize the importance of adequate tissue levels of antibiotics prior to the beginning of surgery.

Oral Antibiotics

Over 30 years ago, the three major requirements for an effective intestinal antiseptic were outlined: (1) rapid, highly bactericidal activity against gastrointestinal pathogenic organisms, (2) low local and systemic toxicity, and (3) limited absorption from the intestine. Two oral regimens are now primarily used: (1) an aminoglycoside agent with erythromycin base, and (2) an aminoglycoside agent with metronidazole. The regimen most often chosen in the United States is neomycin and erythromycin base, which was introduced in 1972 [4, 10, 18, 19]. In Europe and Australia, however, physicians prefer kanamycin and metronidazole or neomycin and metronidazole when oral antibiotics are administered [20].

The timing of the administration of these oral agents is critical, with an elapsed time of 19 h from the first dose to the beginning of the operation being ideal. Therefore, it is recommended that 1 g each of neomycin and erythromycin base be given at 1.00 p.m., 2.00 p.m. and 11.00 p.m. on the day before operation (6 g in total) (table 1) [18, 19, 21]. The procedure should then be scheduled for about 8.00 a.m. the next morning. If the operation is scheduled for a different time, then the times at which the oral agents are administered should be changed accordingly to preserve the 19-hour interval. Giving more than three prophylactic doses of the oral antibiotic drugs is unwarranted, for it may induce the emergence of resistant flora. Authoritative reviews on antibiotic prophylaxis in colon surgery confirm the value of the oral neomycin and erythromycin base regimen in preventing infection after elective colon resection [22–24]. However, there appears to be no convincing evidence to suggest that erythromycin base is superior to metronidazole in this clinical setting. The pharmacokinetic profile of the oral neomycin and erythromycin base preparation has been studied in healthy volunteers [25] and in patients undergoing elective colon resection [26]. Results of these studies suggest that when adequate mechanical bowel preparation is combined with this preoperative antimicrobial bowel regimen, significant intraluminal (local) and serum (systemic) levels of erythromycin and significant local levels of neomycin are present. Therefore, combining both techniques serves to prevent infection after colon operation. Other nonabsorbable, orally administered antibiotics such as rifaximin have been proposed for use in preoperative colon prophylaxis, but larger, double-blind clinical trials are needed to definitely assess their efficacy [27]. In summary, the use of preoperative oral antibiotics is an efficacious and common therapeutic adjuvant as evidenced by the report of Solla and Rothenberger [10] on the clinical regimens utilized by 372 practicing surgeons. Oral antibiotics, most commonly neomycin and erythromycin base, were used in preoperative bowel regimens by almost 92% of the responding surgeons. Furthermore, surgeons who consider oral antibiotics important in the success of a preoperative bowel preparation also continue to realize the necessity of effective outpatient mechanical cleansing of short duration (i.e. 24 h or less) before operation [28, 29]. This combination of mechanical preparation and oral antibiotic preparation is time-tested, and it has yielded excellent clinical results during the past two decades [22, 30].

Parenteral Antibiotics

Parenteral agents that are effective in bowel preparation for elective colon resection, either alone or in combination with an aminoglycoside, include cefoxitin, cefotetan, metronidazole and doxycycline [31]. One study, reported by the Norwegian Study Group for Colorectal Surgery, advocated mechanical cleansing together with a single preoperative intravenous dose of doxycycline for aerobic coverage and tinidazole for anaerobic coverage [32]. Other studies have shown that a single dose of cefotetan is as effective as multiple doses of cefoxitin [33]. For elective operations, most investigators recommend restriction of parenteral antibiotic prophylaxis to no more than five doses during the first 24 h, beginning from the time of surgery. Use of parenteral antibiotic regimens for longer periods of time has been associated with the development of antibiotic-resistant strains of microbes in the colonic lumen [23, 33, 34]. North American surgeons were noted to employ parenteral antibiotics alone in preoperative colonic preparation in about 8% of their patients in a 1990 survey [10], and this percentage increased to roughly 11% of patients in a 1997 survey [4]. Finally, the use of parenteral antibiotic drugs alone is employed in emergency colonic resections.

Combination of Parenteral and Oral Antibiotics

Most North American surgeons now use both oral and parenteral antibiotics along with mechanical cleansing in preoperative preparation for elective colon resection [4, 10]. In a survey of more than 500 surgeons in 1979, only 8% used systemic antibiotics alone, 37% used oral antibiotics alone and 49% used both oral and systemic antibiotics before colon surgery [35]. In a later survey of 372 board-certified colon and rectal surgeons, 88% used both oral and systemic antibiotics in their preoperative preparation, 3% used oral agents alone and 8% used parenteral antibiotics alone [10]. In a more recent survey, 87% of surgeons surveyed used both oral and parenteral antimicrobial agents, while only 11% of respondents utilized parenteral antibiotics alone [4]. Almost 78% of the responding surgeons utilized oral neomycin and erythromycin base or metronidazole combined with a perioperative parenteral antibiotic. Most surgeons start the oral antibiotic preparation in an outpatient situation the day before surgery, and then parenteral agents are added within 2 h from the time that the procedure is to begin. The rate of outpatient antimicrobial bowel preparation is increasing, and patient selection and education is critical in order to reduce the rate of complications. The most commonly used oral and parenteral antibiotics reported in the 1997 North American bowel preparation survey are listed in table 2.

The combined oral and parenteral antimicrobial regimen has obvious appeal in that it theoretically provides both intraluminal bacterial suppression and high serum and tissue antibiotic levels. These theoretical advantages were

Table 2. Most commonly used oral and parenteral antibiotics for preoperative bowel preparations before elective colon and rectal surgery in a North American survey [4]

Oral antibiotic(s)	Number using parenteral antibiotic(s)						
	Cephalosporin			β-lactamase inhibitor combinations	Metro-nidazole	Other	Total
	1st	2nd	3rd				
Neomycin	1	3	0	1	1	0	6
Plus clindamycin	0	2	0	0	0	0	2
Plus erythromycin	22	222	26	30	20	14	334
Plus metronidazole	18	153	8	21	16	3	219
Plus erythromycin and metronidazole	6	21	5	0	0	0	32
Metronidazole	4	7	2	0	0	0	13
Plus erythromycin	4	11	0	3	0	1	19
Total with oral antibiotics	55	419	41	55	37	18	625
Total without oral antibiotics	7	46	7	4	16	6	86
Total	62	465	48	59	53	24	711

Four hundred and seventy-one respondents listed all regimens commonly prescribed by them.

borne out in practical success as evidenced by the metaanalysis performed by Song and Glenny [36]. These authors demonstrated that oral antibiotics alone were not as effective as when they were combined with parenteral antibiotics as well. Furthermore, using this combined antimicrobial chemotherapeutic approach, Coppa and Eng [37] documented that the rates of wound infection, intraabdominal infection and anastomotic leakage were significantly higher in patients who received parenteral cefoxitin alone than in those who received parenteral cefoxitin in addition to oral neomycin-erythromycin base. These investigators also identified the two additional risk factors for an increased infection rate, and these were a surgical resection involving the rectum and an operation that lasted longer than 215 min [37]. When the duration of the procedure was less than 215 min and the resection did not involve the extraperitoneal rectum, infection rates were low: about 3% in both antibiotic groups. Although the evidence is conflicting, it now appears that supplementing mechanical and oral antibiotic preparation with a single parenteral dose of a cephalosporin with aerobic and anaerobic activity (given intravenously within 30 min of incision) may be beneficial, particularly in operations expected to last longer than 3 h. The parenteral antibiotic serves as a fail-safe mechanism when the oral agents have been administered at the wrong times or when the operation has been delayed.

Table 3. Antimicrobial and mechanical bowel preparation in patients with partially obstructing intestinal lesions

Environment	Hospital
Diet	Clear liquids as tolerated, supplemented with parenteral fluids
Preoperative mechanical bowel preparation	Fractional doses of sodium phosphate on days 3 and 2 prior to surgery
Preoperative oral antibiotic bowel preparation	Erythromycin base 1 g, neomycin SO_4 1 g p.o. at 1.00, 2.00 and 11.00 p.m. on the day prior to surgery
Perioperative parenteral antibiotics	Yes: with appropriate aerobic and anaerobic antimicrobial coverage with dose given within 30 min of incision; may be continued 24 h postoperatively

Finally, this combined antibacterial regimen is also frequently utilized in patients with a partial colonic obstruction who can tolerate oral intake (table 3).

Bowel Preparation for Emergency Colon Operation

The clinical conditions that most often necessitate emergency colonic operations are acute hemorrhage, perforation, ischemia, obstruction and trauma. In these circumstances, the operation must be performed without any bowel preparation because oral antibiotic prophylaxis and mechanical cleansing are either impossible or potentially harmful.

Intraoperative Lavage

Several techniques for performing intraoperative lavage have been described [38]. The authors recommend that 8–10 liters of saline irrigation be instilled over 30 min directly into the colon through a balloon-tipped catheter in the distal ileum. The balloon is inflated to occlude the ileocecal valve and prevent reflux of the irrigant into the ileum and jejunum. This technique results in uniform cleansing of the colon, and it has enabled the performance of resections and primary anastomoses in many patients who otherwise would have undergone multiple, staged procedures. However, the most important variable in the success of this intraoperative regimen is a coordinated team approach to prevent spillage of fecal contents or other mishaps.

Table 4. Antimicrobial and mechanical bowel preparation in patients with obstructing intestinal lesions or undergoing emergency colonic surgery

Environment	Hospital
Diet	NPO with parenteral fluids for resuscitation and maintenance
Preoperative mechanical bowel preparation	None with the possible exception of an enema to cleanse the distal rectum
Preoperative oral antibiotic bowel preparation	None
Perioperative parenteral antibiotics	Parenteral antibiotics with appropriate aerobic/anaerobic antimicrobial coverage should be administered preoperatively, intraoperatively and postoperatively depending upon the length of surgery, operative findings and clinical course

NPO = Nothing per os.

Parenteral Antibiotics

Prevention of infectious complications after emergency colon operation depends on a proper operative technique, clinical judgment and the appropriate choice and administration of parenteral antibiotics (table 4). As in elective operations, the antibiotics chosen should be active against both aerobic and anaerobic colonic microflora. They should be given intravenously at appropriate doses, starting shortly before the operation and continuing postoperatively for 1–7 days. The duration of administration is governed by the operative findings and by whether the antibiotic regimen is intended to be preventative (in which case the antibiotics are given for 1 day) or therapeutic in order to manage intraabdominal infections (in which case antibiotics are given for 2 days or more). Many single agents or combinations of agents appear to be equally efficacious and are currently recommended (table 5). The choice of an agent or a combination of agents, therefore, depends on local hospital prices, toxicity profiles and the surgeon's familiarity with the agents.

Topical Antibiotics or Antiseptics

Some surgeons advocate direct application to the wound of or irrigation of the wound with either antibiotics or povidone-iodine during colon resection. Solutions containing povidone-iodine should almost never be placed in the

Table 5. Parenterally administered antimicrobial agents which can be used alone or combined to provide effective coverage of the mixed aerobic-anaerobic infections arising from human colonic bacteria for patients requiring preventive therapy

Aerobics choices	Anaerobic choices	Aerobic-anaerobic choices
Amikacin	Clindamycin	Ampicillin-sulbactam
Aztreonam	Metronidazole	Ertapenem
Ciprofloxacin		Impienem-cilastatin
Gentamicin		Meropenem
Levofloxacin		Piperacillin-tazobactam
Tobramycin		Ticarcillin-clavulanic acid

peritoneal cavity, because they are likely to be absorbed and subsequently to cause toxic effects.

Conclusion

The clinical success of elective colon and rectal surgery as measured by decreased morbidity and mortality rates secondary to infectious complications has changed radically in the last 30 years. Due to the recognition of the importance of appropriate antimicrobial therapy directed at both aerobic and anaerobic species of bacteria, combined oral and parenteral antibacterial agents and mechanical cleansing, surgeons have been able to perform single-stage colonic resections with primary anastomoses routinely. Though recent reports from Europe have called into question the necessity of mechanical cleansing, no clear consensus has been determined, and North American surgeons are steadfast in its continued use. Ultimately, the use of a three-tiered regimen – preoperative mechanical bowel preparation, preoperative oral antibiotic therapy and perioperative parenteral antimicrobial therapy – is a clinical requisite as it has been shown to be efficacious by multiple reports from the last three decades with but a few, recent reports to the contrary.

References

1 Smith WH, Crebb WE: The faecal bacterial flora of animals and man; its development in the young. J Pathol Bacteriol 1961;82:53–66.

2 Nichols RL, Condon RE: Preoperative preparation of the colon. Surg Gynecol Obstet 1971;132:323–337.
3 Ridder MI: A review of the literature on preoperative prophylaxis of the bowel with antibacterial agents. Am J Med Sci 1952;223:301–315.
4 Nichols RL, Smith JW, Garcia RY, Walterman RS, Holmes JWC: Current practices of preoperative bowel preparation among North American colorectal surgeons. Clin Infect Dis 1997;24:609–619.
5 Nichols RL, Gorbach SL, Condon RE: Alteration of intestinal microflora following preoperative mechanical preparation of the colon. Dis Colon Rectum 1971;14:123–127.
6 Smith MB, Baliga P, Sartor WM, Goradia VK, Holmes JWC, Nichols RL: Intraoperative colonic lavage: Failure to decrease mucosal microflora. South Med J 1991;84:38–42.
7 Lindsey JT, Smith JW, McClugage SG, Nichols RL: Effects of commonly used bowel preparations on the large bowel mucosal-associated and luminal microflora in the rat model. Dis Colon Rectum 1990;33:554–560.
8 Tan HL, Liew QY, Loo S, Hawkins R: Severe hyperphosphatemia and associated electrolyte and metabolic derangement following the administration of sodium phosphate for bowel preparation. Anaesthesia 2002;57:478–483.
9 Zmora O, Pikarsky AJ, Wexner SD: Bowel preparation for colorectal surgery. Dis Colon Rectum 2001;44:1537–1549.
10 Solla JA, Rothenberger DA: Preoperative bowel preparation: A survey of colon and rectal surgeons. Dis Colon Rectum 1990;333:154–159.
11 Platell C, Hall J: What is the role of mechanical bowel preparation in patients undergoing colorectal surgery. Dis Colon Rectum 1998;41:875–882.
12 Miettinen RP, Laitinen ST, Markela JT, Paakkonen ME: Bowel preparation with oral polyethylene glycol electrolyte solution vs. no preparation in elective open colorectal surgery: Prospective, randomized study. Dis Colon Rectum 2000;43:669–675.
13 Brownson P, Jenkins SA, Nott D, Ellenbogen S: Mechanical bowel preparation before colorectal surgery: Results of a prospective randomized trial. Br J Surg 1992;79:461–462.
14 Irving AD, Scrimegour D: Mechanical bowel preparation for colonic resection and anastamoses. Br J Surg 1987;74:580–581.
15 Santos JCM, Batista J, Sirimarco MT, Guimaracs AS, Levy CE: Prospective randomized trial of mechanical bowel preparation in patients undergoing elective colorectal surgery. Br J Surg 1994;81:1673–1676.
16 Jansen JO, Kelly TJ, Krukowski ZN, Keenan RA: Right hemicolectomy: Mechanical bowel preparation is not required. J R Coll Surg Edinb 2002;47:557–560.
17 Van Geldere D, Fa-Si-Oen P, Noach LA, Rietra PJ, Peterse JL, Boom RP: Complications after colorectal surgery without mechanical bowel preparation. J Am Coll Surg 2002;194:40–47.
18 Nichols RL, Condon RE, Gorbach SL, Nyhus LM: Efficacy of preoperative antimicrobial preparation of the bowel. Ann Surg 1972;176:227–232.
19 Nichols RL, Broido P, Condon RE, Gorbach SL, Nyhus LM: Effect of preoperative neomycin-erythromycin intestinal preparation on the incidence of infectious complications following colon surgery. Ann Surg 1973;178:453–462.
20 Matheson DM, Arabi Y, Baxter-Smith D, Alexander-Williams J, Keighley MR: Randomized multicentre trial of oral bowel preparation and antimicrobials for elective colorectal operations. Br J Surg 1978;65:597–600.
21 Clarke JS, Condon RE, Bartlett JG, Gorbach SL, Nichols RL, Ochi S: Preoperative oral antibiotics reduce septic complications of colon operations: Results of a prospective, randomized, double-blind clinical study. Ann Surg 1977;186:251–259.
22 Nichols RL: Preventing surgical site infections: A surgeon's perspective. Emerg Infect Dis 2001;7:220–224.
23 Antimicrobial prophylaxis for surgery. Med Lett Drugs Ther 2001;43:92–98.
24 Mangram AJ, Horan TC, Pearson ML, Silver LC, Jarvis WR: Guideline for prevention of surgical site infection, 1999. Hospital Infection Control Practices Advisory Committee. Infect Control Hosp Epidemiol 1999;20:247–280.
25 Nichols RL, Condon RE, DiSanto AR: Preoperative bowel preparation. Erythromycin base serum and fecal levels following oral administration. Arch Surg 1977;112:1493–1496.

26 DiPiro JT, Patrais JM, Townsend RJ, Bowden TA Jr, Hooks VH 3rd, Smith RB, Spiro TE: Oral neomycin sulfate and erythromycin base before colon surgery: A comparison of serum and tissue concentrations. Pharmacotherapy 1985;5:91–94.
27 Gillis JC, Brogden RN: Rifaximin. A review of its antimicrobial activity, pharmacokinetic properties and therapeutic potential in conditions mediated by gastrointestinal bacteria. Drugs 1995;49:467–484.
28 Frazee RC, Roberts J, Symmonds R, Snyder S, Hendricks J, Smith R: Prospective randomized trial of inpatient vs. outpatient bowel preparation for elective colorectal surgery. Dis Colon Rectum 1992;35:223–226.
29 Handelsman JC, Zeiler S, Coleman J, Dooley W, Walrath JM: Experience with ambulatory preoperative bowel preparation at The Johns Hopkins Hospital. Arch Surg 1993;128:441–444.
30 Nichols RL: Antibiotic prophylaxis in surgery. Curr Opin Infect Dis 1994;7:647–652.
31 Nichols RL: Bowel preparation. Sci Am Surg 1995:1–11.
32 Should antimicrobial prophylaxis in colorectal surgery include agents effective against both anerobic and aerobic microorganisms? A double-blind, multicenter study. The Norwegian Study Group for Colorectal Surgery. Surgery 1985;97:402–408.
33 Jagelman DG, Fabian TC, Nichols RL, Stone HH, Wilson SE, Zellner SR: Single-dose cefotetan versus multiple dose cefoxitin as prophylaxis in colorectal surgery. Am J Surg 1988;155 (suppl 5A):71–76.
34 Kager L, Ljungdahl I, Malmborg AS, Nord CE, Pieper R, Dahlgren P: Antibiotic prophylaxis with cefoxitin in colorectal surgery – effect on the colon microflora and septic complications: A clinical model for prediction of the benefit and risks in using a new antibiotic prophylaxis. Ann Surg 1981;193:277–282.
35 Condon RE, Bartlett JG, Nichols RL, Schulte WJ, Gorbach SL, Ochi S: Preoperative prophylactic cephalothin fails to control septic complications of colorectal operations: Results of a controlled clinical trial. Am J Surg 1979;137:68–74.
36 Song F, Glenny AM: Antimicrobial prophylax is in colorectal surgery: A systematic review of randomized controlled trials. Br J Surg 1998;86:1232–1241.
37 Coppa GF, Eng K: Factors involved in antibiotic selection in elective colon and rectal surgery. Surgery 1988;104:853–858.
38 Murray JJ, Schoetz DJ, Coller JA, Roberts PL, Viedenheimer MC: Intraoperative colonic lavage and primary anastomosis in nonelective colon resection. Dis Colon Rectum 1991;34:527–531.

Note Added in Proof

Pursuant to editorial request, an additional literature search of relevant articles pertaining to the need for preoperative mechanical and antimicrobial bowel preparation in colorectal surgery since the time of the initial submission of the article was conducted by the authors. Two studies were encountered, and both lend credence to our argument that the routine use of both antibacterial and mechanical bowel preparation is not only the common practice of American colorectal surgeons, but still has not been scientifically disproven as ineffective or deleterious. Zmora et al. surveyed 1,295 members of the American Society of Colon and Rectal Surgeons as to their preference and bias in regards to preoperative bowel preparation for elective colorectal surgery [1]. 515 responses (40%) were completed, and the tallied results showed that the three-tiered approach to preoperative bowel preparation espoused in our paper is practiced by the majority of the respondents. In fact, 75%, 99%, and 98% of the respondents made routine use of two-drug oral antibiotic prophylaxis, preoperative mechanical preparation, and perioperative intravenous antibiotics, respectively. These data further serve to corroborate our position as outlined in the main body of the manuscript.

The second study by Wille-Jorgensen et al. is a metaanalyis of 6 studies looking at the specific question of whether mechanical bowel preparation changed the rate of anastomotic leakage, mortality, peritonitis, or wound infections [2]. After analysis of the data, the authors found that the rate of anastomotic leakage was greater in the patients prescribed a mechanical bowel preparation over those that were not, and this result was statistically significant. However, there was no statistically significant difference in the rate of death, peritonitis, or wound infections between the two groups of patients. Though this study would refute our claim, an invited editorial concerning the statistical accuracy of this work [3] criticized the paper for using non-homogeneous data and publication bias. Specifically, the author writes that Wille-Jorgenen et al. are 'Comparing apples and oranges and the occasional lemon'.

References

1 Zmora O, Wexner SD, Hajjar L, Park T, Efron JE, Nogueras JJ, Weiss EG: Trends in preparation for colorectal surgery: Survey of the members of the American society of colon and rectal surgeons. Am Surg 2003;69:150–154.

2 Wille-Jorgensen P, Guenaga KF, Castro AA, Matos D: Clinical value of preoperative mechanical bowel cleansing in elective colorectal surgery: A systematic review. Dis Colon Rectum 2003;46(8):1013–1018.

3 Tekkis PP: Invited Editorial. Dis Colon Rectum 2003;46(8):1019–1020.

Ronald Lee Nichols, MD, MS, FACS
Tulane University School of Medicine, Department of Surgery SL22
1430 Tulane Avenue
New Orleans, LA 70112–2699 (USA)
Tel. +1 504 588 5168, Fax +1 504 586 3843, E-Mail Ronald.nichols@tulane.edu

This chapter should be cited as follows:

Nichols RL, Choe EU, Weldon CB: Mechanical and Antibacterial Bowel Preparation in Colon and Rectal Surgery. Chemotherapy 2005;51(suppl 1):115–122.

Scarpignato C (ed): Rifaximin: A Poorly Absorbed Antibiotic.
Pharmacology and Clinical Use.

Rifaximin, a Peculiar Rifamycin Derivative: Established and Potential Clinical Use Outside the Gastrointestinal Tract

Iva Pelosini, Carmelo Scarpignato

Laboratory of Clinical Pharmacology, Department of Human Anatomy, Pharmacology and Forensic Sciences, School of Medicine and Dentistry, University of Parma, Parma, Italy

Abstract

Rifaximin is a poorly absorbed semisynthetic rifamycin derivative with a broad spectrum of antibacterial activity including Gram-positive and Gram-negative bacteria, both aerobes and anaerobes. Although originally developed for the treatment of infectious diarrhea, the appreciation of the pathogenic role of gut bacteria in several organic and functional gastrointestinal diseases has increasingly broadened its clinical use. The availability of a topical formulation (a cream containing 5% of the drug) and the lack of transcutaneous absorption pointed out in both animal and human studies has allowed its topical use in skin infections. Furthermore, since the spectrum of antibacterial action of rifaximin includes many organisms (e.g. *Bacteroides bivius-disiens, Gardnerella vaginalis, Haemophilus ducreyi*) causing genital infections, including *Trichomonas vaginalis* and *Chlamydia trachomatis*, its local application in the treatment of bacterial vaginosis (BV) has been attempted. Finally, since periodontal disease, caused by plaque (an aggregate of various bacteria), can be considered a 'local' infection, intra-pocket rifaximin was tried in the treatment of periodontal infections. While the efficacy in pyogenic infections of the skin has been confirmed by several investigations, which showed an improvement of both subjective and objective parameters significantly better than that of the reference drug (i.e. chlortetracycline or oxytetracycline), the usefulness of rifaximin in BV and periodontal disease needs to be further studied in well-designed clinical trials.

Introduction

Rifaximin, a virtually nonabsorbed antibiotic, is a semisynthetic rifamycin derivative, with a broad antimicrobial spectrum that includes most Gram-positive and Gram-negative bacteria, both aerobes and anaerobes [1, 2]. Unlike systemically available antibiotics, this antimicrobial allows localized targeting (e.g. enteric or cutaneous) of pathogens and is associated with a minimal risk of systemic toxicity or side effects [3, 4]. Provided that nonabsorbed antibiotics are as effective as systemically absorbed drugs for the target illness, their safety and tolerability profiles may render them more appropriate for certain patient groups, such as young children, pregnant or lactating women, and the elderly, among whom side effects are a particular concern.

Taking into account its excellent activity against a broad range of enteropathogens, the first 'logical' indication for this gastrointestinal (GI)-targeted antibiotic was the treatment of infectious diarrhea in both adults and children [5]. The appreciation of the pathogenic role of gut bacteria in several organic and functional GI diseases [6, 7] has increasingly broadened its clinical use [2]. However, the availability of a topical formulation (a cream containing 5% of the drug) and the lack of transcutaneous absorption pointed out in both animal [8] and human [9] studies have allowed its topical use in skin infections. Furthermore, since the spectrum of antibacterial action of rifaximin includes many organisms (e.g. *Bacteroides bivius-disiens, Gardnerella vaginalis, Haemophilus ducreyi*) causing genital infections [10], including *Trichomonas vaginalis* [10] and *Chlamydia trachomatis* [11], its local application in the treatment of bacterial vaginosis (BV) has been attempted. Finally, since periodontal disease, caused by plaque (an aggregate of various bacteria), can be considered a 'local' infection [12], intrapocket rifaximin was tried out in the treatment of periodontal infections.

All these extra-GI clinical uses of rifaximin will be reviewed below.

Skin Infections

Human skin provides a great living environment for the growth of microbes. The types and numbers of microorganisms vary according to the part of the body and the age and gender of the individual [13]. Despite this, normal healthy skin presents a natural physical barrier to bacterial invasion. An intact stratum corneum layer provides a barrier to a wide variety of pathogens. The natural resistance of the skin to bacterial penetration and multiplication is not completely understood, but elements involved include the following factors [14]: (1) the inability of organisms to penetrate the keratinized stratum corneum, (2) desquamation, which sheds bacteria as it sloughs keratinocytes, (3) natural acidity of the skin (pH 5.5), (4) presence of antibacterial substances in sebaceous secretions and intracellular lipids of the stratum corneum, (5) relatively low moisture content of the skin, and (6) normal cutaneous microflora.

Changes in any of these factors can greatly influence an individual's susceptibility to infection, as can changes in the overall ability of the host to mount an inflammatory response. Nonpathogenic microbes are capable of becoming disease-producing pathogens in individuals with reduced cellular or humoral defenses or defects (e.g., immunocompromised or nutritionally compromised individuals).

Staphylococcus aureus and group A streptococci are the two most dominant pathogens involved in primary and secondary infections of the skin and minor skin wounds in outpatient settings [15]. Dominant pathogens in the hospital setting are tracked through the SENTRY Antimicrobial Surveillance ProGram established in 1997, which follows skin and soft tissue infections reported through a worldwide network of more than 100 hospitals. There is a remarkable consistency over the years that *S. aureus* is the most common hospital-acquired pathogen followed by *Pseudomonas aeruginosa.*

In order for bacteria to be pathogenic, they must be able to adhere to, grow on, and invade the host [16]. Bacteria possess numerous virulence genes that allow for growth in these privileged niches. Epidermal infections caused by *S. aureus* and *Streptococcus pyogenes* include impetigo and ecthyma. Dermal infections consist of erysipelas, cellulitis, and necrotizing fasciitis. The pilosebaceous unit is involved in folliculitis, furunculosis, and carbunculosis. Moreover, *S. aureus* and *S. pyogenes* produce toxins that may elicit a superantigen response, causing massive release of cytokines. The staphylococcal scalded skin syndrome, toxic shock syndrome, and scarlet fever are all superantigen-mediated.

Systemic therapy with a variety of β-lactams, macrolides and lincosamides (clindamycin) has been the cornerstone of skin infection therapy for many years [17]. However, topical antibiotics can play an important role in both treatment and prevention of many primary cutaneous bacterial infections commonly seen in the dermatological practice [18]. Indeed, while systemic antimicrobials are needed in the complicated infections of skin and skin structure, the milder forms can be successfully treated with topical therapy alone [18]. The topical agents used most often in the treatment of superficial cutaneous bacterial infections are tetracyclines, mupirocin, bacitracin, polymyxin B, and neomycin.

Due to the frequent difficulty of doing cultures before giving an antibacterial drug, topical treatment often requires the use of broad-spectrum antibiotics. However, the selection of resistant strains, especially via the use of broad-spectrum antimicrobials with marked systemic diffusion even after topical application, represents a continuous challenge also in the field of skin infection [19]. *S. aureus* strains have developed worldwide a resistance to penicillin due to β-lactamase production in >90% of cases, and methicillin resistance is now a major problem with resistance levels of >50% in certain areas of the world.

These resistant strains are often multiresistant, being not sensitive to erythromycin and tetracycline, with resistance to quinolone developing rapidly. Group A streptococci are still susceptible to penicillin, but increasing problems with erythromycin and tetracycline have been reported [19].

Rifaximin is broad-spectrum antibiotic, which covers many skin pathogens, whose lack of transcutaneous absorption has been well documented by both animal [8] and human [9] studies. On these grounds, a topical formulation (i.e. cream) containing 5% of the active compound was developed and tested in the treatment of pyogenic skin infections. Some open trials [20, 21] showed the efficacy and safety of the formulation and pointed out the lack of selection of resistant strains after topical application of rifaximin. In any event, drug delivery from the topical formulation is orders of magnitude higher than the 'breakpoint' level set for resistance, allowing to overcome even a resistant-defined strain.

Randomized, controlled studies (some of which were single blinded) compared rifaximin to chlortetracycline or oxytetracycline [22–30] in the therapy of skin infections caused by different pyogenic bacteria. In almost all these trials the clinical efficacy of rifaximin was significantly better than that of the reference drug. Indeed, the improvement of both subjective (i.e. itching, burning, pain) and objective (i.e. erythema, edema, papules, blebs, erosions, scabs) parameters was generally more rapid with the rifamycin derivative (fig. 1), which often led to a reduction in the duration of treatment [26]. In many studies (table 1) a bacteriological investigation was performed before and after therapy: on average, bacterial eradication at the infection site was achieved in 96.5% of the rifaximin-treated patients and in 79.2% of the tetracycline-treated ones, the overall odd ratio being 6.51 (95% CI 2.71–15.64, $p < 0.0001$).

The dogma of antibiotic-associated contact dermatitis has been perpetuated and generally accepted throughout the dermatological and general medical community over the past decades. The acceptance of this dogma has in part been fueled by surveys of identified allergens from contact allergy clinics [31, 32]. For example, the most recent study conducted by the North American Contact Dermatitis Group [32] showed a positive patch test response to neomycin (20% formulation) of 11.6% in a population of 3,104 patients referred for diagnostic patch testing. In this connection, being rifaximin unabsorbed, sensitization phenomena with this antibiotic are virtually unlikely. As a matter of fact, sensitization was never observed in clinical trials. One study [26] also examined whether photosensitization occurred after topical application of the drug. To this end, a skin area, where rifaximin cream had been applied, was exposed to medium and long UV rays and a photopatch test was performed. In no patient was photosensitization observed.

These data, taken together, demonstrate that topical application of rifaximin represents an effective and safe treatment of pyogenic skin infections. An additional application of this dermatological formulation would be infection

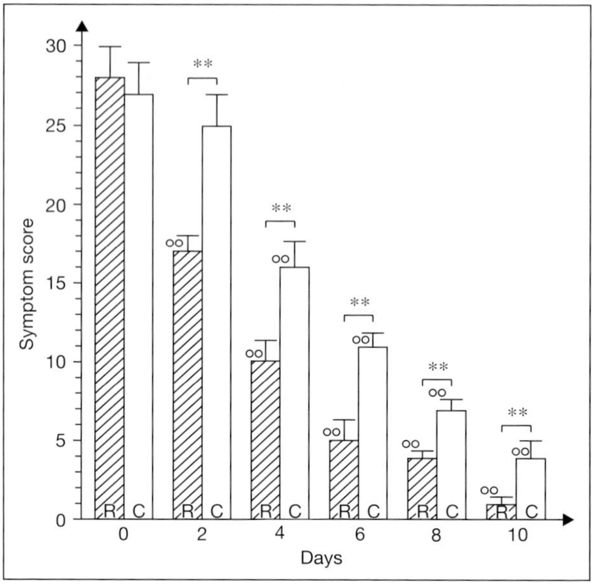

Fig. 1. Cumulative subjective plus objective symptom score after 10-day topical application of rifaximin (5% cream, n = 30, R) or chlortetracycline (3% cream, n = 30, C) of patients with pyogenic skin infections (from Della Marchina et al. [30]). °°$p < 0.01$ versus basal value (day 0); **$p < 0.01$ between the two groups.

Table 1. Bacterial eradication at the infection site in patients with pyogenic skin infections after short-term treatment with topical rifaximin or either chlortetracycline (C) or oxytetracycline (O)

Authors, year	Ref. no.	Rifaximin	Reference drug	
Lazzaro et al., 1988	22	30/30 (100)	25/30 (83.4)	C
Marincola Cattaneo et al., 1988	23	31/32 (98.8)	21/31 (67.7)	C
Lazzaro et al., 1992	24	12/12 (100)	11/12 (91.7)	C
Palazzini and Palmerio, 1993	25	13/14 (91.7)	4/7 (57.1)	O
Moroni et al., 1993	26	16/16 (100)	11/15 (73.4)	O
Pasi and Palazzini, 1993	27	11/11 (100)	9/10 (90)	O
Cannata and Piccardo, 1993	28	7/7 (100)	11/11 (100)	C
Rafanelli et al., 1993	29	16/19 (84.2)	14/20 (70)	O
Total		136/141 (96.5)	106/136 (79.2)	

Figures in parentheses represent percentage.

prophylaxis in superficial skin wounds, particularly when used with a dressing that occludes the wound. Prophylactic topical antibiotic use makes particular sense for wounds in which the risk of infection is high, such as those that are likely to be contaminated (accidental wounds, lacerations, abrasions, and burns). Because all traumatic wounds should be considered contaminated, topical antibiotics are a logical measure to prevent wound infection [33]. Thanks to its pharmacokinetic and pharmacodynamic properties, rifaximin would be particularly suitable for preventing wound infection.

Bacterial Vaginosis

BV, previously known as nonspecific vaginitis or *Gardnerella* vaginitis, is the most common cause of vaginal discharge in women of childbearing age [34]. Estimates of its prevalence depend on the population studied, but include 17–19% in family planning clinics and 4–10% in student health clinics [35], increasing to 24–40% in sexually transmitted disease clinics. BV has been observed in 16–29% of pregnant women and is more frequently detected (30%) in women attending infertility clinics. It predominantly affects young, sexually active females but can occur in the absence of sexual intercourse.

This clinical syndrome is now recognized as polymicrobial superficial vaginal infection involving a loss of normal hydrogen peroxide (H_2O_2)-producing lactobacilli and an overgrowth of anaerobes [34]. While commonly found in increased numbers in women with BV, *G. vaginalis* is not invariably present [36]. The massive overgrowth of vaginal anaerobes is accompanied by an increased production of proteolytic carboxylase enzymes, which act to break down vaginal peptides to a variety of amines (especially trimethylamine) which, in high pH, become volatile and malodorous. The amines are associated with increased vaginal transudation and squamous epithelial cell exfoliation, creating the typical discharge [37]. Indeed, an increased pH (greater than 4.5 units) of the vaginal secretion, a fishy odor of the vaginal discharge before or after the addition of 10% KOH (the so-called whiff test) and the presence of clue cells (epithelial cells with adherent coccobacilli) are, together with the symptoms, the main diagnostic criteria for BV [34, 37]. The term vaginosis is used because of the superficial nature of the infection. The wet mount usually does not show the increased number of leukocytes seen in other types of vaginitis. Although lactobacilli are essential for normal vaginal acidity, they are themselves acidophilic and hence attracted to an acid environment. The more anaerobic vaginal milieu of BV is not conducive to lactobacillary growth and dominance. What remains unknown, however, is whether the loss of lactobacilli precedes or follows this massive upheaval in flora [37].

BV is associated with an increased risk of several pathological conditions, including postoperative infection following hysterectomy and postabortion pelvic inflammatory disease [34]. In addition, 7 published studies (2 case-control and 5 cohort studies) have reported an increased risk of preterm birth in women with BV [37]. An appropriate diagnosis and treatment of BV may, therefore, lower a patient's risk of associated pelvic inflammatory disease, endometritis and adverse pregnancy outcomes. In this connection, a Cochrane systematic review [38] did show that eradicating BV significantly decreases the risk of preterm prelabor rupture of membranes without lowering that of preterm birth.

BV being an infectious disease, antibiotics represent the logical therapeutic approach [39]. However, a high spontaneous cure rate in some patients without symptoms has been found [40]. For this reason, placebo-controlled groups are recommended for antibiotic effectiveness trials. Besides systemic toxicity [4], antibiotic treatment of BV can also lead to vulvovaginal yeast infections [41]. The benefit of antimicrobial therapy should, therefore, be weighed against the potential risks. Metronidazole and clindamycin are the most effective antimicrobial agents [34, 37, 39]. Erythromycin fails, because macrolide antibiotics are not effective at the acidic pH level of the vagina [42]. Ampicillin too is ineffective, probably because of poor activity against anaerobes, especially those producing of β-lactamases [43]. Other newer antimicrobials, such as ciprofloxacin [44] and amoxicillin/clavulanate [43, 45], show some effectiveness but appear to be less efficacious than metronidazole or clindamycin. Topical therapy with 2% clindamycin once daily for 7 days or 0.75% metronidazole gel once daily for 5 days has been shown to be as effective as oral metronidazole [46]. More recently, abbreviated 3-day courses of topical clindamycin and metronidazole have achieved comparable early cure rates, but long-term follow-up suggests higher rates of early recurrence [47]. Vaginal antimicrobials obviously result in minimal risk to the fetus in pregnant women.

Although metronidazole represents the most effective therapy of BV, no single treatment is completely successful in either cure or prevention. This is why several attempts have recently been made to use alternative and safer treatments [48]. The absence of lactobacilli in the vagina, a specific feature of BV, raised the question as to whether the restoration of lactobacilli by probiotic therapy can restore the normal flora and improve the chances of having a healthy term pregnancy. As a matter of fact, certain lactobacilli strains can safely colonize the vagina after oral and vaginal administration, displace and kill pathogens including *G. vaginalis* and *Escherichia coli*, and modulate the immune response to interfere with the inflammatory cascade that leads to preterm birth [49]. During pregnancy, local treatment restoring the normal acidity and vaginal flora, without systemic effect, is of course preferable to any other approach.

Table 2. Efficacy of two different rifaximin formulations in the treatment of BV in nonpregnant women (from Palazzini and Desai [52])

Rifaximin formulation	Positive vaginal cultures		Microbiological and clinical success rates, %	
	Before treatment	After treatment	Eradication rate	Cure rate
Foam	15/15 (100)	2/15 (13.4)	86.7	86.7
Cream	16/16 (100)	7/16 (46.7)	56.2	56.2

Rifaximin (5% cream or foam) was applied vaginally from the delivery system at bedtime for 5 consecutive nights. Figures in parentheses represent percentage.

The very fact that several alternative therapies have been tried in BV is evidence that no single treatment provides the symptomatic and bacteriological cure rate the physician requires. Thanks to its antibacterial activity [10, 11], covering *G. vaginalis* and other pathogens responsible for urogenital infections, as well as its 'topical' antimicrobial action, rifaximin could be a suitable alternative for the local treatment of BV even in pregnant women. To this end, a 5-day and a 28-day toxicological study [50, 51] were performed in rabbits. Animals were given 1 ml of rifaximin 20% in K-Y® lubricating jelly applied deep into the vagina using a rubber catheter. All rabbits survived throughout the study and were free of signs of systemic toxicity. No signs of drug-related vaginal irritation were seen either by macroscopic observation or microscopic examination. A randomized, open-label pilot study [52] was performed in Italy to compare the effectiveness of two rifaximin formulations specifically developed for vaginal use (5% vaginal cream and 5% vaginal foam) in the treatment of BV. As shown in table 2, patients treated with the foam delivery system had a cure rate, which was higher than that achieved with the cream formulation. Only 1 patient in the cream arm experienced local irritation resulting in discontinuation of the treatment. The foam delivery system was, therefore, selected for further development.

Since a high spontaneous cure rate has often been observed [40], double-blind, placebo-controlled trials are needed to definitely assess the efficacy of rifaximin in the treatment of BV.

Periodontal Disease

Chronic inflammatory periodontitis occurs frequently in the adult population. The exact prevalence of the disease in the US and worldwide has been estimated to be 20% of the adult population, but has not been definitively determined because studies lack a consistent definition of the disease and a consistent methodology [53]. To this end, the American Academy of Periodontology [54] updated its classification system for periodontal diseases in 1999 to create a common terminology compatible with current scientific knowledge of periodontal diseases. Gingivitis and periodontitis are classified as separate diseases. Gingivitis is an inflammation of the marginal gingiva that does not produce attachment loss or loss of bone. Pockets that may occur with gingivitis are actually 'pseudopockets', and are due to gingival enlargement and do not involve apical migration of the gingival attachment or bone loss [55]. Periodontitis occurs when the junctional epithelium and periodontal attachment move apically along the tooth root. Alveolar bone also resorbs towards the apex of the tooth during the disease process (fig. 2). It is believed that pathogenic bacterial plaque induces an inflammatory immune response, which may compromise periodontal structures. The plaque would be comprised of pathogenic organisms, predominantly Gram-negative anaerobic bacteria [56], large enough in numbers to effect a response in a susceptible host. Genetic and systemic factors may affect these events [55]. Disease severity ranges along a continuum of slight to severe, and localized to generalized, depending upon the amount, location and rate of attachment loss. Chronic periodontitis often affects different areas of the mouth to different degrees. It is usually progressive, characterized by bursts of disease progression followed by periods when the disease is more quiescent. If left untreated, tooth loss may result due to the progressive nature of the disease [55, 57].

It is now well accepted that the goal of all periodontal therapies is to reduce, eliminate and/or repair the damage to the periodontal structures resulting from the deleterious effects of the host response to pathogenic organisms [55]. The nature and severity of chronic periodontitis are a result of the interactions between microbial factors and a susceptible host. Pathogenic bacteria in the gingival sulcus or periodontal pocket are necessary for periodontitis to occur, but bacteria alone are only part of the picture. It is well known that the body's local and systemic response to bacteria and their toxins determines the extent and severity of the disease. Controlling pathogenic bacterial colonization minimizes the host response. This is best accomplished by routine brushing, flossing and otherwise disrupting plaque and biofilm. The recommendations of dental professionals to the patient for plaque control procedures and products are essentially to achieve a healthy periodontal attachment for life. Likewise, nonsurgical approaches such as scaling and root planing (SRP) as well as the antimicrobial use have all been proven to improve periodontal health [58]. Several different surgical therapies have been evaluated as a last resort, but clinical

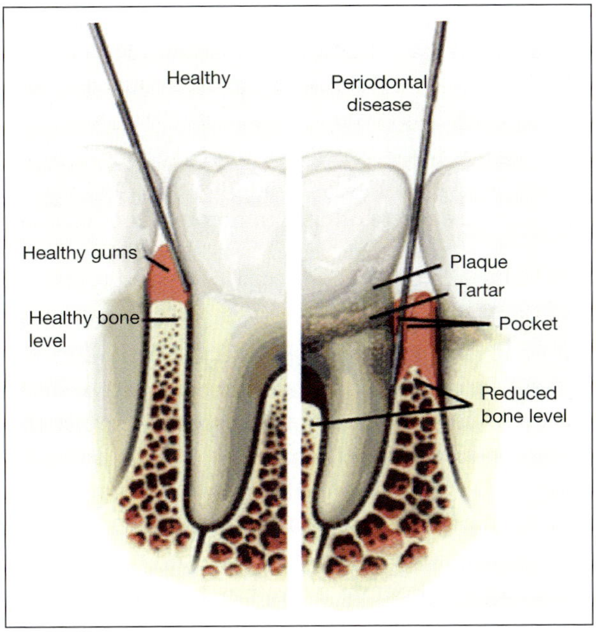

Fig. 2. Pathophysiological sequence of events in periodontal disease. Bacteria produce byproducts (e.g. toxins or enzymes) which, along with mucus, constantly form a sticky, colorless 'plaque' on teeth. If not removed, plaque can harden and form bacteria-harboring 'tartar' around teeth. Tissue that attaches the gums to the teeth can be destroyed by the irritants of plaque. If this is the case, gums pull away from the teeth and small pockets arise between the teeth and gums. The pockets then become filled with more plaque, deepen, and it becomes impossible to clean plaque out. At this stage the bone structure supporting teeth can actually be destroyed (courtesy of Drs J. Chavez and S.E. Zaragoza, El Paso Community College, Texas, USA).

outcomes are less predictable due to a variability in factors such as the dental surgeon's skill, experience, bias, procedures, and reproducibility of outcome measures [59].

Although the mechanical periodontal treatment alone is adequate to ameliorate or resolve the clinical condition in most cases, adjunctive antimicrobial agents, delivered either systemically or locally, can enhance the effect of therapy. In this connection, two recent meta-analyses [60, 61] have shown that systemic antimicrobials in conjunction with SRP can offer an additional benefit over SPR alone in the treatment of periodontitis both in terms of change in the clinical attachment level and probing pocket depth. When examining the effect of individual antibiotics, it was found that there were statistically significant improvements in clinical attachment level with tetracycline and metronidazole [61].

The advantages of systemic antibiotics include the ability of the drug to control pathogens in all periodontal tissues and other sites where they may have an impact. However, systemic antibiotics may not reach the needed concentrations in the periodontal pocket, may have side effects and interactions, may be subject to compliance issues and may actually select resistant strains. Due to all these concerns, they are not routinely used in chronic periodontitis but reserved for selected patients, such as refractory cases, where often antimicrobial combinations are used [62].

Over the past 20 years, locally delivered, anti-infective pharmacological agents, most recently employing sustained-release vehicles, have been introduced. As outlined in a recent systematic review [63], controlled clinical trials have consistently shown that these formulations, along with SRP, have resulted in a clinically and statistically significant increase in the percentage of patients achieving predetermined periodontal benefits compared to scaling and SPR alone. Some trials have also shown that an antimicrobial agent alone can reduce probing depths as much as SRP alone [63]. Here again, tetracyclines [64] and metronidazole [65] are the most widely used antimicrobials.

The broad antibacterial activity of rifaximin as well as its 'topical' action make this antibiotic suitable for intra-pocket administration in periodontal disease. As a matter of fact, local application of rifaximin compares well with tetracyclines and metronidazole in other extra-GI diseases, i.e. skin infections and BV, respectively (see above). On the other hand, rifampicin (rifampin), another rifamycin derivative, has been successfully used in the treatment of some dental infections, including chronic periodontitis [66–69].

In a preliminary study [70], intrapocket administration of rifaximin in patients with periodontal disease was studied from both microbiological and clinical points of view. The activity of this antibiotic against the microorganisms isolated from periodontal pockets is shown in table 3. The high local concentration of rifaximin should likely exceed the observed MIC values. Indeed, its topical application was followed by a quick disappearance of anaerobic bacteria and a marked reduction of aerobic microorganisms. This was accompanied by a significant clinical improvement.

In the above trial [70] rifaximin was dissolved in chloroform and applied by repeated painting. After the solvent had dried a red sludge persisted over the dental structures allowing a continuous antimicrobial effect. Better delivery systems, such as subgingival controlled release preparations [12], are, however, needed to fully exploit the rifaximin potential in periodontal disease. In this connection, a gum-like device [71] has been developed that allows a controlled and continuous release of the antibiotic within the oral cavity. Large double-blind controlled trials using this and other formulations are now needed to establish the best therapeutic regimen for this indication.

Table 3. Inhibitory activity of rifaximin on microorganisms isolated from periodontal pockets in patients with periodontal disease (from Mangiante et al. [70])

	MIC_{50}, μg/ml	MIC_{90}, μg/ml	Range, μg/ml
Bacteroides fragilis	0.1	12.5	0.025–100
Bacteroides spp.	0.1	50	0.025–100
Clostridium spp.	0.4	50	0.0125–100
Fusobacterium spp.	0.4	50	0.05–100
Bifidobacterium spp.	0.8	6.2	0.4–50
Eubacterium spp.	0.2	0.4	0.05–6.2
Propionibacterium spp.	0.2	12.5	0.025–12.5
Peptococcus spp.	0.1	3.1	0.025–100
Peptostreptococcus spp.	0.2	25	0.025–100
Streptococcus spp.	0.2	32	0.025–100
Veillonella spp.	0.1	6.0	0.025–100

Conclusions

Due to its excellent activity against a broad range of enteropathogens as well as its lack of absorption after oral administration the first 'topical' application of rifaximin was within the GI tract [1, 2]. The appreciation of the pathogenic role of gut bacteria in several organic and functional GI diseases [6, 7] has broadened its clinical use, which now goes beyond the original indication, i.e. GI infections.

It was later realized that rifaximin can be applied directly to the skin and the vaginal and gingival mucosae without absorption and without any risk of irritation. The spectrum of antimicrobial activity being large enough to cover many of the pathogens involved in skin infection, BV and periodontal disease, topic application of this antibiotic was attempted in these clinical conditions. While the efficacy in pyogenic infections of the skin has been confirmed by several investigations, the usefulness of rifaximin in BV and periodontal disease needs to be further studied in well-designed clinical trials. No doubt, new clinical applications of this peculiar antibiotic will appear in the future.

References

1 Gillis JC, Brogden RN: Rifaximin. A review of its antibacterial activity, pharmacokinetic properties and therapeutic potential in conditions mediated by gastrointestinal bacteria. Drugs 1995;49: 467–484.

2 Scarpignato C, Pelosini I: Rifaximin, a poorly absorbed antibiotic: Pharmacology and clinical potential. Chemotherapy 2005;51(suppl 1):36–66.

3 DuPont HL: Community-acquired diarrheal disease in western countries: Applications of nonabsorbable oral antibiotic therapy. Adv Stud Med 2003;3(suppl A):S945–S950.
4 Cunha BA: Antibiotic side effects. Med Clin North Am 2001;85:149–185.
5 Ericsson CD, DuPont HL: Rifaximin in the treatment of infectious diarrhea. Chemotherapy 2005; 51(suppl 1):73–80.
6 Hart AL, Stagg AJ, Frame M, Graffner H, Glise H, Falk P, Kamm MA: The role of the gut flora in health and disease, and its modification as therapy. Aliment Pharmacol Ther 2002;16:1383–1393.
7 Guarner F, Malagelada JR: Gut flora in health and disease. Lancet 2003;361:512–519.
8 Venturini AP, Bertoli D, Marchi E: Transcutaneous absorption of a topical rifamycin preparation: Rifaximin (L/105). Drugs Exp Clin Res 1987;13:231–232.
9 Berlö JA, Debruyne HJ, Gortz JP: A prospective study in healthy volunteers of the topical absorption of a 5% rifaximin cream. Drugs Exp Clin Res 1994;20:205–208.
10 Hoover WW, Gerlach EH, Hoban DJ, Eliopoulos GM, Pfaller MA, Jones RN: Antimicrobial activity and spectrum of rifaximin, a new topical rifamycin derivative. Diagn Microbiol Infect Dis 1993; 16:111–118.
11 Prasad ES, Wenman WM: In vitro activity of rifaximin, a topical rifamycin derivative, against *Chlamydia trachomatis*. Diagn Microbiol Infect Dis 1993;16:135–136.
12 Minabe M, Suzuki F, Umemoto T: Intra-pocket antibiotic therapy using resorbable and non-resorbable slow-release devices containing tetracycline. Periodontal Clin Investig 2000;22:14–21.
13 Roth RR, James WD: Microbiology of the skin: Resident flora, ecology, infection. J Am Acad Dermatol 1989;20:367–390.
14 Swartz MN, Weinberg AN: General considerations of bacterial diseases; in Freedberg IM, Eisen AZ, Wolff K, Austen KF, Goldsmith LA, Katz SI (eds): Fitzpatrick's Dermatology in General Medicine (book on CD-ROM), ed 5. New York, McGraw-Hill, 1999.
15 Update on topical antibiotic therapy: Changing antibiotic susceptibility patterns and clinical implications. Proceedings from a clinical roundtable. November 9, 2002, Scottsdale, Arizona, USA. Cutis 2003;71(3 suppl):2–24.
16 Chiller K, Selkin BA, Murakawa GJ: Skin microflora and bacterial infections of the skin. J Investig Dermatol 2001;6:170–174.
17 Guay DR: Treatment of bacterial skin and skin structure infections. Expert Opin Pharmacother 2003;4:1259–1275.
18 Spann CT, Taylor SC, Weinberg JM: Topical antimicrobial agents in dermatology. Dis Mon 2004; 50:407–421.
19 Espersen F: Resistance to antibiotics used indermatological practice. Br J Dermatol 1998; 139(suppl 53):4–8.
20 Tempera G, Pinizzotto MR, Oliveri S: Microbiological-clinical study on the selection of resistant bacterial strains during topical treatment pyodermatitis with rifaximin cream. Stampa Med Eur (Rome) 1993;13:29–36.
21 Ena P, Zanetti S, Sechi L, Fadda G: Open study on rifaximin topical treatment for skin infections due to pyogenic bacteria. NAM (Milan) 1993;9:325–328.
22 Lazzaro C, Calaciura C, Spitalieri S, Lazzaro GC: Treatment of pyogenic skin infections: Results of a controlled trial with a new topica preparation (in Italian). Aggiornamenti Med Chir (Rome) 1989;13:1–11.
23 Marincola Cattaneo V, Attania A, Palazzini E, Monti A: Topic use of rifaximin in the treatment of pyodermitis (in Italian). Biol Med (Rome) 1988;10:69–78.
24 Lazzaro C, Salanitri T, Spitaleri S, Lazzaro Danzuso GC: Effectiveness and tolerance of topical rifaximin treatment for pyodermatosis. Clinical controlled trial vs chlortetracycline. Med Praxis (Milan) 1992;13:1–11.
25 Palazzini E, Palmerio B: Treatment of pyogenic skin infections with rifaximin cream. Eur Rev Med Pharmacol Sci 1993;15:87–92.
26 Moroni P, Da Valli R, Carboni G: Controlled clinical trial of topical rifaximin treatment for pyodermatitis. Aggiornamenti Med Chir (Rome) 1993;11:506–517.
27 Pasi F, Palazzini E: Assessment of efficacy and tolerance of rifaximin in the topical treatment of pyodermia: Controlled study vs. oxytetracy-cline. Derm Exper (Rome) 1993;8:13–20.

28 Cannata G, Piccardo G: Single-blind study of rifaximin effectiveness and safety for the topical treatment of bacterial skin infections. Biol Med (Rome) 1993;15:7–19.
29 Rafanelli A, Rafanelli G, Palazzini E: Effectiveness and safety of a new topical antibiotic cream for use in patients with bacterial skin infection. Prog Rep (Rome) 1993;5:21–29.
30 Della Marchina M, Renzi G, Renzi C, Palazzini E: Rifaximin in the local treatment of pyodermia: A controlled clinical trial versus oxytetracycline. Biol Med (Rome) 1993;15:21–34.
31 Morris SD, Rycroft RJ, White IR, Wakelin SH, McFadden JP: Comparative frequency of patch test reactions to topical antibiotics. Br J Dermatol 2002;146:1047–1051.
32 Marks JG Jr, Belsito DV, DeLeo VA, Fowler JF Jr, Fransway AF, Maibach HI, Mathias CG, Pratt MD, Rietschel RL, Sherertz EF, Storrs FJ, Taylor JS: North American Contact Dermatitis Group patch test results for the detection of delayed-type hypersensitivity to topical allergens. J Am Acad Dermatol 1998;38:911–918.
33 Dire DJ, Coppola M, Dwyer DA, Lorette JJ, Karr JL: Prospective evaluation of topical antibiotics for preventing infections in uncomplicated soft-tissue wounds repaired in the ED. Acad Emerg Med 1995;2:4–10.
34 Majeroni BA: Bacterial vaginosis: An update. Am Fam Physician 1998;57:1285–1289.
35 Hillier SL, Holmes KK: Bacterial vaginosis; in Holmes KK, Mardh PA, Sparling PF, et al (eds): Sexually Transmitted Diseases. New York, McGraw-Hill, 1999, pp 563–587.
36 Hill GB: The microbiology of bacterial vaginosis. Am J Obstet Gynecol 1993;169:450–454.
37 Sobel JD: Bacterial vaginosis. Annu Rev Med 2000;51:349–356.
38 McDonald H, Brocklehurst P, Parsons J, Vigneswaran R: Antibiotics for treating bacterial vaginosis in pregnancy. Cochrane Database Syst Rev 2003;2:CD000262.
39 Joesoef M, Schmid G: Bacterial vaginosis. Clin Evid 2003;9:1712–1720.
40 Bump RC, Zuspan FP, Bueschling WJ 3rd, Ayers LW, Stephans TJ: The prevalence, six-month persistence, and predictive values of laboratory indicators of bacterial vaginosis (nonspecific vaginitis) in asymptomatic women. Am J Obstet Gynecol 1985;150:917–924.
41 Redondo-Lopez V, Meriwether C, Schmitt C, Opitz M, Cook R, Sobel JD: Vulvovaginal candidiasis complication bacterial vaginosis. Sex Transm Dis 1990;17:51–53.
42 Durfee MA, Forsyth PS, Hale JA, Holmes KK: Ineffectiveness of erythromycin for treatment of *Haemophilus* vaginalis-associated vaginitis: Possible relationship to acidity of vaginal secretions. Antimicrob Agents Chemother 1979;16:635–637.
43 Symonds J, Biswas AK: Amoxicillin, Augmentin, and metronidazole in bacterial vaginosis associated with *Gardnerella vaginalis* (letter). Genitourin Med 1986;62:136.
44 Carmona O, Hernandez-Gonzale S, Kobelt R: Ciprofloxacin in the treatment of nonspecific vaginitis. Am J Med 1987;82(suppl 4A):321–323.
45 Vander Meijden WI, Piot P, Loriax SM, Stolz E: Amoxycillin, amoxycillin-clavulanic acid, and metronidazole in the treatment of clue cell-positive discharge: A comparative clinical and laboratory study. J Antimicrob Chemother 1987;20:735–742.
46 Ferris DG, Litaker MS, Woodward L, Mathis D, Hendrich J: Treatment of bacterial vaginosis: A comparison of oral metronidazole, metronidazole vaginal gel and clindamycin vaginal cream. J Fam Pract 1995;41:443–449.
47 Ahmed-Jushuf IH, Shahmanesh M, Arya OP: The treatment of bacterial vaginosis with a 3-day course of 2% clindamycin cream: Results of a multicenter, double-blind, placebo-controlled trial. Genitourin Med 1995;71:254–266.
48 Neri A, Rabinerson D, Kaplan B: Bacterial vaginosis: Drugs versus alternative treatment. Obstet Gynecol Surv 1994;49:809–813.
49 Reid G, Bocking A: The potential for probiotics to prevent bacterial vaginosis and preterm labor. Am J Obstet Gynecol 2003;189:1202–1208.
50 Blaszcak DL: Five day vaginal irritation pilot study in rabbits with rifaximin. East Milstone, Bio-Dynamics, 1991.
51 Blaszcak DL: A 28 day vaginal toxicity study of rifaximin in the rabbit. East Milstone, Bio-Dynamics, 1992.
52 Palazzini E, Desai S: Pilot study on the in vivo efficacy of two formulations of rifaximin for the treatment of bacterial vaginosis. Bologna, Alfa Wassermann/Schiapparelli Searle, 1992.

53 Brown LJ, Oliver RD, Loe H: Evaluating periodontal status of US employed adults. J Am Dent Assoc 1990;121:226–232.
54 Armitage GC: Development of a classification system for periodontal diseases and conditions. Ann Periodontol 1999;4:1–6.
55 Mailhot JM, Fried SL: Oral health and wellness: Understanding periodontal health, recognizing disease states and choices in treatment strategies. J Contemp Dent Pract 2003;4:110–121.
56 Lovegrove JM: Dental plaque revisited: Bacteria associated with periodontal disease. J NZ Soc Periodontol 2004;87:7–21.
57 Jeffcoat MK, Reddy MS: Progression of probing attachment loss in adult periodontitis. J Periodontol 1991;62:185–189.
58 Cobb CM: Non-surgical pocket therapy: Mechanical. Ann Periodontol 1996;1:443–490.
59 Wilson TG: Can surgery be justified for patients with periodontitis? Curr Opin Periodontol 1997;4:64–68.
60 Herrera D, Sanz M, Jepsen S, Needleman I, Roldan S: A systematic review on the effect of systemic antimicrobials as an adjunct to scaling and root planing in periodontitis patients. J Clin Periodontol 2002;29(suppl 3):136–159.
61 Haffajee AD, Socransky SS, Gunsolley JC: Systemic anti-infective periodontal therapy. A systematic review. Ann Periodontol 2003;8:115–181.
62 Haffajee AD, Uzel NG, Arguello EI, Torresyap G, Guerrero DM, Socransky SS: Clinical and microbiological changes associated with the use of combined antimicrobial therapies to treat 'refractory' periodontitis. J Clin Periodontol 2004;31:869–877.
63 Hanes PJ, Purvis JP: Local anti-infective therapy: Pharmacological agents. A systematic review. Ann Periodontol 2003;8:79–98.
64 Pavia M, Nobile CG, Bianco A, Angelillo IF: Meta-analysis of local metronidazole in the treatment of chronic periodontitis. J Periodontol 2004;75:830–838.
65 Knoll-Kohler E: Metronidazole dental gel as an alternative to scaling and root planing in the treatment of localized adult periodontitis. Is its efficacy proved? Eur J Oral Sci 1999;107:415–421.
66 Chanchus PA: The rifomycin. Its use in endodontics – Clinical results (in French). Chir Dent Fr 1965;25:69–74.
67 Picchi N, Pizzoni D: Clinical and pharmaco logical study of rifampicin in dentistry (in Italian). Rass Int Stomatol Prat 1970;21:265–272.
68 Fabris U: First therapeutic results obtained with the use of rifampicin in apical parodontosis (in Italian). Arcisp S Anna Ferrara 1970;23:505–510.
69 Montana Ramonet JM: Rifomycin in dentistry (in Spanish). Rev Esp Estomatol 1970;18:25–34.
70 Mangiante PE, Eftimiadi C, Balbi G, Cortella P, Della Casa P: Rifaximin: A new antibiotic for the topical treatment of periodontal disease (in Italian); in Pierleoni P (ed): Proceedings of the 21st National Congress of the Italian Society of Dentistry and Maxillo-Facial Surgery. Bologna, Monduzzi Editore, 1987, pp 643–646.
71 Dalseno R, Chiarelli P: Controlled and continued delivery of rifaximin and/or other substances. Patent No. WO200441240, 2003.

Prof. Carmelo Scarpignato, MD, DSc, PharmD, FCP, FACG
Laboratory of Clinical Pharmacology, School of Medicine and Dentistry
University of Parma, Via Volturno, 39
IT–43100 Parma (Italy)
Tel. +39 0521 903863, eFax +1 603 8435621, E-Mail scarpi@tin.it

This chapter should be cited as follows:

Pelosini I, Scarpignato C: Rifaximin, a Peculiar Rifamycin Derivative: Established and Potential Clinical Use Outside the Gastrointestinal Tract. Chemotherapy 2005;51(suppl 1):122–130.

Author Index

Subject Index